RNA PROCESSING

Edited by **Paula Grabowski**

RNA Processing
Edited by Paula Grabowski

Published by InTech
Janeza Trdine 9, 51000 Rijeka, Croatia

Publishing Process Manager Marija Radja

Technical Editor Teodora Smiljanic

Cover Designer InTech Design Team

Additional hard copies can be obtained from orders@intechopen.com

RNA Processing, Edited by Paula Grabowski
p. cm.
ISBN 978-953-307-557-0

For EU product safety concerns:
IN TECH d.o.o., Prolaz Marije Krucifikse Kozulić 3, 51000 Rijeka, Croatia,
info@intechopen.com or visit our website at intechopen.com.

Meet the editor

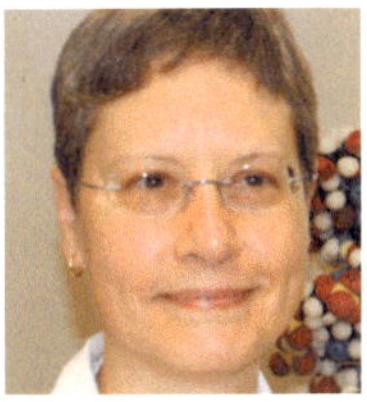

My laboratory has had a longstanding interest in the regulation of alternative pre-mRNA splicing in mammalian cells. As a graduate student with Thomas Cech at the University of Colorado, I characterized the splicing and autocyclization reactions of the Group I intron of the pre-ribosomal RNA of Tetrahymena, which was the first example of a self-splicing ribozyme. As a postdoctoral fellow working with Phillip Sharp at MIT, I developed an affinity selection approach to purify the constituents of the human spliceosome, which provided insights into its dynamic assembly pathway and chemical reaction mechanism. At Brown University, my laboratory provided novel support for the exon definition hypothesis by demonstrating the proportionality of the strength of base pairing of U1 small nuclear ribonucleoprotein complex at the 5′splice site on the rate of branch point formation at the upstream intron. At the University of Pittsburgh, my group has focused on the tissue specific regulation of alternative splicing. We have studied the mechanisms of several splicing factors in depth, including Polypyrimidine Tract Binding protein (PTB), hnRNP A1 and CUGBP2. To gain insights into the underlying splicing codes for each of these factors, we have used bioinformatics to expand the identification and testing of additional candidate target RNAs in the genome. Our current work aims to understand the plasticity of alternative splicing as this relates to the observed changes in splicing patterns that occur when cells are exposed to conditions of stress or stimulation. Current model systems involve neuronal cells subject to stimulation and cells undergoing viral infection. We are interested in understanding the mechanisms by which the plasticity of splicing can be modulated by cellular events, and how imbalances in its fine-tuned regulation can lead to neurodegenerative disease, aging, cancer and viral pathogenesis.

Contents

Preface

RNA functions broadly as informational molecule, genome, enzyme and machinery for RNA processing. While these functions reflect ancient activities, they also remain vital components of contemporary biochemical pathways. In eukaryotic cells RNA processing impacts the biogenesis of RNA molecules of essentially every shape and function from cleavage at the 5′ and 3′ ends to the removal of intronic sequences by splicing. The processing and modification of ribosomal RNAs are essential for the assembly of the protein synthesis machinery.

RNA processing is an integral part of the life cycle that gives rise to infectious HIV-1 particles. The processing of informational mRNAs is integrated into the flow of gene expression during co-transcriptional splicing, 3′-end formation and transport. Alternative splicing and 3′ end formation diversifies protein functions, and varies with the developmental stage and cell type. RNA processing allows for the coordination of mRNA production and quality control enforcement through micro RNAs regulatory contributions fine-tuning gene expression' throughout the genome.

The collection of chapters in this volume describes the current state of understanding of the broad array of RNA processing events in animal and plant cells, key unanswered questions, and cutting edge approaches available to address these questions. Some questions discussed in this volume include, how viruses subvert the RNA processing machinery of the host cell, how the coordination of co-transcriptional RNA processing is regulated at the level of chromatin, the status of RNA processing in plant organelles, and how micro RNA machinery is biosynthesized and regulated.

Paula Grabowski
Dept of Biological Sciences
University of Pittsburgh
USA

Part 1

RNA Processing and Chromatin

1

Chromatin Remodelling and RNA Processing

Stefanie Böhm and Ann-Kristin Östlund Farrants
Dept of Cell Biology, The Wenner-Gren Institute, Stockholm University, Stockholm Sweden

1. Introduction

RNA processing is an essential process in eukaryotic cells, creating different RNA species from one and the same gene. RNA processing occurs on nearly all kinds of RNAs, including mRNA that codes for proteins, ribosomal RNA, tRNA, snRNAs, and μRNA. RNA processing usually occurs co-transcriptionally, and many factors are recruited by the RNA polymerase itself. This stimulates RNA processing by enhancing the correct assembly of factors as the RNA is being produced. Some factors, such as splice factors and cleavage factors for rRNA, are also recruited by the growing RNA-chain. A further link has been established by the transcription rate itself: the low processivity of the RNA polymerase, where it pauses a lot, favours inclusion of alternative splice sites, for instance.

1.1 RNA processing in RNA polymerase II transcription

RNA processing of the mRNA, 5' capping (addition of a methyl-guanosine at the 5' end), splicing (removal of internal introns) and polyadenylation (cleavage and polyadenylation of the 3′ end), are tightly coupled to transcription, and take place mainly co-transcriptionally (for review see Moore and Proudfoot, 2009; Wahl et al., 2009). The factors required for these processing events are recruited to the growing RNA chain during transcriptional elongation by specific sites or structures on the nascent RNA, the transcription machinery and the chromatin environment (for review see Moore and Proudfoot, 2009; Alexander and Beggs, 2010; Luco et al., 2011; Schwartz and Ast, 2010; Carillo Oesterreich et al., 2011). Some of the factors necessary for RNA processing are also recruited by the RNA polymerase itself. RNA polymerase II has a C-terminal domain (CTD) with a repeated sequence of seven amino acids on the largest subunit, (Rbp1). The CTD forms a platform to which many different proteins involved in transcription may associate. The repeated sequence is conserved, YSPTSPS, in different organisms, whereas the length of the CTD is different, 52 residues in human cells and 26 in yeast. The CTD goes through a series of phosphorylations depending on where in the transcription cycle the polymerase is: unphosphorylated at the recruitment to the promoter, serine-5 phosphorylation (Ser-5) at promoter clearance (the first 20-40 nucleotides) and serine-2 (Ser-2) phosphorylation on the elongating RNA polymerase II (for review see Meinhart et al. 2005; Buratowsky, 2009). Other modifications exist; Ser-7 phosphorylation and the recently found argenine-3 phophorylation play roles in snRNA and snoRNA transcription (Egloff et al., 2007; Kim et al., 2009; Sims et al., 2011), and Ser-7 phosphorylation was recently found to be more abundant in intronic sequences (Hyunmin et al., 2010). The CTD cycle relies on kinases and phosphatases acting at the right moment during transcription (review in Phatnani and Greenleaf 2006; Bukowski 2009). First the CTD is phosphorylated at Ser-5 at the promoter by the cdk7/kin28 in the RNA polymerase II auxiliary factor TFIIH, and this promotes promoter clearance. The shift into elongating mode is, at least partly, made by the dephosphorylation of Ser-5 by specific phosphatases, Rtr1 and Ssu72 and the phosphorylation of Ser-2 by cdk9 in the active P-Tefb complex in metazoan (ctk1 performs a similar task in yeast). Fpc1 is the phosphatase connected to dephosphorylation of Ser-2 of the CTD of RNA polymerase II. Recent studies have questioned these static events, and now a dynamic turnover of the phosphorylations is put forward, in which an elongating RNA polymerase is predominantly Ser-2 phosphorylated but the Ser-5 is also phosphorylated to some extent (Burkowsky et al., 2009).

1.1.1 The CTD of the RNA polymerase in RNA processing – recruitment versus elongation rate

The concepts that the transcriptional elongation rate and recruitment of RNA processing factors through the CTD of RNA polymerase II are important for RNA processing have been known for some time (McCracken et al., 1997). Several proteins are recruited to transcription sites via association with the CTD, often depending on phosphorylation state (reviewed in Perales and Bentley, 2009). Capping of the nascent transcript occurs co-transcriptionally, as soon as the growing RNA leaves the exit channel of the RNA polymerase II. The enzymes involved in the capping machinery, at least Ceg1 in yeast, associate with the Ser-5-P CTD of the initiating RNA polymerase II (Komaninsky et al., 2000; Schroeder et al., 2000). The recruitment of 5′ capping machinery to the RNA polymerase enhances the capping reaction (Moteki et al. 2002), but it also has an influence on transcription. It has been suggested that the capping machinery or capping of the nascent transcript stabilises the RNA polymerase, which helps to convert the initiating polymerase to an elongating polymerase (Moore and Proudfoot, 2009; Perales and Bentley, 2009)). Termination and polyadenylation are also enhanced by the polyadenylating machinery associating with the Ser-2 phosphorylated CTD (Komanisnky et al., 2000; Adamson et al., 2002; Lunde et al., 2010).

The spliceosome is assembled by different snRNPs being recruited by cis-acting sequences on RNA, the 5′ splice site and the 3′ splice site around introns. The recruitment of splicing factors occurs stepwise, with U1 snRNPs assembling on the 5′ splice site and U2 snSNP at the 3′ splice site, before the tri snRNP U4-U5/U6, assemble and the intron is removed (for review see Wahlet al., 2009; Moore and Proudfoot, 2009). The recruitment and assembly process of the different snRNPs is enhanced by transcription, and the complexes are further stabilised by the cap-binding complex (Lacardie et al., 2006; Listerman et al, 2006; Görnemann et al., 2005). A close coupling of the splicing to the transcriptional process has been seen also in several *in vitro* studies (Hicks et al., 2006, Das et al., 2006) in which transcription enhances splicing if the RNA polymerase II is transcribing and not T7 polymerase, lacking the CTD. It has also been shown that some of these snRNPs and splicing factors associate with the RNA polymerase II itself, in particular U1 snRNPs and some SR proteins (Morris et al., 2000; Das et al., 2007) (Figure 1A). The U1 snRNP was recently shown to associate with the RNA polymerase II early in the transcription cycle, independently of whether the gene contains introns or not, an interaction that would allow the U1 snRNP to scan the growing RNA for splice sites (Brody et al., 2011). It can be seen that the amount of spliceosomes increases in intron-containing genes (Brody et al., 2011), most likely being recruited to the pre-mRNA by splice sites. These studies have led to the proposal that spliceosomes are efficiently loaded onto the nascent transcript if recruited by RNA polymerase early in the transcription process, since the factors do not have to compete with inhibitory RNA-binding factors. However, the interactions between the CTD or other subunits of the RNA polymerase II and splice factors vary from study to study, which has questioned the generality of the results. It is possible that the interactions only occur on specific genes or in specific cell types (discussed in Carillo Oesterreich et al., 2011).

It has also been shown that different promoters affect splicing differently, suggesting that different transcription factors at the promoter recruit specific splice factors. In particular, co-regulators to nuclear receptors associate with splice factors, which in turn also act as transcription factors, regulating transcriptional initiation and elongation (Auboeuf et al., 2004; Auboeuf et al, 2007). Splicing also enhances transcription, in particular at splice sites near the promoter (Furger et al,. 2002; Damgaard et al., 2008). Promoter proximal splice sites increase the binding of TFIID, TFIIB and TFIIH, all important general transcription factors for transcriptional initiation, and thereby increase loading and initiation of RNA polymerase II. Furthermore, the splice factor SC35, which is a splicing enhancer, associates with RNA polymerase and the cdk9 in the P-Tefb complex (Lin et al. 2008). Depletion of SC35 results in a transcription block, most likely caused by a lack of P-Tefb at the transcription site, which in turn leads to a severe reduction in Ser-2 phosphorylation of the CTD necessary for the switch to the elongating form of RNA polymerase II. Another example of a splice factor that interacts with P-Tefb is SKIP (prp45 in yeast) (Brès et al. 2005), which in this way influences transcriptional elongation.

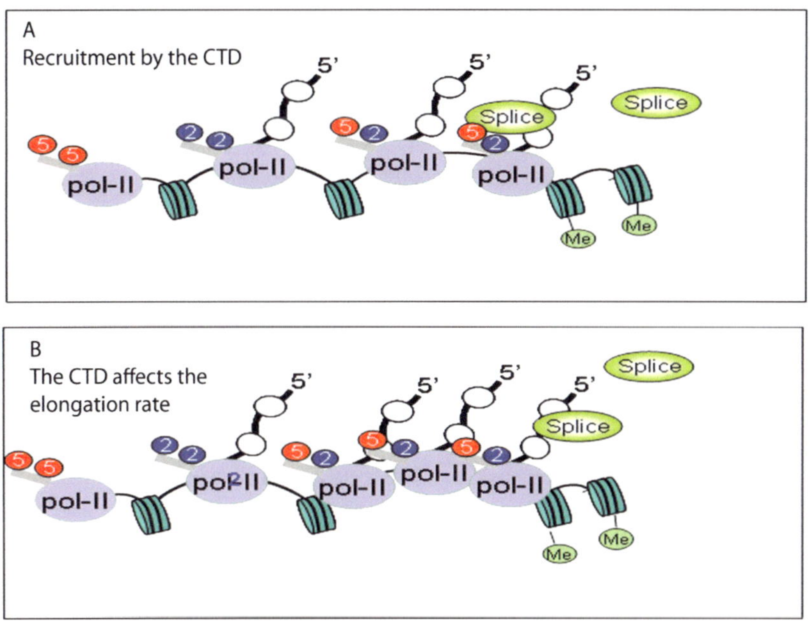

"5" denotes Ser-5 phosphorylation, "2" denotes Ser-2 phosphorylation, "splice" is splice factor.

Fig. 1. The CTD affects splicing outcome, two models. A) The phosphorylation state of the CTD recruits splice factors. B) The phosphorylation state of the CTD affects the elongation rate of RNA polymerase II.

The RNA polymerase pauses during transcription, both near the transcription start site and locally inside the gene body. It is well established that the RNA polymerase II stalls proximal to the promoter, before switching from an initiation Ser-5 phosphorylated CTD mode to Ser-2 phosphorylated elongating mode (Brodsky et al., 2005). This is achieved by the recruitment of P-Tefb by the Ser-5 phosphorylated CTD, but also by histone modifications, such as H3K4me3 and H3Bub (for review Brés et al., 2008; Lenasi and Barboric, 2010) Pausing of RNA polymerases also occurs in the gene body (Figure 1B), local pausing, which may be achieved by a number of mechanisms: intrinsic features of the RNA polymerase II, such as backtracking, when the RNA polymerase II slides, elongation factors, and features in gene architecture, such as DNA sequences and structures formed in the growing RNA (review in Carillo Oesterrich et al,. 2011; Perales and Bentley, 2009). Several genome wide studies of the distribution of RNA polymerases have observed an accumulation at exons, suggesting a slower rate when the RNA polymerase meets an exon. It has been shown that paused RNA polymerase II is hyperphosphorylated, both Ser-5 and Ser-2 phosphorylation are present on the CTD (Munoz et al., 2008). Since both mutation of the CTD mimicking constant phosphorylation and inhibition of CDK9 induced a slower rate, it was suggested that homogenous phosphorylation is required achieved by altering the phosphorylation/dephosphorylation cycle (Munoz et al. 2008). The slower elongation rate often occurs at the 3′ splice site of introns, concomitant with hyperphosphorylation of the CTD and splice factor recruitment, as was shown in UV-damaged cells (Munoz et al. 2008). Recent studies have also shown that the splicing event induces transcriptional pausing. The RNA polymerase accumulates in the Ser-5 CTD form at 3′ splice sites in the gene body (Alexander et al., 2010). Alexander et al. (2010) used a model gene in yeast with introns to map RNA polymerases with high resolution. The stalling of RNA polymerase II was not observed in intronless genes or in genes with mutated splice sites. Alexander et al. (2010) suggest a check point control, related to splicing, in which such splice factors as SC35, Skip or DExD/H-box RNA helicases or even base-pairing between the snoU12 and the mRNA are involved. A similar mechanism has also been shown at the terminal exon in yeast, where an accumulation of RNA polymerase II is found (Carrillo Oesterrieich et al, 2010). Intronless genes or genes with mutated splice sites do not have stalled RNA polymerases (Alexander et al. 2010; Carrillo Oesterreich et al., 2010).

1.1.2 Alternative splicing – Recruitment versus the transcriptional elongation rate

Splicing is a regulated process, and exons can be included or excluded giving different mRNAs, which generates a diversity of protein products. Alternative splicing is regulated by splice factors, such as specific SR protein and hnRNP proteins, which bind to specific sequences on RNA. Both splicing enhancer elements and splicing silencers exist and these sequences are found both in introns and exons (for review see Wahl et al., 2009). The splice factors can be expressed in a tissue-specific manner or can be activated by signalling pathways. In addition, core splice components are involved in alternative splicing, which has in some cases been attributed to production of different isoforms with specific function (Dredge et al, 2005) and in others to autoregulation coupled to degradation by the nonsense mediated decay pathway (Saltzman et al, 2008). Although a general splice factor is alternatively spliced and autoreguated, not all splicing events are affected. Recently, it was shown that the U1 core factor SmB7B′ is autoregulated, and its downregulation affects alternative splicing of several RNA processing proteins resulting in the reduction of snRNPs

(Saltzman et al., 2011). Another mechanism that affects splicing outcome is the transcription rate; pausing of the RNA polymerase favours inclusion of exons (Kornblihtt et al., 2004). This was shown by using a slow transcribing RNA polymerase II, which produced transcripts with more included exons (de la Mata et al., 2002). The slower rate gives time for splice factors to find the splice site, in particular the weak 3′ splice site upstream of alternative exons. Regulation of alternative splicing has therefore been suggested to rely on elongation rate, with pausing of the RNA polymerase II resulting in exon inclusion. It has been hard to find one general mechanism for alternative splicing, which sometimes is an all or nothing event, sometimes several alternative splice forms exist in the same cell. Many different factors are involved in splice site choice, many only being involved in a subset of genes. The complex regulation, both by specific alternative splice regulators, general splice factors and the transcription elongation rate, is a challenge. In addition, transcription occurs in a chromatin environment, with nucleosomes being present along the gene. This provides a further layer of regulation, in addition to splice factors and the transcription rate.

1.2 Chromatin influences RNA processing

Co-transcriptionally RNA processing occurs in a chromatin environment. Chromatin constitutes a barrier for transcription, both initiation and elongation. Several ways of changing the structure occurs upon transcription; the nucleosomes are moved and histones in nucleosomes are modified. Histone acetylation and H3K4me3 are particularly abundant at promoters, creating an open chromatin structure so that TFIIB and the RNA polymerase can bind. These modifications drop towards the 3′ end of the gene. Instead H3K36me3 appears.

1.2.1 Nucleosome distribution at exons

Several studies have suggested that the chromatin architecture influences RNA processing of RNA pol II genes. Based on DNA sequencing, Baldi et al. (1996) and Kogan and Trifinov (2005) suggested that exons have nucleosomes positioned at intron-exon junctions. Genome-wide analyses using Mn-digested chromatin of CD4+ T cells before deep Solexa sequencing (presented in Schones et al., 2008) have shown that exons are more prone to harbour positioned nucleosomes than intronic regions (Tilgner et al., 2009; Schwartz et al., 2009: Andersson et al., 2009; Hon et al., 2009; Speis et al., 2009; Nahkuri et al., 2009; Chodavarapu et al., 2010). If the exon is longer than 147 bp (the number of nucleotides wrapped around the histone core), the positioned nucleosome has a position at the 3' end in chromatin from *C. elegans* (Kolasinska-Twister et al., 2009). The distribution observed in human cells differs; however, the peak observed is at the 5′ end of exons (Hon et al., 2009). The average exon length in human cells is approximately 150 bp, fitting the length of one nucleosome, but both shorter and longer exons exist. The discrepancy between studies may be attributed to the definition of exon length used. When analysing both shorter and longer exons a consensus arises: short exons (50 bp or shorter) do not contain a positioned nucleosome, long exons (more than 300 bp) have positioned nucleosomes at both the 5′ end and the 3′ end of exons (Schwartz et al., 2009; Andersson et al., 2009; Hon et al., 2009). The positioned nucleosomes are stronger in exons with weak splice sites, but pseudo-exons (with strong splice sites which are not used) are depleted of nucleosomes (Tilgner et al., 2009; Spies et al., 2009). Schwartz et al. (2009) found that the occupancy was related to exon usage, with less nucleosomes on low-abundant alternative exons, and more in high abundant, constitutive exons. The higher nucleosome occupancy in exons is a conserved feature, found in both Mn-seq from *C. elegans*, *Drosophila*, mice, man, and in a number of other eukaryotes, such as fungi and plants. The position of the nucleosomes is explained by the DNA sequence, the higher GC-content of exons producing a favourable curvature in the DNA (Tilgner et al., 2009; Schwartz et al., 2009; Speis et al., 2009). This has been suggested to be caused by codon bias to exclude long stretches of A-tracts in exons (Cohanif and Haran, 2009). Another explanation is provided by Schwartz et al. (2009), who found nucleosome exclusion sequences at the 3′ splice site, thereby shoving the nucleosome into the exon. The fact that transcription does not affect the position of the nucleosomes suggests that the underlying sequence determines the nucleosome pattern and form a mechanism to mark exons (Anderson et al., 2009; Chodavarapu et al., 2010). However, a study investigating three cell types, the erythroid K562, the monocytic U937 and CD14+ monocytes, showed that the pattern of positioned nucleosomes varies - a higher density over exons of expressed genes is seen in primary CD14+ cells, whereas the cell lines K562 and U937 displayed a lower density (Dahrma et al., 2010). More cell types must be investigated to resolve these matters; these results may reflect differences in cell type.

The nucleosome distribution at polyadenylation site is also set, with a region around the polyadenylation signal being depleted of nucleosomes, and a region downstream with a higher enrichment of nucleosomes (Speis et al., 2009; Carrillo Oesterreich, 2010). The depletion of nucleosomes is not linked to the level of transcription, but the downstream nucleosomes depend on the level of usage of the polyadenlylation site: high-level usage has more nucleosomes 76-375 bp downstream of the polyadenylation site.

1.2.2 Histone modifications at exons

The nucleosome position is only markedly increased at exons compared to introns (1.5 fold) and this is not affected by transcription (discussed in Schwartz and Ast, 2010), which has lead to several studies correlated the nucleosome occupancy data with genome-wide ChIP-seq of several histone modifications. Histone modifications are involved in the regulation of transcription initiation and elongation, where they change both the nucleosome structure and recruit factors. The connection of the nucleosome distribution data with data from histone modifications along genes identified the H3K36-me3 as a specific modification accumulated at exons, and more pronounced at exons in the 3′ end of the gene (Kolasinska-Zwierz et al., 2009; Schwartz et al., 2009; Andersson et al., 2009; Hon et al., 2009). Tilgner et al. (2009) could not find a clear accumulation of H3K36me3 at exons, however, when adjusted to the distribution of nucleosomes. The conflicting results reported, mainly based on the same data, could be due to different normalisation criteria and different algorithms used when correlating data obtained with different techniques; MN-seq with ChIP-seq and ChIP-Chip data (discussed in Ringrose, 2010). Nevertheless, most studies identified H3K36-me3 as a mark for exons, together with several other modifications, forming a modification code along genes (Table 1). H3K36me3 accumulation at exons in the gene body was also seen in expressed genes when Dhami et al. (2010) investigated the three different cell types. In this study, some histone modifications were excluded from exons in expressed genes; H3K9me2/3, H3K27me2/3. These cell types also display a specific modification pattern for exons in non-expressed genes, H3K27me3. A recent study has further examined the nucleosomal architecture at exon-intron junctions, based on published genome-wide MN digestion-seq and ChIP-seq surveys (Huff et al., 2010). A specific histone modification pattern was identified in the 5′ end of the gene, different from the 3′ end of the gene. The genes were therefore divided into three parts; promoter region, 5′ end of the gene (up until the internal exons), and the 3′ end of the gene, to further map the chromatin landscape. The 5′ intron-rich region had higher levels of H3K79me2, and also peaked in H2Bub. The H3K36me3 was higher in the 3′ exon-rich part of the gene, and peaked near exons and extended downstream.

Promoter	Exon 5′	Exon 3′	Alternative exons	Silent exons	Excluded from exons	introns	pol II accumul.	Ref.
H3K4me3	H2Bub H3K79me2 H3K4me2	H3K36me3				H3K79me2?		Huff el al. CD4+
H3K4me3		H3K36me3	H3K36me3			H3K9me3? H3K4me3?		Kolasinksa et al. C.elegans
		H3K36me3 H3K27me1	H3K36me3 (H3K27me1 /3 H3K36me1 H3K4me1 H3K9me1)	H3K27me3 H3K36me1	H3K9me2/3	H3K9me2/3 H3K27me2/3		Dhami et al. three cell lines
H3K4me3 at TSS	H3K4me3	H3K36me3 H3K27me2			H3K9me3		no	Speis et l. CD4+
		H3K36me3 H3K79me1 H4K20me1 H2BK5me1	H3K36me3				At exons	Schwartz et al. C.elegans
		H3K36me3 Before normalisatio n			H4K20me1			Tilgner et al. CD4+
H3K4me3 H3K9me1	H3K36me3 H2BK5me1 H4K20me1	H3K36me3	H3K36me3	H3K9me3 in excluded exons				Hon et al. CD4+
		H3K36me3 H3K79me1 H2BK5me1	H3K36me3	H3K27me2 /3				Andersson et al. CD4+
							At exons	Chodavarapu et al. Plants etc

Table 1. Histone modifications found in different part of RNA polymerase II genes. Underlined modification means that it changes with level of transcription. Font size represents level of the histone modification relative to others in the same study. The predominant cell type used in the study is found under the reference.

1.2.2.1 How are the histone modifications achieved and maintained?

The distribution of the nucleosomal exon–intron pattern is mainly explained by the underlying DNA sequence, but the histone modifications varies along the gene, indicating that active mechanisms also apply to set and maintain the pattern. Nucleosome modifications at exon-introns follow the level of transcription, but not completely. Histone modifications are loaded onto the histone tails by modifying enzymes recruited to the site of action (reviewed in Gardner et al., 2011; Murr, 2010). Modifications associated with promoters, acetylated histones and H3K4me3 are set by histone acetyl transferases (HATs) and the SET1/MLL/COMPAS methyl transferases, respectively. These modifications are then removed by histone deacetylases (HDACs) and demethylases (HMTs). HATs are often co-regulators at the promoter, and MLL is recruited to the promoter by Ser-5 CTD on the RNA polymerase II. However, sometimes histone modifications at the promoter do not depend on transcription, instead they prime the genes for transcription (Raisner et al., 2005; Kouskouti and Talianidis, 2005; Liber et al., 2010: Min et al., 2011). Other histone marks are more abundant in the gene body (Murr et. al., 2010; Bannister and Kouzarides, 2011). H3K36 tri-methylations are achieved by HypB/setd2 (Set2 in yeast) methyl transferases (Edmunds et al., 2008), which in turn are recruited to the transcribed gene most likely by Ser-2 CTD on the elongating RNA polymerase II (Eissenberg et al. 2007). The occurrence of modifications specifically at exons raises the question of how these patterns are set. By comparing the patterns of genes at different expression levels in the three cell types investigated, Dhami et al. (2010) identified a priming event consisting of H3K27me3 and H3K36me1 at non-expressed genes. These marks were then replaced by H3K36me3 and H3K27me1 during transcription, and the levels reflected the expression level of the gene. This study also demonstrated a difference in alternatively spliced exons, showing less H3K36me3 at less-included exons. This suggests that some of the modifications are set not only by events during transcription, such as the elongation rate of RNA polymerase II, but also by events in splicing.

Huff et al. (2010) addressed the question of whether splicing *per se* can affect the nucleosome modification pattern, by investigating two genes that are alternatively spliced upon stimuli, YPEL5 and CD45. No effect on the H3K36me3 levels could be seen upon inclusion of the alternative exons, ruling out that splicing events are setting the marks. Instead, these marks are relatively stable, similar to histone marks at promoters where marks are present without active transcription. Based on these results, a model in which exons are defined, or primed, by histone marks can be put forward. In this model the basic marks can shift according to a set pattern, H3K27me3 to H3K36me3, by active transcription, but not splicing. However, this model is based on only two studies and needs verification. It is also worth noting that exons have a higher degree of DNA methylation, both in plants and in human cells (Chodavarapu et al., 2010). Whether this is a result of a higher DNA methylation of nucleosomal DNA or an active recruitment of DNA-methylation enzymes at exons remains to be resolved. In addition, the question of how the priming of exons in non-transcribed exons is achieved remains to be investigated.

1.2.2.2 The functional significance of the chromatin pattern

The next question to be addressed is whether the nucleosome distribution and histone modifications associated with exon-introns play a functional role in splicing? Two ideas have been proposed: The nucleosomes form "speed bumps" for the RNA polymerase or the histone modifications on nucleosomes form recruitment platforms for splice factors (Figure 2A and 2B). The "speed bump" model is related to the "kinetic model", and presumes that nucleosomes constitute a barrier for the elongating RNA polymerase II, in particular that nucleosomes at exons make the polymerase pause more. An accumulation of RNA pol II is seen also over exons (Schwartz et al., 2009; Dhami et al., 2010; Chodavarapu et al., 2010), indicating that the higher nucleosome density at exons (Schwartz et al., 2009) or the identity of the specific modifications provides a barrier for the RNA polymerase and makes it pause (Dhama et al., 2010). The pausing of the RNA polymerase II will then allow for splice factors to assemble onto the growing mRNA. The "recruitment model" instead proposes that the chromatin architecture, with different histone modifications, is involved in recruiting components of the spliceosome and splice factors, such as SR-proteins and hnRNPs. These proteins will then decide the splicing outcome by binding to the nascent RNA and direct the spliceosome to the right place. These two models will be discussed below.

1.2.2.3 RNA polymerase rate in a chromatin environment and alternative splicing

RNA polymerase II processivity has an affect on splice site choice, as can be seen in alternative splicing. Alternative exons are included with a slower moving elongating RNA polymerase II (de la Mata et al. 2003). Inclusion of alternative splice sites can also be seen in cells by using different inhibitors of transcription, such as 5,6-dichlorobenzimidazole, 1-b-D-ribofuranoside (DRB), which inhibits b-Tefb from phosphorylating elongating RNA polymerase II, and camptothecin (CPT), an inhibitor of topoisomerase I (reviewed in Kornblihtt 2004; Kornblihtt 2007). The slower rate gives time for splice factors not only to find the strong splice site, but also weak splice sites surrounding alternative exons, and assemble the U2 snRNP before the appearance of a strong splice site (Figure 2A). However, the result of a slow RNA polymerase II may not always result in inclusion of alternative exons as also specific inhibitors of alternative splicing have time to be recruited to splicing silencers (Pagani et al. 2003). Whether changes in the elongation rate of RNA polymerase along a gene are a general mechanism to affect splicing outcome is still unclear. It is not yet established whether the elongation rate of RNA polymerase II changes at alternative exons at all genes, or whether this is a local effect seen in only a subset of genes. It has been shown that the processivity of RNA polymerase II is consistent during transcription, at approximately 3. 8 kb/min, independently of whether intron-rich regions or exon-rich regions are transcribed. This was measured on a few endogenous genes with long introns by qPCR coupled to the alleviation a DRB block of elongation by RNA polymerase II (Singh and Padgett, 2009). In a separate study using FRAP of GFP-RNA polymerase II on a model gene, Brody et al. (2011) found that the RNA polymerase rate is similar on intronless genes as it is on genes harbouring several exons/introns. On the other hand, unspliced polyadenylated mRNA remains at the gene locus until properly spliced. These studies did not address the question of RNA processivity on genes with alternatively included exons. Recently, Ip et al. (2011) showed that the elongation rate affects the inclusion of alternative splice sites in a subset of genes. From a mechanistic point of view, the exons affected displayed an accumulation of RNA polymerase II upstream of the exon, in agreement with paused polymerases. These exons were surrounded by weaker splice sites than other alternative exons, and followed by a strong 3′ splice site at the downstream exon. The genes harbouring alternative exons sensitive to a slower elongation rate were mainly involved in RNA processing and apoptosis, and the alternative exon usage often introduced a premature termination codon, marking the transcript for nonsense-mediated decay.

The processivity or pausing of the RNA polymerase depends on several factors: the architecture of the gene, DNA sequences, and factors bound to DNA and chromatin. Nucleosomes affect the RNA polymerase rate, but depending on which histone modifications they carry, the effects are of different magnitudes. Acetylated nucleosomes, for example, increase the rate of elongation by increasing the accessibility of DNA, whereas repressive methylation modifications reduce the RNA polymerase processivity. It has been shown that histone modifications alter the splice site choice, for instance that inhibiting histone deacetylases (HDACs) , creating hyperacetylated nucleosomes, results in the exclusion of alternative exons at the 5′ end of the gene (Kornblihtt 2003; Allo 2011). This was attributed to an increase in H3-Ac at the 5′ end of genes. Recently, it was shown that an increase in H4-Ac at alternative splice sites in the gene body increases RNA polymerase II processivity, which in turn favours exclusion of the alternative exons (Hnilicavá et al. 2011). The HDAC inhibitor also reduces the association of the SR-protein SRp40 with chromatin/RNP, maybe also affecting splice factor acetylation. It has also been shown that inducing repressive histone marks, H3K9me2, by siRNA slows RNA polymerase II, and exons in the proximity of the recessive mark are included (Allo et al. 2010; Allo et al. 2011). The kinetic model connected to the genome-wide results predicts that H3K36me3, maybe together with other modifications or factors, decreases the RNA polymerase II processivity and leads to exon inclusion. The higher density of RNA polymerases at exons would favour such a model, but most studies find a lower H3K36me3 level at alternatively used exons than constitutively used exons. H3K36me3 is found on actively transcribed genes and follows the transcription level, which indicates that other factors must operate in addition to RNA processivity to determine exon usage.

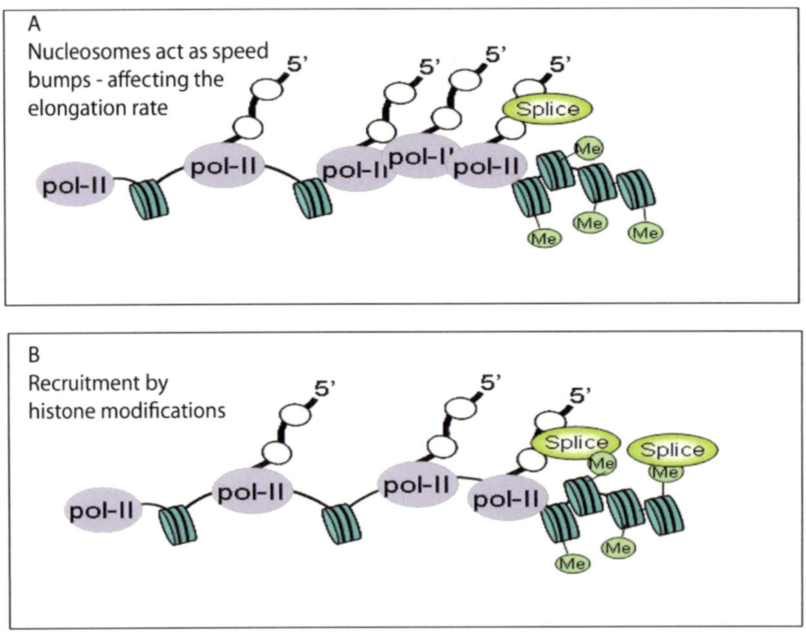

Fig. 2. **Chromatin affects the splicing outcome, two models.** A) Nucleosomes with modifications act as speed bumps affecting the elongation rate of RNA polymerase II. B) Histone modifications recruit splicing factors to splice sites.

1.2.2.4 Splicing factor recruitment to chromatin in alternative splicing

The recruitment model suggests that histone modifications constitute a platform for specific proteins to bind (Figure 2B). These proteins are chromatin-binding proteins that adopt an adapter function to recruit splice factors or they are splice factors that bind histone modifications directly. The capping machinery, for instance, binds not only to the CTD of the RNA polymerase, but also to the H3K4me3 found close to the promoters (Perales and Bentley, 2009). Four examples of chromatin factors functioning in splicing and possessing the adapter function have been described, and these examples will be discussed below. The first one is a protein that is recruited to chromatin by binding to H3K36me3, MORF-related gene 15 (MRG15). The H3K36me3 is the major histone modification observed in transcribed exons, and it is tempting to suggest that the function is to attract specific factors to exons. H3K36me3 is recognised by MRG1, which interacts with the TIP60 HAT complex and HDACs. The yeast orthologue is involved in preventing promiscuous transcriptional initiation inside genes by removing acetyl groups formed around the elongating RNA polymerase II. The MRG15 protein also interacts with the H3K4me3 demethylase RBD2 (retinoblastoma binding protein 2) on certain genes. Luco et al. (2010) connected MRG15 with the PTB protein (polypyrimidine tract binding protein), which regulates the alternative splicing of certain transcripts by binding to a splicing silencer sequence on the RNA. MRG15 interacts with PTB, and this interaction is used to recruit the PTB to alternative exons on a subset of genes. However, H3K36me3 is located at all exons, and also at included alternative spliced exons, so a splice-enhancing protein must exist that couples H3K36me3 to inclusion of exons. It is also hard to reconcile a model in which H3K36me3 is a marker for alternative exons with the pattern identified in genome-wide surveys, where all exons exhibited the mark.

The chromatin remodelling ATPase CHD1 is recruited to active genes by binding to H3K4me3, and in turn interacts with the ATPase SNF2h and U2 spliceosome components (Sims et al. 2007). The CHD1 protein and H3K4me3 are not involved in changing splicing outcome, but rather the efficiency of the splicing reaction, suggesting that the recruitment of splicing factors is enhanced to splice sites. The H3K4me3 appears mainly at the 5′ end of genes and is not abundant in the 3′exon-rich part, (Spies et al. 2009), which suggests that the impact on splicing is restricted to the exons proximal to the promoter. However, H3K4me3 has been identified on isolated exons in the 3′ end of genes in highly transcribed genes (Spies et al. 2009), and the question is whether the effects seen by CHD1 and H3K4me3 are on these exons.

Acetylated histones have been correlated to an increased RNA processivity, but genome-wide studies have also shown a peak of H3K9-Ac just prior to exons in active genes (Dharma et al. 2010). The SAGA complex, with the HAT GCN5, interacts with acetylated histones, and recruits U2 snRNP proteins in yeast (Gunderson and Johnson 2009). Recently it was shown in yeast that deleting HDAC causes mis-regulation of the U2 snRNP along the gene body, suggesting that the dynamic acetylation-deacetylation cycle along the gene regulate spliceosome assembly (Gunderson et al. 2011). The deacetylation in the gene body is essential not only to prevent internal initiation of transcription but also to restrict splicosome assembly to exons.

The fourth example of a chromatin protein that interacts with splice factors is the heterochromatin protein 1 (HP1). HP1, which associates with H3K9me3 in repressive chromatin, associates with hnRNPs in *Drosophila* cells, both in actively transcribed genes and in heterochromatin (Piacentini et al. 2009). It has been suggested that the role of HP1α in transcribed genes is not to affect the splicing reaction, but to be involved in the packaging and export of RNPs for a subset of genes. Recently, it was shown that phosphorylated HP1γ interacts with H3K9me3 in alternative exons in the CD44 gene in human cells (Saint-André et al. 2011). Activation of PKC, which phosphorylates HP1γ, results in the inclusion of the variable exons, a process that is reduced when HP1γ is silenced. Simultaneously with the targeting of HP1γ, the RNA polymerase II and the splice factor U2AF65 are enriched at the variable spliced region of the gene. It has been proposed that HP1γ acts as an adapter for splicing factors, but the accumulation of RNA polymerase II suggests that it also reduces the processivity of RNA polymerase II. The histone modification pattern over this region contains peaks of H3K9me3, with low levels of H3K36me3. Most genome-wide studies show that H3K9me3 is excluded from exons in transcribed genes, but a genome-wide screen of histone methylations found a peak of H3K9me in the gene body (Barski et al., 2007). The discrepancy between the genome-wide studies and the CD44 gene regarding the presence of H3K9me3 could also be explained by the genome-wide surveys missing subsets of genes that exhibit a different histone modification pattern than the most prevalent ones, and also that cell type specific differences may exist.

1.2.2.5 Chromatin remodelling factors in alternative splicing

Chromatin remodelling complexes have also been implicated in RNA processing. Biochemically purified SWI/SNF complex interacts with several snRNP proteins and splice factors, such as Prp4 (Delaire et al. 2001) and Prp8 (Patrik Asp and Ann-Kristin Östlund Farrants, unpublished data). A functional role of the mammalian SWI/SNF ATPase proteins, BRM and BRG1, affects the splicing of specific genes. The SWI/SNF complexes are mainly involved in transcriptional initiation, remodelling the structure of nucleosomes at the promoter (for review Hargreaves and Crabtree, 2011). In addition, they have an effect on the splicing patterns of the CD44 gene and the telomerase gene (Batsche et al., 2006; Ito et al. 2008). The mechanism behind the splicing effect has been attributed to an effect on the elongation rate of RNA polymerase II at the region containing various exons. The expression of BRM is to reduce the processivity of RNA polymerase by inducing a Ser-5 phosphorylation of the CTD, while at the same time BRM interacts with the splicing regulator protein SAM68. SAM68 requires to be phosphorylated by PKC to bind to the nascent RNA and to BRM, which couples BRM and its effect on splicing to activation by external signals. The ATPase activity, which is required for chromatin remodelling, is not essential for the splicing effect. A number of genes have been identified, all of which rely on BRM for inclusion of alternative exons. However, the BRM on polytene chromosomes from the diphterian *Chironomus tentans* has been observed not only on chromatin but also on the growing mRNP (Figure 3A) (Tyagi et al., 2009), suggesting that the SWI/SNF complexes can influence splicing on several levels.

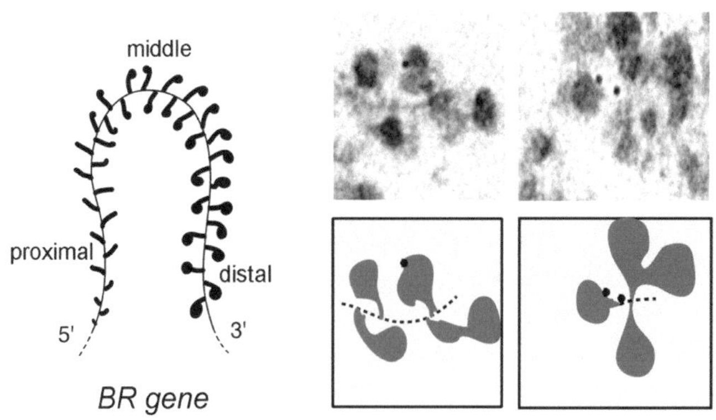

Fig. 3. **The ATPase BRM associates with both chromatin and the growing RNA.** Left panel) Schematic view of a Balbiani ring gene in *C. tentans*, with growing RNP-particles. Right panel) EM images showing gold labelled BRM on Balbiani ring genes on the top, with drawings below.

The BRM also fractionates with the RNA fraction, as do the human BRG1 and BRM. Similar to BRM in human cells, SiRNA silencing of the *Drosophila* BRM affects the splice pattern of a subset of genes. Closer examination of these genes did not reconcile the splicing outcome on all genes affected with a slow transcription elongation rate. These variations led to the model presented in Figure 4A and 4B, which proposes that SWI/SNF complexes operate on two levels, one on chromatin by affecting the transcription elongation rate and one on RNA, most likely by associating to splice factors. A similar mechanism has been proposed for other chromatin proteins, such as the HATs PD20 and PCAF (Sjölinder et al., 2005; Obrdlik et al., 2008).

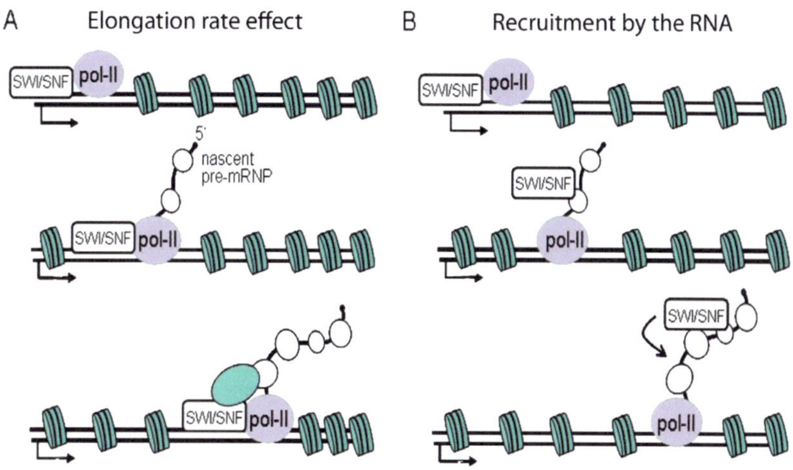

Fig. 4. **Models of chromatin remodelling in alternative splicing.** A) SWI/SNF works at the chromatin level, slowing down the elongation rate. B) SWI/SNF associates with the growing mRNA.

1.3 Summary

It is clear that RNA processing is coordinated with transcription and chromatin environment. Firstly, several processing factors associate with the RNA polymerase II, or with chromatin proteins, suggesting that the processes are interlinked. Secondly, the transcriptional elongation rate affects splicing outcomes; several lines of evidence show that a pausing RNA polymerase II results in inclusion of exons, in particular at alternative exons with weak splice sites. One open question that still remains to be answered is how the RNA polymerase is slowing down at exons. One possible way of slowing down the elongating RNA polymerase is to change the phosphorylation state of its CTD, increasing its Ser-5 phosphorylation. The mechanism behind this is not known, however. Is a Ser-5 kinase recruited at internal exons or is a phosphatase inactivated? The Ser-5 kinase TFIIH is found at the promoter, but it has been suggested that CDK9 in the p-Tefb functions as a Ser-5 kinase in the gene body (Munoz et al., 2009). The yeast orthologue ctk1 has both Ser-5 and Ser-2 kinase activity (Jones et al., 2004). It has also been suggested that a change in the phosphorylation/dephosphorylation cycle contributes to the altered elongation rate (Munoz et al., 2009). Or is the phosphorylation secondary to sequences in the DNA, or backtracking

of the RNA polymerase? Moreover, the effect of chromatin and the histone modifications specific to exons and introns, on the elongation rate needs to be elucidated.
The elongation rate of RNA polymerase II does not explain all splicing outcomes, and other mechanisms, such as recruitment of splicing enhancers and silencers to nascent RNA also contribute. In addition, chromatin remodelling proteins can be recruited to the nascent RNA and influence splice site choice. Recent studies have shown that chromatin landscape is involved in splicing; exons are denser in nucleosomes than introns and the histones at exons carry specific histone modifications. In particular H3K36me3 are abundant in exons, the level is dependent on transcription. This mark is not affected by splicing events, suggesting a preset state, marking exons in a particular manner depending on exon usage, resulting in different patterns in different cell types. This raises several important questions. How are exon-intron histon marks set: by H3K36me3 specific methyl transferases or by demethylases being recruited? How are these modification enzymes recruited? The finding that expressed exons carry H3K36me3, whereas exons in non-expressed genes carry H3K27me3 suggests that the regulation of histones mark is even more complex. The studies presented show that chromatin and histone modifications constitute a further level of regulation of gene expression.

2.1 Chromatin and ribosomal processing

Ribosomal biogenesis employs a specific RNA polymerase machinery, employing specific processing and assembly factors. A large gene, the 47/45S rRNA gene, is transcribed by the RNA polymerase I, in the nucleolus, and from this transcript three of the four ribosomal RNAs in ribosomes; 18S, 5.8S and 28 S, are produced. The 4th rRNA is transcribed from a separate, small gene, by RNA polymerase III, in the nucleolus in yeast but in the nucleoplasm in metazoans. The nucleolus is the location also of rRNA processing and assembly. The ribosomal genes are present in tandem repeats, around 200 in yeast and 400 in human cells, spread out on five chromosomes (for review Grummt and McStay, 2008). These gene loci constitute the nucleolar organisation centres (NORs) around which the nucleoli are formed after exit from mitosis when actively transcribed. RNA polymerase I transcription requires specific auxiliary factors, such as the UBF (upstream binding factor) and SL1 (selectivity factor 1), a TBP-containing complex. UBF binds to the rDNA promoter and recruits SL1, which in turn recruits the RNA polymerase I. The assembly of the transcription imitation complex is regulated by phosphorylation and acetylation of UBF and SL1 throughout the cell cycle through signalling pathways. UBF is a high motility group protein (HMG), which bends DNA in a similar manner to a nucleosome. UBF is found not only at the promoter but also along actively transcribed genes. The major fraction of the genes is not transcribed, however, and do not have UBF bound, or very low levels bound. Instead, these genes are organised into heterochromatin.

2.1.1 RNA processing in RNA polymerase I transcription - rRNA processing

The processing of the rRNAs involves cleavage of the transcripts and covalent modifications, such as pseudouridylation, 2′-O ribose methylation and base methylations (Decatur and Fournier, 2003; Henras et al., 2008). The processing of the rRNAs is initiated co-transcriptionally with the assembly of a "terminal knob", which comprises the growing pre-rRNA with snoRNPs and modifying proteins. The pre-RNA is subsequently cleaved into the separate rRNAs by a number of exonucleases and endonucleases, which are helped by snoRNA and RNA helicases, GTPases and kinases (Strunk and Karbstein, 2010; Kressler et al., 2010). The 47/45S is assembled with the snoRNPs U3, U8 and U13 (U14, snR30) and processing proteins, such as RNA helicases, cotransciptionally into the 90S pre-ribosomal particle (also called the "small subunit processome", SSU). The essential snoRNA most likely binds to RNA and produces the right structure to the pre-RNA for further processing: the snoU3 binds to the ETS and ITS1 surrounding the 18S rRNA module by complementary base pairing, helicases are then required to dissociate the snoRNA during the maturation process (Bohnsack et al., 2008). SnoU3 binds early to the pre-RNA, together with several proteins important for the cleavage and modification of the 18S rRNA, and this part will later assemble into the 40S ribosome. The distal part of the rRNA, which will after cleavage of the 90S SSU form the LSU, large subunit processome, assembles later when the 5.8 and 28S appears.

Some proteins that assemble into the SSU are directly bound to the snoU3 RNP, the UTP (U three proteins). Seven UTPs in yeast form a separate subcomplex, t-UTP, which is associated with chromatin, affects transcription and is necessary for processing (Wery et al. 2009). A homologous complex is present in human cells, with six identified proteins (Prieto and McStay, 2007). The function of the t-UTPs on transcription and chromatin has not been fully worked out. It has been proposed that the t-UTP in yeast is involved in pre-RNA stabilisation rather than in RNA polymerase I transcription (Wery et al. 2009).

2.1.2 The link between transcription and pre-RNA processing

The pre-RNA processome contains proteins that affect both transcription and processing. This has led to the proposal that transcription and processing are coordinated and influence each another. The t-UTP complex would then be the first level of coordinating these events during transcription, since it is recruited early in the process. Schneider et al. (2007) showed that transcriptional defects can affect processing. A mutant RNA polymerase I, which exhibited a slow initiation and elongation, was produced in yeast and these cells have severe defects in pre-RNA processing and assembly. It was proposed that a slower elongation rate produces improper recruitment of processing proteins and snoRNA. It has long been unclear how t-UTPs affect transcription, but recently a t-UTP, 1A6/DRIM (t-UTP20), was found to associate with a histone acetyltransferase-like protein, hALP, in human cells (Peng et al., 2010, Kong et al., 2011). The hALP is involved in acetylating UBF, and by being recruited to 1A6/DRIM, the processome promotes transcriptional initiation and, possibly, elongation.

2.1.3 Chromatin and RNA processing

The chromatin structure at the RNA polymerase I genes is complex. The silent copies are tightly packaged with nucleosomes, with features characteristic for heterochromatin, such as the repressive marks H3K9me3, H4K20me3 and DNA methylated CpGs at the promoter. The setting of the repressive state is caused by a chromatin remodelling complex, the NoRC (Santoro et al., 2002; Zhao et al. 2009). The active copies are heavily transcribed and whether canonical nucleosomes are present is debated. Studies in yeast show that no histones or very small nucleosomes are present on genes that have RNA polymerase I (Merz et al., 2008; Jones et al., 2007). Similarly, it has been proposed that mammalian cells are devoid of nucleosomes. UBF, which binds to the DNA as a dimer, resembles a nucleosome and may be the major chromatin protein in active rDNA in (Sanij and Hannan, 2009). However, histone chaperones in the FACT complex, which function as elongation factors in RNA polymerase II transcription, also influence RNA polymerase I transcription (Birch et al., 2009). Whether the chromatin structure constitutes a barrier for RNA polymerase I is unclear. A number of chromatin remodelling proteins have been associated with active genes, such as the CSB (Cockayes syndrome protein B) (Bradsher et al., 2002; Yuan et al., 2007; Lebedev et al., 2008) and B-WICH (Cavellán et al. 2006, Percipalle et al., 2006, Vintermist et al., 2011). Chromatin remodelling factors have been also isolated with the p32 (splicing factor 2–associated protein p32), which has been identified as a regulator of the transformation of the 90S particle to a 40S and a 60S pre-RNA particle. The p32 is also involved in RNA polymerase II splicing, so it is unclear whether the interaction with 13 chromatin remodelling proteins stems from p32 in RNA polymerase I or RNA polymerase II transcription. The CSB and B-WICH are involved in active transcription of ribosomal genes affect histone modification. CSB recruits the histone methyltransferse G9a, which results in H3K9me2 histones at actively transcribed genes (Yuan et al., 2007). The B-WICH, composed of the WSTF (William syndrome transcription factor), the ATPase SNF2h and nuclear myosin 1 (NM1), remodels chromatin at the promoter, and allows HAT to associate. The HATs subsequently acetylate histone H3, in particular H3K9-Ac. Both H3K9me2 and H3-Ac lead to increased transcription. Interestingly, the B-WICH complex also contains RNA processing proteins, such as RNA helicase Guα and the Myb-binding protein, and the 45S rRNA (Cavellán et al. 2006). Further analysis has shown that also the snoU3 associates with the complex (Figure 5A) and the B-WICH subunits can be linked to the 45S rRNA on the gene (Figure 5B). NMI binds RNA and is important for the export of the 60S subunit (Obrdlik et al., 2010), indicating that it is loaded onto the RNA via a chromatin-remodelling complex at the promoter and along the gene. It then follows the 60S pre-ribosome, when the 90S pre-18S-processome is cleaved off, through assembly and export.

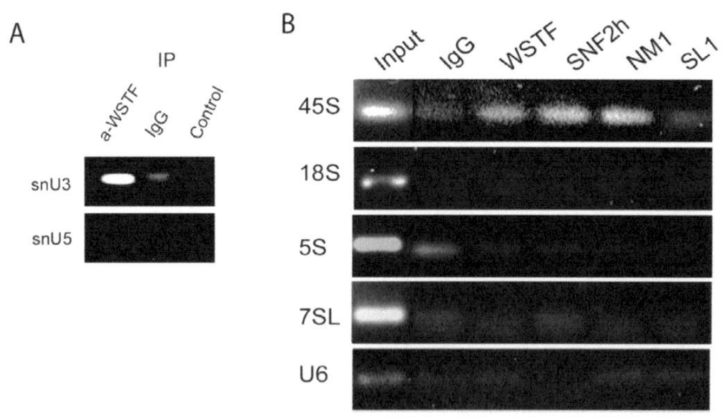

Fig. 5. **B-WICH associates to RNA.** A) IP of WSTF from HeLa cell nuclear extract, from which RNA was purified, converted to cDNA using random primers, and analysed by PCR with primers specific of U3-RNA and U5-RNA. (Control is no Antibody). B) RNA immunoprecipitation of cross-linked chromatin, antibodies against the proteins indicated above the lanes. PCR was performed at the genes indicated to the left.

Even though the B-WICH is not regarded as a t-UTP, some aspects resemble such a complex, a model has been proposed, where the complex affects transcription by chromatin remodelling, whereas other components are acting on processing (Figure 6).

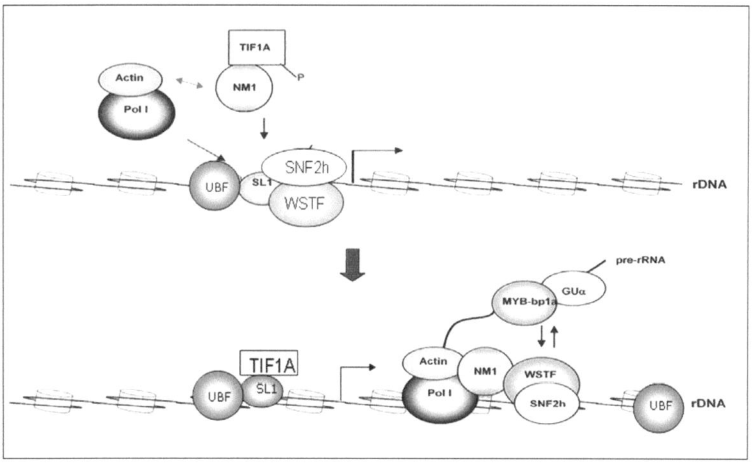

Fig. 6. **Chromatin remodelling in ribosomal transcription.** The chromatin remodelling complex B-WICH assembles at the promoter and interacts with RNA processing factors and RNA during transcription.

2.2 Summary

The different steps, transcription, processing and export, in ribosomal biogenesis are tightly linked. The assembly of the processing factors, such as RNA helicases and snoRNP, are important, recognising structures in the rRNA and other proteins. An increasing number of "processing" factors are recruited at the promoter and these affect both processing and transcription. Even chromatin remodelling factors act as processing factors, function to remodel chromatin at the promoter and provide processing and export factors to the processomes. The B-WICH is one such example, with the main function in chromatin remodelling, but associates with several RNAs and processing proteins. Another is the hALP t-UTP. The function of the t-UTP is still unknown, so more factors with functions both in chromatin remodelling and RNA processing may exist.

3. Conclusions

Nuclear processes are tightly coupled and coordinated. Several lines of evidence now show that most RNA processing, both the action of RNA polymerase I and that of RNA polymerase II, is performed co-transcriptionally (Staley and Woolford, 2009). Both processes comprise RNA polymerases producing RNP particles, in which the RNA is to be matured. The machineries are different but many principles of action resemble one another. Transcription and RNA processing are influencing one another, conducted in the vicinity of one another, and some proteins bind to polymerases and the growing RNA at the same time, influencing both transcription and processing. Many of these interactions, such as interactions with proteins recruited to the RNA polymerase II, are dynamic and need changing for the next step to proceed. The organisation of the chromatin structure at the transcribed genes has now emerged as a further component in the network, both in RNA polymerase I and RNA polymerase II transcription. In RNA polymerase I transcription, it is likely that UBF, together with histone proteins, takes on the role of nucleosomes in RNA polymerase II transcription. Recent results demonstrate that histone modifications regulate both the elongation rate and the recruitment of processing proteins to the RNA. Furthermore, the RNA can also recruit chromatin proteins, making RNA processing a complex network of protein and RNA interactions regulated by phosphorylations, acetylation, methylation and small GTPases.

4. Acknowledgements

This work is supported by the Swedish Cancer foundation, Carl Trygger Foundation and Magnus Bergvall Foundation.

5. References

Alló M, Buggiano V, Fededa JP, Petrillo E, Schor I, de la Mata M, Agirre E, Plass M, Eyras E, Elela SA, Klinck R, Chabot B, & Kornblihtt AR. (2009) Control of alternative splicing through siRNA-mediated transcriptional gene silencing. *Nat Struct Mol Biol.* 16(7):717-724.

Alló M, Schor IE, Muñoz MJ, de la Mata M, Agirre E, Valcárcel J, Eyras E, & Kornblihtt AR. (2011) Chromatin and Alternative Splicing. *Cold Spring Harb Symp Quant Biol.* Feb 2.

Alexander R, & Beggs JD. (2010) Cross-talk in transcription, splicing and chromatin: who makes the first call? *Biochem Soc Trans.* 38(5):1251-1256.

Alexander RD, Innocente SA, Barrass JD, & Beggs JD. (2010) Splicing-dependent RNA polymerase pausing in yeast. *Mol Cell* 40(4):582-593.

Andersson R, Enroth S, Rada-Iglesias A, Wadelius C, & Komorowski J. (2009) Nucleosomes are well positioned in exons and carry characteristic histone modifications. *Genome Res.* Oct;19(10):1732-41.

Adamson TE, Shutt DC & Price DH. (2005) Functional coupling of cleavage and polyadenylation with transcription of mRNA. *J. Biol. Chem.* 280(37):32262-32271.

Auboeuf D, Dowhan DH, Kang YK, Larkin K, Lee JW, Berget SM, & O'Malley BW. (2004) Differential recruitment of nuclear receptor coactivators may determine alternative RNA splice site choice in target genes. *Proc Natl Acad Sci U S A.* 101(8):2270-2274.

Auboeuf D, Batsché E, Dutertre M, Muchardt C, O'Malley BW. (2007) Coregulators: transducing signal from transcription to alternative splicing. *Trends Endocrinol Metab.* 18(3):122-129.

Baldi P, Brunak S, Chauvin Y, & Krogh A. (1996) Naturally occurring nucleosome positioning signals in human exons and introns. *J Mol Biol.* 263(4):503-510.

Barski A, Cuddapah S, Cui K, Roh TY, Schones DE, Wang Z, Wei G, Chepelev I, & Zhao K. (2007) High-resolution profiling of histone methylations in the human genome. *Cell.* 129(4):823-837.

Birch JL, Tan BC, Panov KI, Panova TB, Andersen JS, Owen-Hughes TA, Russell J, Lee SC, & Zomerdijk JC. (2009) FACT facilitates chromatin transcription by RNA polymerases I and III. *EMBO J.* 28(7):854-65.

Bannister AJ, & Kouzarides T. (2011) Regulation of chromatin by histone modifications. *Cell Res.* 21(3):381-95.

Batsché E, Yaniv M, & Muchardt C. (2006) The human SWI/SNF subunit Brm is a regulator of alternative splicing. *Nat Struct Mol Biol.* 13(1):22-9.

Bohnsack MT, Kos M, & Tollervey D. (2008) Quantitative analysis of snoRNA association with pre-ribosomes and release of snR30 by Rok1 helicase. *EMBO Rep.* 9(12):1230-6.

Bradsher J, Auriol J, Proietti de Santis L, Iben S, Vonesch JL, Grummt I,& Egly JM. (2002) CSB is a component of RNA pol I transcription. *Mol Cell* 10: 819-829.

Brès V. Gomes N. PickleL, & Jones K.A. (2005) A human splicing factor, SKIP, associates with P-TEFb and

enhances transcription elongation by HIV-1 Tat. *Genes Dev.* 19(10):1211-26.

Brès V, Yoh SM, & Jones, KA. (2008) The multi-tasking P-TEFb complex. *Curr Opin Cell Biol.* 20(3): 334–340.

Brody Y, Neufeld N, Bieberstein N, Causse SZ, Böhnlein EM, Neugebauer KM, Darzacq X, & Shav-Tal Y. (2011) The in vivo kinetics of RNA polymerase II elongation during co-transcriptional splicing. *PLoS Biol.* 9(1):e1000573.

Buratowski S. (2009) Progression through the RNA polymerase II CTD cycle. *Mol Cell.* Nov 25;36(4):541-6.

Carrillo Oesterreich F, Preibisch S, & Neugebauer KM. (2010) Global analysis of nascent RNA reveals transcriptional pausing in terminal exons. *Mol Cell.* 40(4):571-81.

Carrillo Oesterreich FC, Bieberstein N, & Neugebauer KM. (2011) Pause locally, splice globally. *Trends Cell Biol.* Apr 27.

Cavellán E, Asp P, Percipalle P, & Östlund Farrants A-K (2006) The WSTF-SNF2h chromatin remodeling complex interacts with several nuclear proteins in transcription. *J Biol Chem* 281: 16264-16271.

Chodavarapu RK, Feng S, Bernatavichute YV, Chen PY, Stroud H, Yu Y, Hetzel JA, Kuo F, Kim J, Cokus SJ, Casero D, Bernal M, Huijser P, Clark AT, Krämer U, Merchant SS, Zhang X, Jacobsen SE, & Pellegrini M. (2010) Relationship between nucleosome positioning and DNA methylation. *Nature.* 466(7304):388-392.

Cohanim AB, & Haran TE. (2009) The coexistence of the nucleosome positioning code with the genetic code on eukaryotic genomes. *Nucleic Acids Res.* 37(19):6466-6476.

Damgaard CK, Kahns S, Lykke-Andersen S, Nielsen AL, Jensen TH, & Kjems J. (2008) A 5' splice site enhances the recruitment of basal transcription initiation factors in vivo. *Mol Cell.* 29(2):271-278.

de la Mata M, Alonso CR, Kadener S, Fededa JP, Blaustein M, Pelisch F, Cramer P, Bentley D, & Kornblihtt AR. (2003) A slow RNA polymerase II affects alternative splicing in vivo. *Mol Cell.* 12(2):525-532.

Dhami P, Saffrey P, Bruce AW, Dillon SC, Chiang K, Bonhoure N, Koch CM, Bye J, James K, Foad NS, Ellis P, Watkins NA, Ouwehand WH, Langford C, Andrews RM, Dunham I, & Vetrie D. (2010) Complex exon-intron marking by histone modifications is not determined solely by nucleosome distribution. *PLoS One.* 5(8):e12339.

Decatur WA, & Fournier MJ. (2003) RNA-guided nucleotide modification of ribosomal and other RNAs. *J Biol Chem.* 278(2):695-698.

Dellaire G, Makarov EM, Cowger JJ, Longman D, Sutherland HG, Lührmann R, Torchia J, & Bickmore WA. (2002) Mammalian PRP4 kinase copurifies and interacts with components of both the U5 snRNP and the N-CoR deacetylase complexes. *Mol Cell Biol.* 22(14):5141-5156.

Edmunds JW, Mahadevan LC, & Clayton AL. (2008) Dynamic histone H3 methylation during gene induction: HYPB/Setd2 mediates all H3K36 trimethylation. *EMBO J.* 27(2):406-420.

Egloff S, O'Reilly D, Chapman RD, Taylor A, Tanzhaus K, Pitts L, Eick D, & Murphy S. (2007) Serine-7 of the RNA polymerase II CTD is specifically required for snRNA gene expression. *Science.* 318(5857):1777-1779.

Egloff S, & Murphy S. (2008) Cracking the RNA polymerase II CTD code. *Trends Genet.* 24(6):280-288.

Eissenberg JC, Shilatifard A, Dorokhov N, & Michener DE. (2007) Cdk9 is an essential kinase in Drosophila that is required for heat shock gene expression, histone methylation and elongation factor recruitment. *Mol Genet Genomics.* 277(2):101-114.

Fox-Walsh K, & Fu XD. (2010) Chromatin: the final frontier in splicing regulation? *Dev Cell* 18(3):336-338.

Furger A, O'Sullivan JM, Binnie A, Lee BA, & Proudfoot NJ. (2002) Promoter proximal splice sites enhance transcription. *Genes Dev.* 16(21):2792-2799.

Gardner KE, Allis CD, & Strahl BD. (2011) OPERating ON Chromatin, a Colorful Language where Context Matters.*J Mol Biol.* 409(1):36-46

Görnemann J, Kotovic KM, Hujer K, & Neugebauer KM. (2005) Cotranscriptional spliceosome assembly occurs in a stepwise fashion and requires the cap binding complex. *Mol Cell.* 19(1):53-63.

Granneman S, & Baserga SJ. (2005) Crosstalk in gene expression: coupling and co-regulation of rDNA transcription, pre-ribosome assembly and pre-rRNA processing. *Curr Opin Cell Biol.* 17(3):281-286.

Gunderson FQ, & Johnson TL. (2009) Acetylation by the transcriptional coactivator Gcn5 plays a novel role in co-transcriptional spliceosome assembly. *PLoS Genet.*5(10):e1000682.

Gunderson FQ, Merkhofer EC, & Johnson TL. (2011) Dynamic histone acetylation is critical for cotranscriptional spliceosome assembly and spliceosomal rearrangements. *Proc Natl Acad Sci U S A.*108(5):2004-2009.

Ip JY, Schmidt D, Pan Q, Ramani AK, Fraser AG, Odom DT, & Blencowe BJ. (2011) Global impact of RNA polymerase II elongation inhibition on alternative splicing regulation. *Genome Res.* 21(3):390-401.

Ito, T, Watanabe, H., Yamamichi, N., Kondo, N., Tando T, Haraguchi T, Mizutani T, Sakurai K, Fujita S, Izumi T, Isobe T, & Iba H. (2008) Brm transactivates the telomerase reverse transcriptase (TERT) gene and modulates the splicing patterns of its transcripts in concert with p54nrb. *Biochem. J.* 411, 201-209.

Hargreaves DC, & Crabtree GR. (2011) ATP-dependent chromatin remodeling: genetics, genomics and mechanisms. *Cell Res.* 21(3):396-420.

Henras AK, Soudet J, Gérus M, Lebaron S, Caizergues-Ferrer M, Mougin A, & Henry Y. (2008) The post-transcriptional steps of eukaryotic ribosome biogenesis. *Cell Mol Life Sci.* 65(15):2334-2359.

Hnilicová J, Hozeifi S, Dušková E, Icha J, Tománková T, Staněk D (2011) Histone deacetylase activity modulates alternative splicing. PLoS One 6(2):e16727.

Hon G, Wang W, & Ren B. (2009) Discovery and annotation of functional chromatin signatures in the human genome. *PLoS Comput Biol.* 5(11):e1000566

Huff JT, Plocik AM, Guthrie C, & Yamamoto KR. (2010) Reciprocal intronic and exonic histone modification regions in humans. *Nat Struct Mol Biol.* 17(12):1495-1499.

Jones HS, Kawauchi J, Braglia P, Alen CM, Kent NA,& Proudfoot NJ (2007) RNA polymerase I in yeast transcribes dynamic nucleosomal rDNA. *Nat Struct Mol Biol* 14: 123–130.

Kim M, Suh H, Cho EJ, & Buratowski S. (2009) Phosphorylation of the yeast Rpb1 C-terminal domain at serines 2, 5, and 7. *J Biol Chem.*284(39):26421-26426.

Kogan S, & Trifonov EN. (2005) Gene splice sites correlate with nucleosome positions. *Gene.*352:57-62.

Kolasinska-Zwierz P, Down T, Latorre I, Liu T, Liu XS, & Ahringer J. (2009) Differential chromatin marking of introns and expressed exons by H3K36me3. *Nat Genet.* 41(3):376-381.

Komarnitsky P., Cho, E.J., and & Buratowski, S. (2000) Different phosphorylated forms of RNA polymerase II and associated mRNA processing factors during transcription. *Genes & Dev.* 14: 2452-2460.

Kong R, Zhang L, Hu L, Peng Q, Han W, Du X, & Ke Y. (2011) hALP, A Novel Transcriptional U Three Protein (t-UTP),Activates RNA Polymerase I Transcription by Binding and Acetylating the Upstream Binding Factor (UBF). *J Biol Chem.* 286(9):7139-7148.

Kouskouti A, & Talianidis I. (2005) Histone modifications defining active genes persist after transcriptional and mitotic inactivation.*EMBO J.* 24(2):347-357.

Kressler D, Hurt E, & Bassler J. (2010) Driving ribosome assembly. Biochim Biophys Acta. Jun; 1803(6):673-83.

Lacadie SA, & Rosbash M. (2005) Cotranscriptional spliceosome assembly dynamics and the role of U1 snRNA:5'ss base pairing in yeast. *Mol Cell.* 19(1):65-75.

Lavigne M, Eskeland R, Azebi S, Saint-André V, Jang SM, Batsché E, Fan HY, Kingston RE, Imhof A, & Muchardt C. (2009) Interaction of HP1 and Brg1/Brm with the globular domain of histone H3 is required for HP1-mediated repression. *PLoS Genet.* 5(12):e1000769.

Lenasi T, & Barboric M. (2010) P-TEFb stimulates transcription elongation and pre-mRNA splicing through multilateral mechanisms. *RNA Biol.* 7(2):145-150.

Liber D, Domaschenz R, Holmqvist PH, Mazzarella L, Georgiou A, Leleu M, Fisher AG, Labosky PA, & Dillon N. (2010) Epigenetic priming of a pre-B cell-specific enhancer through binding of Sox2 and Foxd3 at the ESC stage. *Cell Stem Cell.* 7(1):114-126.

Lin S, Coutinho-Mansfield G, Wang D, Pandit S, & Fu XD. (2008) The splicing factor SC35 has an active role in transcriptional elongation. *Nat Struct Mol Biol.* 15(8):819-826.

Listerman I, Sapra AK, & Neugebauer KM. (2006) Cotranscriptional coupling of splicing factor recruitment and precursor messenger RNA splicing in mammalian cells. *Nat Struct Mol Biol.* Sep;13(9):815-22.

Lebedev A, Scharffetter-Kochanek K, & Iben S (2008) Truncated Cockayne syndrome B protein represses elongation by RNA polymerase I. *J Mol Biol* 382: 266-274.

Luco RF, Pan Q, Tominaga K, Blencowe BJ, Pereira-Smith OM, & Misteli T. (2010) Regulation of alternative splicing by histone modifications. *Science.* 327(5968):996-1000.

Luco RF, Allo M, Schor IE, Kornblihtt AR, & Misteli T. (2011) Epigenetics in alternative pre-mRNA splicing. *Cell.* 144(1):16-26.

Lunde BM, Reichow SL, Kim M, Suh H, Leeper TC, Yang F, Mutschler H, Buratowski S, Meinhart A, & Varani G. (2010) Cooperative interaction of transcription termination factors with the RNA polymerase II C-terminal domain. *Nat Struct Mol Biol.* 17(10):1195-1201.

McCracken S, Fong N, Yankulov K, Ballantyne S, Pan G, Greenblatt J, Patterson SD, Wickens M, & Bentley DL. (1997) The C-terminal domain of RNA polymerase II couples mRNA processing to transcription. *Nature.* 385(6614):357-361.

McStay B, & Grummt I. 2008) The epigenetics of rRNA genes: from molecular to chromosome biology. *Annu Rev Cell Dev Biol.*24:131-57.

Meinhart A, Kamenski T, Hoeppner S, Baumli S, & Cramer P. (2005) A structural perspective of CTD function. *Genes Dev* 19(12):1401-1415.

Merz K, Hondele M, Goetze H, Gmelch K, Stoeckl U, & Griesenbeck J (2008) Actively transcribed rRNA genes in S. cerevisiae are organized in a specialized chromatin associated with the high-mobility group protein Hmo 1 and are largely devoid of histone molecules. *Genes Dev* 22: 1190–1204.

Min IM, Waterfall JJ, Core LJ, Munroe RJ, Schimenti J, & Lis JT. (2011) Regulating RNA polymerase pausing and transcription elongation in embryonic stem cells. *Genes Dev.* 25(7):742-754.

Moore M, & Proudfoot N. (2009) Pre-mRNA processing reaches back to transcription and ahead to translation. *Cell* 136;688-700.

Morris DP, & Greenleaf AL. (2000) The splicing factor, Prp40, binds the phosphorylated carboxyl-terminal domain of RNA polymerase II. *J Biol Chem.*275:39935–39943.

Moteki S & Price D. (2002) Functional coupling of capping and transcription of mRNA. *Mol. Cell* 10(3):599-609.

Muñoz MJ, de la Mata M, & Kornblihtt AR. (2010) The carboxy terminal domain of RNA polymerase II and alternative splicing. *Trends Biochem Sci.* 35(9):497-504.

Murr R. (2010) Interplay between different epigenetic modifications and mechanisms. *Adv Genet.* 70:101-41.

Nahkuri S, Taft RJ, & Mattick JS. (2009) Nucleosomes are preferentially positioned at exons in somatic and sperm cells. *Cell Cycle.* 8(20):3420-3424.

Obrdlik A, Kukalev A, Louvet E, Östlund Farrants A-K, Caputo L, & Percipalle P. (2008) The histone acetyl transferase PCAF associates with actin and hnRNP U for RNA polymerase II transcription. *Mol. Cell. Biol.* 28:6342-6357.

Obrdlik A, Louvet E, Kukalev A, Naschekin D, Kiseleva E, Fahrenkrog B, & Percipalle P. (2010) Nuclear myosin 1 is in complex with mature rRNA transcripts and associates with the nuclear pore basket. *FASEB J.* 24(1):146-157.

Pagani F, Buratti E, Stuani C, Bendix R, Dörk T, & Baralle FE. (2002) Promoter architecture modulates CFTR exon 9 skipping. *Nat Genet.* ;30(4):426-429.

Pandit S, Wang D, & Fu XD. (2008) Functional integration of transcriptional and RNA processing machineries. *Curr Opin Cell Biol.* 20(3):260-265.

Perales R , & Bentley D (2009) "Cotranscriptionality": the transcription elongation complex as a nexus for nuclear transactions. *Mol Cell* 36(2):178-191.

Percipalle P, Fomproix N, Cavellán E, Voit R, Reimer G, Krüger T, Thyberg J, Scheer U, Grummt I, & Östlund Farrants A-K (2006) The chromatin remodelling complex WSTF-SNF2h interacts with nuclear myosin 1 and has a role in RNA polymerase I transcription. *EMBO Rep* 7: 525530.

Peng Q, Wu J, Zhang Y, Liu Y, Kong R, Hu L, Du X, & Ke Y. (2010) 1A6/DRIM, a novel t-UTP, activates RNA polymerase I transcription and promotes cell proliferation. *PLoS One.* ;5(12):e14244.

Prieto JL, & McStay B. (2007) Recruitment of factors linking transcription and processing of pre-rRNA to NOR chromatin is UBF-dependent and occurs independent of transcription in human cells. *Genes Dev.* 21(16):2041-54.

Raisner RM, Hartley PD, Meneghini MD, Bao MZ, Liu CL, Schreiber SL, Rando OJ, & Madhani HD. (2005) Histone variant H2A.Z marks the 5' ends of both active and inactive genes in euchromatin. *Cell.* 123(2):233-248.

Reyes-Reyes M, & Hampsey M. (2007) Role for the Ssu72 C-terminal domain phosphatase in RNA polymerase II transcription elongation. *Mol Cell Biol.* 27(3):926-936.

Ringrose L. (2010) How do RNA sequence, DNA sequence, and chromatin properties regulate splicing? *F1000 Biol Rep.* 12;2:74.

Saint-André V, Batsché E, Rachez C, & Muchardt C. (2011) Histone H3 lysine 9 trimethylation and HP1γ favor inclusion of alternative exons. *Nat Struct Mol Biol.* 18(3):337-344.

Saltzman AL, Pan Q, & Blencowe BJ. (2011) Regulation of alternative splicing by the core spliceosomal machinery. *Genes Dev.* 25(4):373-384.

Saltzman AL, Kim YK, Pan Q, Fagnani MM, Maquat LE, & Blencowe BJ. (2008) Regulation of multiple core spliceosomal proteins by alternative splicing-coupled nonsense-mediated mRNA decay. *Mol Cell Biol.* 28(13):4320-30.

Sanij E, & Hannan RD. (2009) The role of UBF in regulating the structure and dynamics of transcriptionally active rDNA chromatin. *Epigenetics.* ;4(6):374-382.

Santoro R, Li J, & Grummt I. (2002) The nucleolar remodeling complex NoRC mediates heterochromatin formation and silencing of ribosomal gene transcription. *Nat Genet.* 32(3):393-396.

Schones DE, Cui K, Cuddapah S, Roh TY, Barski A, Wang Z, Wei G, & Zhao K. (2008) Dynamic regulation of nucleosome positioning in the human genome. *Cell.* 132(5):887-898.

Schwartz S, Meshorer E, & Ast G. (2009) Chromatin organization marks exon-intron structure. *Nat Struct Mol Biol.* 16(9):990-995.

Schroeder SC, Schwer B, Shuman S, & Bentley D. (2000) Dynamic association of capping enzymes with transcribing RNA polymerase II. *Genes Dev.* 14(19):2435-2440.

Singh S, & Padgett, RA. (2009) Rates of in situ transcription and splicing in large human genes. *Nat Struct Mol Biol.* 16(11):1128–1133.

Schneider, D.A., French, S.L., Osheim, Y.N., Bailey, A.O., Vu, L., Dodd, J., Yates, J.R., Beyer, A.L.,& Nomura, M. (2006). RNA polymerase II elongation factors Spt4p and Spt5p play roles in transcription elongation by RNA polymerase I and rRNA processing. *Proc. Natl. Acad. Sci. USA* 103:12707–12712.

Schneider DA, Michel A, Sikes ML, Vu L, Dodd JA, Salgia S, Osheim YN, Beyer AL, & Nomura M. (2007). Transcription elongation by RNA polymerase I is linked to efficient rRNA processing and ribosome assembly. *Mol Cell* 26(2):217-229.

Sims RJ 3rd, Millhouse S, Chen CF, Lewis BA, Erdjument-Bromage H, Tempst P, Manley JL, & Reinberg D. (2007) Recognition of trimethylated histone H3 lysine 4 facilitates the recruitment of transcription postinitiation factors and pre-mRNA splicing. *Mol Cell.* 28(4):665-676.

Sims RJ 3rd, Rojas LA, Beck D, Bonasio R, Schüller R, Drury WJ 3rd, Eick D, & Reinberg D. (2011) The C-terminal domain of RNA polymerase II is modified by site-specific methylation. *Science.* 332(6025):99-103.

Sjölinder M, Björk P, Söderberg P, Sabri N, Östlund Farrants A-K, & Visa N. (2005) The growing pre-mRNA recruits actin and chromatin-modifying factors to transcriptionally active genes. *Genes Dev* 19:1871-1884.

Smith ER, Lee MG, Winter B, Droz NM, Eissenberg JC, Shiekhattar R, & Shilatifard A. (2008) Drosophila UTX is a histone H3 Lys27 demethylase that colocalizes with the elongating form of RNA polymerase II. *Mol Cell Biol.* 28(3):1041-1046.

Solier S, Barb J, Zeeberg BR, Varma S, Ryan MC, Kohn KW, Weinstein JN, Munson PJ, & Pommier Y. (2010) Genome-wide analysis of novel splice variants induced by topoisomerase I poisoning shows preferential occurrence in genes encoding splicing factors. *Cancer Res.* 70(20):8055-8065.

Spies N, Nielsen CB, Padgett RA, & Burge CB. (2009) Biased chromatin signatures around polyadenylation sites and exons. *Mol Cell.* 36(2):245-254.

Spiluttini B, Gu B, Belagal P, Smirnova AS, Nguyen VT, Hébert C, Schmidt U, Bertrand E, Darzacq X, & Bensaude O. (2010) Splicing-independent recruitment of U1 snRNP to a transcription unit in living cells. *J Cell Sci.* ;123(Pt 12):2085-2093.

Staley JP, & Woolford JL Jr. (2009) Assembly of ribosomes and spliceosomes: complex ribonucleoprotein machines. *Curr Opin Cell Biol.* 21(1):109-18.

Strunk BS, & Karbstein K. (2009) Powering through ribosome assembly. RNA. Dec; 15(12):2083-104

Tilgner H, Nikolaou C, Althammer S, Sammeth M, Beato M, Valcárcel J, Guigó R. 2009) Nucleosome positioning as a determinant of exon recognition. *Nat Struct Mol Biol.* 16(9):996-1001.

Tyagi A, Ryme J, Brodin D, & Östlund Farrants A-K, Visa N. (2009) SWI/SNF associate with nascent pre-mRNPs and regulates alternative pre-mRNA processing. *PLoS Genetics* May 5:e1000470.

Vintemist A, Böhm S, Sadeghifar F, Lovet E, Mansén A, Percipalle P, & Östlund Farrants A-K. (2011) The chromatin remodelling complex B-WICH is required for maintaining an open chromatin structure during ribosomal transcription. *PLoS ONE,* 6(4):e19184.

Wahl MC, Will CL, & Lührmann R. (2009) The spliceosome: design principles of a dynamic RNP machine. *Cell.* 136(4):701-718.

Wery,M., Ruidant,S., Schillewaert,S., Lepore,N. & Lafontaine,D.L. (2009) The nuclear poly(A) polymerase and Exosome cofactor Trf5 is recruited cotranscriptionally to nucleolar surveillance. *RNA,* 15:406–419.

Yoshikawa H, Komatsu W, Hayano T, Miura Y, Homma K, Izumikawa K, Ishikawa H, Miyazawa N, Tachikawa H, Yamauchi Y, Isobe T, & Takahashi N. (2011) Splicing factor 2-associated protein p32 participates in Ribosome biogenesis by regulating the binding of Nop52 and fibrillarin to pre-ribosome particles. *Mol Cell Proteomics.* May 2.

Yuan X, Feng W, Imhof A, Grummt I, & Zhou Y (2007) Activation of RNA polymerase I transcription by Cockayne syndrome group B protein and histone methyltransferase G9a. *Mol Cell* 27: 585–595.

Zhang L, Schroeder S, Fong N, & Bentley DL. (2005) Functional interaction of yeast pre-mRNA 3' end processing factors with RNA polymerase II. *EMBO J.* 24(13):2379-2390.

Zhou Y, Schmitz KM, Mayer C, Yuan X, Akhtar A, & Grummt I. (2009) Reversible acetylation of the chromatin remodelling complex NoRC is required for non-coding RNA-dependent silencing. *Nat Cell Biol.* 11(8):1010-1016.

2

Hide and Go Seek: Activation of the Secretory-Specific Poly (A) Site of *Igh* by Transcription Elongation Factors

Christine Milcarek
University of Pittsburgh / Department of Immunology
United States of America

1. Introduction

The regulation of the immunoglobulin heavy chain (Igh) alternative RNA processing has served as a model system for revealing the competition between *cis* and *trans*-acting RNA factors influencing splicing and polyadenylation, reviewed in (Peterson 2007) and (Borghesi and Milcarek 2006). This review will explore recent studies on the role of transcription elongation factors in the super elongation complex (SEC) including ELL2 (eleven-nineteen lysine rich leukemia factor) on driving poly(A) site choice. Elongation factors impel high levels of Igh mRNA production and alternative processing at the promoter proximal, secretory-specific poly(A) site (sec) in plasma cells by enhancing RNA polymerase II modifications and downstream events. The sec poly(A) site, essentially hidden in B cells, is found by SEC factors in plasma cells.

Most mRNAs have a poly(A) tail and it has been estimated that up to 20% of the human genes may be arranged with a competition of splicing and polyadenylation sites as seen in the Igh (Tian, Pan et al. 2007; Rigo and Martinson 2008). Numerous genes contain multiple poly(A) sites (Tian, Hu et al. 2005); many subject to regulation (Edwalds-Gilbert, Veraldi et al. 1997) and (Lutz and Moreira 2011). Advancing developmental stage is generally correlated with use of promoter distal poly(A) sites (Ji, Lee et al. 2009; Ji and Tian 2009). Yet the opposite situation applies as B-cells terminally differentiate into plasma cells; elongation factors may hold the key to understanding this apparent paradox.

Transcriptional pausing and subsequent elongation are emerging as important check points for gene regulation. Phosphorylation of the carboxyl-terminal domain of RNAP-II by initiation and elongation factors directs the correct associations to ultimately drive mature mRNA output. The SEC, composed of nine proteins including pTEFb and ELL (see key), kick starts elongation by facilitating the phosphorylation of both the negative acting factors that have stalled the polymerase and polymerase itself. The mPAF is recruited by the action of the pTEFb through phosphorylation of the serine-2 of the RNA polymerase carboxyl-terminal domain heptad repeat; mPAF brings along with it the polyadenylation factors. The factors that polyadenylate mRNA are more strongly associated with the polymerase transcription complex on highly active promoters and/ or through up-regulation of the polyadenylation and elongation factors, especially CstF (cleavage stimulatory factor), pTEFb, and ELL2. Polymerases deficient in the appropriate factors may transit the gene, but if these pauci-polymerases proceed, they lack sufficient concentrations of factors to efficiently process the nascent RNA. Information from the literature on the linkages between elongation and alternative processing as well as TAR:TAT mediated RNA output and pTEFb interactions in HIV infected T-cells inform the search for understanding the mechanisms operative in the Igh locus.

Frequently used abbreviations: CPSF, *Cleavage Polyadenylation Specificity Factor with subunits of 160, 100, 73 & 30 kDa;* CstF, *Cleavage stimulatory factor. Subunits of 77, 64 and 50 kDa;* CTD, *the carboxyl-terminal domain of eukaryotic RNA polymerase II;* ELL2, *eleven-nineteen lysine rich leukemia factor, RNA polymerase elongation factor 2, similar but not identical to ELL1; Igh, immunoglobulin heavy chain;* mPAF, *Human/ mammalian analog of yeast complex, polymerase II associated factors that coordinate setting of histone marks associated with active transcription;* Mediator, *Large, variable complex of proteins associated with DNA-bound transcription factors aiding RNAP-II binding to transcription start site. Composition may depend on promoter;* pTEFb, *positive transcription elongation factor b, composed of cyclin T and cdk9;* RNAP-II, *RNA Polymerase II of eukaryotic cells, composed of multiple subunits;* SEC, *super elongation complex for transcription elongation;* Sec:mb, *Ratio of secretory-specific polyadenylated to M1 spliced Igh mRNA; >20:1 in plasma cells;* SR proteins, *Serine and Arginine rich proteins that tend to enhance splicing (eg. SF2/ASF) of the pre-mRNA exons to which they bind. In contrast, SRp20 seems to suppress exon inclusion;* U1A, *Protein A (35 kDa) found with the U1 small nuclear RNP (U1 snRNP).*

2. Igh and plasma cell gene regulation, an RNA processing problem

The mature B-cell has an exquisitely specific antigen receptor, the membrane form of the Immunoglobulin of the mu or delta type, paired with Ig light chain, expressed on its surface. The V region of the Ig is the result of a series of gene rearrangements generating specificity in the development of that B cell. This B cell can be activated by antigen association directly or be assisted in its differentiation by T-cells to start to secrete the Ig in the terminally differentiated B cell, i.e. the plasma cell. There are seven immunoglobulin heavy chain genes (Igh) in mice. The mouse heavy-chain genes (isotypes) are named mu, delta, gamma 1, gamma 2a, gamma 2b and gamma 3, and alpha; they are clustered together in an array on the chromosome in that order. The name of the heavy chain designates the name of the H2:L2 molecule; for example μ2:L2, i.e. mu heavy chains plus light chains, are designated IgM while and δ2:L2 are called IgD. The heavy chains encode secreted proteins of approximately 55,000 kDa, with mu producing the largest H chain. The light chains (kappa or lambda) produce approximately 25,000 kDa proteins and the genes undergo no alternative RNA processing. Each Igh gene has the capability to produce both membrane-specific and secreted forms of the protein, as encoded in the alternatively processed heavy chain mRNAs. Plasma cells express only one of the Igh isotypes as a secreted protein.

Blimp-1, (B-lymphocyte inducer of maturation) a transcription repressor, turns off a number of early B-cell transcription factors like pax-5 and bcl-6 while it indirectly activates production of the secreted form of the Igh mRNA and a family of gene products leading to plasma cell terminal differentiation. Among the blimp-inducible genes are ELL2 and EAF2 (Kuo and Calame 2004; Shaffer, Shapiro-Shelef et al. 2004); these are two transcription elongation factors previously isolated in transcription studies. Activation of the blimp-1 gene occurs both in T-dependent and T-independent pathways for B-cell development, as

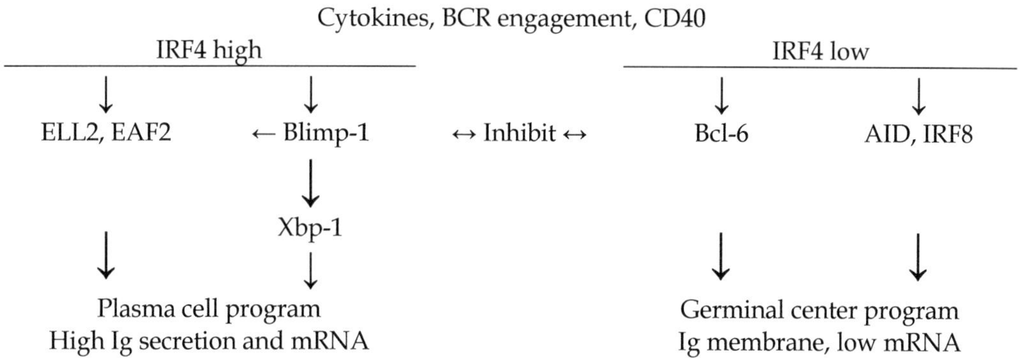

Fig. 1. A proposed schema of plasma cell versus germinal center cell development adapted from (Lu 2008) and (Sciammas, Shaffer et al. 2006) with roles for ELL2 and EAF2 added. Blimp-1 and Bcl-6 have been shown to inhibit each other (Shaffer, Yu et al. 2000). Xbp-1 is also involved in the unfolded protein response in plasma cells (Shaffer, Shapiro-Shelef et al. 2004).

recently reviewed (Martins and Calame 2008). Blimp-1 is low or absent in memory B-cells; meanwhile IRF-4 levels are key to the activated/ memory/ plasma cell transition; the role for each gene, as well as Xbp-1, is still under active investigation, see review (Martins and Calame 2008); one synthesis of all the information is presented in (Lu 2008). It is also notable that ELL2 expression is influenced directly by expression of IRF4, a transcription factor that modulates plasma cell differentiation; IRF4 was found bound to the ELL2 promoter by chromatin immune-precipitation studies (Shaffer, Emre et al. 2008).
The Igh transcripts of any isotype are subject to alternative RNA processing, summarized in (Borghesi and Milcarek 2006) and (Peterson 2007) and diagrammed in Figure 2. The various Igh genes have different numbers of CH regions so the last secretory exon is labeled CH4 in the mu Igh or CH3 in the gamma genes. When the secretory specific poly(A) site is used, the pre-mRNA is cleaved so that splicing between the site embedded in the last secretory-specific exon and M1 does not occur. This is the preferred but not exclusive mode in plasma cells. The spacing between the weak M1 splicing and sec-specific poly (A) sites in the various Igh genes is highly conserved at ~300 nts. When the splice in CH3 (γ) or CH4 (μ) is

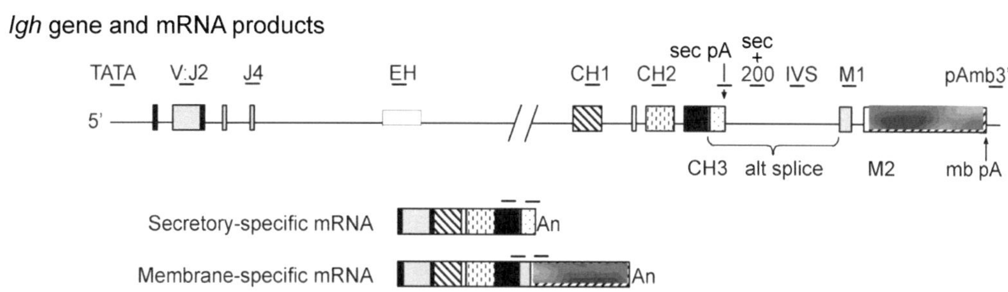

Fig. 2. **The Igh chain.** Mouse IgG2a heavy chain gene is shown with sites for primers used for QPCR (Shell, Martincic et al. 2007). The identical IgG2a gene is expressed in the A20 mouse B cells and AxJ plasma cells; the VH used is a single copy gene. The two mRNAs, secretory (sec) and membrane-specific (mb) are shown.

completed to M1, the secretory specific poly(A) site is removed from the pre-mRNA and unavailable and the mb poly(A) site is used. This is the predominant pathway in mature and memory B-cells. The sec poly(A) and splice to M1 are therefore mutually exclusive in any one transcript, while within the population of RNAs the sec:mb ratio is ~1:1 in B-cells and in plasma cells sec:mb is >20:1. The tendency to use the first poly(A) site in plasma cell development for the Igh gene reverses the trend seen in many developmentally regulated genes where it is the downstream site not the upstream site favored as development proceeds, perhaps caused by a weakening of mRNA polyadenylation activity (Ji, Lee et al. 2009). ELL2 may be induced to reverse this trend in plasma cells and thus alleviating a transcriptional pause may lead to alternative mRNA processing. We will explore the regulation of the alternative processing of the Igh RNA in the course of this review.

3. Differential expression of factors in a number of pathways seen between B cells and plasma cells

The entire ~11 kb gamma 2a or 2b Igh gene is transcribed ~2kb past the membrane poly(A) site regardless of which poly(A) site is used; this occurs in both B-cells and plasma cells (Flaspohler and Milcarek. 1990; Flaspohler and Milcarek 1992; Flaspohler, Boczkowski et al. 1995). The plasma cell phenotype dominates over that seen in the mature/memory B-cell when somatic cell hybrids were created and influences the nuclear versus cytoplasmic accumulation of many RNAs; Igh chain is the most profoundly affected. Igh protein levels are directly proportional to Igh mRNA levels (Milcarek, Hartman et al. 1996).

Weak poly(A) sites are used more efficiently in plasma cells than in B/ memory cells even in constructs in which there is no splicing between the sites. Polyadenylation therefore tips the balance towards secretory poly(A) site use in plasma cells (Milcarek and Hall 1985; Kobrin, Milcarek et al. 1986; Lassman, Matis et al. 1992; Lassman and Milcarek 1992; Matis, Martincic et al. 1996). Differences between plasma and memory B-cells are found in the polyadenylation machinery. These changes occur in the binding efficiency of basal factors Cleavage Stimulatory Factor CstF-64 and Cleavage Polyadenylation Specificity Factor CPSF-100 (Edwalds-Gilbert and Milcarek 1995; Edwalds-Gilbert and Milcarek 1995). LPS induction of splenic B-cells increases CstF-64 and introduction of CstF-64 into chicken DT40 B-cells results in Ig secretion (Takagaki, Seipelt et al. 1996), see Table 1.

Both the Igh 5′ splice site in the last sec exon and the sec poly(A) sites are weak and in competition (Peterson and Perry 1989); overall splicing is decreased in plasma cells (Bruce, Dingle et al. 2003). A shift in the SR-proteins is seen from the activating type (ASF/SF2) in B-cells to the repression type (SRp20) in plasma cells. The factors hnRNP F and U1A, both of which block the secretory-specific poly(A) site from functioning, are reduced in plasma cells (Veraldi, Arhin et al. 2001; Milcarek, Martincic et al. 2003; Alkan, Martincic et al. 2006) and (Ma, Gunderson et al. 2006) which would allow the secretory site to function better. The major effectors in the alternative processing in B versus plasma cells are summarized in Table 1.

The OCA-B transcription factor is up-regulated in plasma cells (Qin, Reichlin et al. 1998); it binds to oct2 at the Igh promoter. The CCNC complex of cyclin C and cdk8 along with PC4/ sub1 are induced by IRF4 in multiple myeloma a tumor of the plasma cells (Shaffer, Emre et al. 2008) and could act on the Igh gene to regulate transcription.

We re-examined the micro-array data on gene expression in B versus plasma cells that we published previously (Martincic, Alkan et al. 2009) to concentrate on transcription elongation factors. The data are shown Table 1. The robust up-regulation of blimp-1 and IRF4 are presented as controls to show that the plasma cells are at the fully differentiated stage, as expected. The ELL2 and PC4 mRNA are the next most highly induced in plasma cells, increased approximately 6-fold over B cells. Most of the other factors like cdk8, cyclin C and eaf2 are moderately induced in our test plasma cells (<2-fold). But it is of interest that supt5h (a DSIF subunit) and pTEFb subunits cdk9 and cyclin T are also induced ~2-fold as is the relA subunit of NF-kB, a transcription factor that binds to the Igh enhancer region.

Factors, function	5′ splice favored (B and memory cells)	Sec poly(A) site favored (Plasma cells/ myeloma)
Igh mRNA form	Mb> sec	Sec>>mb
Igh mRNA abundance	1	20-100 greater
OCA-B, Igh promoter binding	Low	Higher
Blimp-1, IRF4, general transcription factors	Low	6-300 X
relA, NF-kB transcription factor	Low	~2X
Cdk8, cyclin C. PC4, CTD phosphorylation	Low	~4X in myeloma
RNA polymerase loading on Igh	Low	High
Ser-2, ser-5 P on CTD RNAP-II Igh promoter	Low	~8X
LPS induced CstF-64, polyadenyation	-	~6X
ELL2, transcription elongation	Low	~6X
pTEFb, Supt5h, elongation	Low	~2X
hnRNP F, polyadenylation inhibitor	~4X	Low
U1A, polyadenylation inhibitor	~4X	Low
ASF/SF, splicing	High	Low
SRp20, splicing	Low	High
Pausing at sec poly(A) site	yes	same

Table 1. Expression levels in B versus plasma cells, see text for references

Taking all this information into account, it is clear that the plasma cell program for expression of the secreted form of the Igh mRNA is indeed complex. Transcription and elongation are a unifying theme for many of the changes seen. There is up-regulation of a number of transcription factors including the NF-kB subunit relA. There are changes to the phosphorylation of the CTD of RNAP-II and the enzymes that do this. Transcription elongation factors like ELL2 are up-regulated. Each of these aspects of gene expression will be discussed in turn, below.

3.1 Do factors bound at the Igh promoter or enhancer influence alternative Igh RNA processing?

The original studies of the Igh gene showed only a small enhancement of transcription activity in plasma cells over that seen in B-cells (Kelly and Perry 1986). Those studies used the incorporation of radioactive nucleotides and filter hybridization. Our studies using chromatin immunoprecipitation showed only a 2-fold change in the amount of RNA polymerase II on the Igh TATA region (see Figure 2). Meanwhile, the modifications of polymerases differ between the cell types and may contribute significantly to processing changes; this will be discussed in a subsequent section. But the alternative processing of the Igh gene appears to obey the same rules with respect to alternative processing whether the gene is intact (Kobrin, Milcarek et al. 1986) or if the CH1 exon to the 3′ end are placed as a cassette linked to an SV40 promoter (Peterson and Perry 1986). Therefore most studies have ignored the contribution of the Igh promoter to regulation. However, recent studies linking elongation and pausing to alternative processing of RNA implicate the promoter; the changes we saw in polymerase modifications also suggest a re-examination of factors that might act the Igh promoter.

Neither blimp-1 nor IRF-4 has any mapped interactions with the Igh promoter. But TAF105 is a lymphocyte specific "general transcription factor" found in a small fraction of TFIID complexes (Dikstein, Zhou et al. 1996; Wolstein, Silkov et al. 2000). TAF105 is dispensable for B-cell differentiation (Freiman, Albright et al. 2002); its role in immunoglobulin heavy chain (Igh) expression is unknown. Meanwhile, OCA-B (OBF-1/Bob1) is a transcription factor that binds indirectly to the octamer sequence in the Igh promoter through oct2, interacts with TAF105 (Wolstein, Silkov et al. 2000) and is up-regulated in plasma cells (Qin, Reichlin et al. 1998). OCA-B deficient mice show strain-specific, partial blocks at multiple stages of B-cell maturation and a complete disruption of germinal center formation in all strains. IgM secretion (an early event) may be normal while IgG+ cell expansion (a later event) is disrupted but not isotype switching (Teitell 2003). Gene array studies show that OCA-B may act on genes for cell expansion, like cyclin D3 (Kim, Siegel et al. 2003), not Igh secretion *per se*, although its role in alternative processing has not been extensively studied. Oct2 was originally believed to work on Igh expression but studies with knock-out mice reveal that its major role is on regulation of the IL-5 receptor (Emslie, D'Costa et al. 2008). But these factors may direct RNAP-II modifications.

The subunits cdk8 and cyclin C (CCNC) are involved in modification of the RNA polymerase and might possibly thus serve a regulatory role in alternative Igh mRNA processing. These two are up-regulated in the condition known as multiple myeloma (Shaffer, Emre et al. 2008) a tumor of a plasma cell, along with PC4 (aka sub1 in yeast). Both cdk8 and cyclin C have been shown to be associated with the mediator complex. Mediator is a co-activator of transcription; the composition of this large complex may vary with the promoter in response to different DNA-bound activators, acting as a link between them and the transcription start-site (Sato, Tomomori-Sato et al. 2004). The order of addition of mediator vs RNAP-II may vary for different genes (Lewis and Reinberg 2003). Transcriptional enhancers like p53 and VP16 target different mediator subunits (Taatjes, Marr et al. 2004) and other general transcription factors like TFIIB and TFIIA ; meanwhile herpes virus 1 ICP4 targets TFIID, another general transcription factor bound at the promoter (Grondin and DeLuca 2000). CPSF, a subunit of the polyadenylation complex, was found associated with TFIID at the promoter and subsequently transferred to the elongating polymerase (Dantonel, Murthy et al. 1997). Transcriptional activators like GAL4-VP16 enhance the polyadenylation of mRNA precursors through interaction with elongation factors (Nagaike, Logan et al. 2011). It will be interesting to determine if CCNC functions in alternative Igh RNA processing. The role of CTD phosphorylation is discussed below.

The nuclear factor kappa B (NF-kB) was first discovered in B-cells but subsequently found in most other cells. It has been shown to regulate a number of important processes including the cell cycle (Hinz, Krappmann et al. 1999). The relA and p50 subunits are released from an inhibitor and allowed to enter the nucleus on activation of NF-kB; expression is constitutive in mature B-cells (Fields, Seufzer et al. 2000). There are binding sites for NF-kB throughout the Igh gene (Horowitz, Zalazowski et al. 1999). We see an increase in relA in plasma cells. What role NF-kB plays in the differential expression of the Igh mRNAs is not known but may provide insights into the role of activation of promoters and increased polyadenylation.

The nuclear transcription factor C/EBPβ , also called NF-IL6, regulates a variety of genes involved in diverse functions such as acute phase response,(Poli 1998) immune function,(Screpanti, Romani et al. 1995; Tanaka, Akira et al. 1995; Poli 1998) inflammation,(Lekstrom-Himes and Xanthopoulos 1999) and hematopoiesis (Calkhoven, Muller et al. 2000). Binding sites for factor C/EBPβ are found in the Igh enhancer and a variety of genes important in lymphocytes and multiple myeloma (Pal, Janz et al. 2009). Deletion of the C/EBPβ gene in mice results in impaired generation of B lymphocytes (Chen, Liu et al. 1997). Therefore it is a candidate for up-regulating Igh transcription leading ultimately to Ig secretion.

The composition of transcription complexes assembled on different core promoters has been shown to affect splice site selection during pre-mRNA splicing (Cramer, Caceres et al. 1999; Zhao, Hyman et al. 1999). The promoter sequence motif in the Simian Virus 40 (SV40) early core promoter influences alternative splicing presumably by influencing both the composition of the transcription complex that assembles and the processivity of transcription elongation (Gendra, Colgan et al. 2007). Thus the common theme between the Igh and SV40 promoters, both of which were used to drive first poly(A) site use in the Igh locus, is that they are strong promoters in plasma cells. The Igh gene may get that way by the up-regulation of *trans* acting factors like cdk8 and cyclin C or something else while the SV40 promoter is inherently strong and something may be lacking or inhibitory in B cells which does not allow it to function optimally. There is still much to learn about this.

The presence or absence of the TATA element in the core promoter can change the way the NF-kB gene itself engages elongation and pausing factors (Amir-Zilberstein, Ainbinder et al. 2007). Thus there is a tight link between the promoter, initiation, elongation and polyadenylation in NF-kB. Interestingly, different Igh V regions vary with respect to the presence or absence of the TATA box (Johnston, Wood et al. 2006) so this linkage of TATA to elongation seen in NF-kB may not be applicable to the Igh family.

3.2 RNA polymerase II phosphorylation is altered on the Igh gene in plasma cells

Productive metazoan gene expression involves recruitment of RNAP-II to the promoter region, subsequent initiation of transcription, followed by, in many cases, a pause which is then released to allow elongation and RNA processing. The resulting mature mRNA is spliced and polyadenylated as a part of the transcription elongation "machine". At least 50 proteins are involved in DNA recognition and assembly of a transcription complex on a promoter. RNAP-II, general transcription factors, gene-specific DNA binding proteins, the mediator complexes and nucleosome-modifying factors are involved. Modifications occur in the chromatin, the RNA polymerase II itself, elongation and processing factors; this is a concerted, multifaceted transformation, reviewed in (Selth, Sigurdsson et al. 2010) and (Hargreaves, Horng et al. 2009). Many excellent reviews have been published that deal with the transition from initiation to elongation, for example (Nechaev and Adelman 2011) and the linkage of elongation to RNA processing, DNA repair, Ig gene hypermutation, nuclear export and sister chromatid cohesion (Akhtar, Heidemann et al. 2009; Perales and Bentley 2009).

The RNA polymerase large subunit contains a carboxyl-terminal domain (CTD) which can be phosphorylated in multiple positions of the 52 repeats of the heptad consensus: Tyrosine-Serine-Proline-Threonine-Serine-Proline-Serine, reviewed in (Muñoz, de la Mata et al. 2010). Phosphorylations of Ser-2, ser-5 and ser-7 of the CTD are the major modifications but *cis-trans* isomerization (Xu and Manley 2007) as well as serine and threonine glycosylation can occur. The multilayered phosphorylation of the CTD is brought about by a series of enzymatic activities during initiation and elongation. Near the promoter, TFIIH (Kin28/cdk7) phosphorylates ser-5 and ser-7 of the heptad consensus (Akhtar, Heidemann et al. 2009; Glover-Cutter, Larochelle et al. 2009). Associated with mediator complex are cyclin C and cdk8 which also phosphorylate primarily ser-5 although some activity on ser-2 has been noted. In a plasma cell tumor cdk8, cyclin C and PC4 the mammailian homolog of the yeast sub1 are up-regulated (Shaffer, Emre et al. 2008); this is highly suggestive of a role for them in Igh mRNA production. Yeast sub1 has been shown to interact with all the CTD kinases and it may have multiple actions throughout the transcription cycle (Garcia, Rosonina et al. 2010). Surprisingly, our experiments did not show a role for PC4/ sub1 in directing alternative Igh mRNA expression (Martincic, Alkan et al. 2009) and below.

The primary phosphorylation of ser-2 occurs through the action of positive transcription elongation factor b, aka pTEFb (composed of Cyclin T1 or 2 & cdk9). The pivotal role of pTEFb in elongation has been described in numerous studies, reviewed in (Pirngruber, Schhebet et al. 2009), and discussed below. Whole genome studies of CTD phosphorylation in *S. cerevisiae* reveal a complex pattern of the three ser-phosphorylations that are gene specific with the ser-7 marks being dynamic, i.e. placed anew most likely by bur1, the yeast cyclin dependent kinase (Tietjen, Zhang et al. 2010). Thus the myriad combinations of these three modifications on 52 repeats, alone or together, allows for tremendous multiplicity in the association of factors with the CTD.

These phosphorylations of the CTD allow for the associations of histone modifying enzymes primarily to histone H3; activating modifications include acetylation at K9 and K14 and methylations at K4, K36 and K79 to link the CTD to processing factors and possibly help unwind the DNA from the histone core.

Kinases	TFIIH Yeast Kin28/cdk7	Cyclin C/cdk8 aka CCNC	Cyclin T/cdk9 aka pTEFb	?
RNAP-II CTD phosphorylation	Ser-5, ser-7	Ser-5> ser-2	Ser-2>>ser-5	?
Co-factor?	..........................Sub1/PC4 ??..................................			
Interactions/enzymes	MLL, SMYD2 yeast set1, set7/9	NSD1 Yeast set2		Dot1L
Activating Histone H3 methylations	Lysine 4	Lysine 36		Lysine 79

Table 2. Linkage between the activation of RNA polymerase II and histone H3 modifications.

With this in mind, we investigated the patterns of polymerase loading and serine phosphorylation of CTD on the Igh gene in two cell lines representing either B-cells or plasma cells, which are noteworthy in that they carry the identical IgG2a heavy chain gene (Shell, Martincic et al. 2007). Using chromatin immunoprecipitation and real time PCR across the Igh locus (probes illustrated in Figure 2) we found that there is a large increase in both ser-5 and ser-2 phosphorylation of CTD near the 5′ end in plasma cells concomitant with high Ig heavy chain secretory-specific mRNA production. Factors for polyadenylation (CPSF-160, CstF-50 and -64), transcription elongation (ELL2), and co-transcription activation (PC4) can be found in much greater abundance near the 5′ start site in the plasma cells than in B-cells, See Figure 3 for summary of those data. We concluded that increased phosphorylation of RNA polymerase II at the start of transcription and the increased association of polyadenylation, and elongation/ co-transcription factors are important in influencing alternative mRNA processing of the Ig heavy chain gene. Using siRNA to ELL2 reduced the binding of ELL2 and CstF-64 to the Igh TATA region (Figure 3) implying a sequential relationship among those factors.
The drug D-ribo-furanosyl-benzimidazole (DRB) can be used to inhibit the action of pTEFb on its targets (Yamaguchi, Wada et al. 1998). We showed that treatment of plasma cells with DRB inhibits ser-2 phosphorylation and causes the unmodified RNAP-II on the Ig heavy chain in plasma cells to stall near the 5′-end of the Ig gene (Shell, Martincic et al. 2007) and Figure 3. DRB also causes the decreased association of ELL2, PC4 and the polyadenylation factor CstF-64, suggesting that their binding to RNAP-II require the ser-5 and ser-2

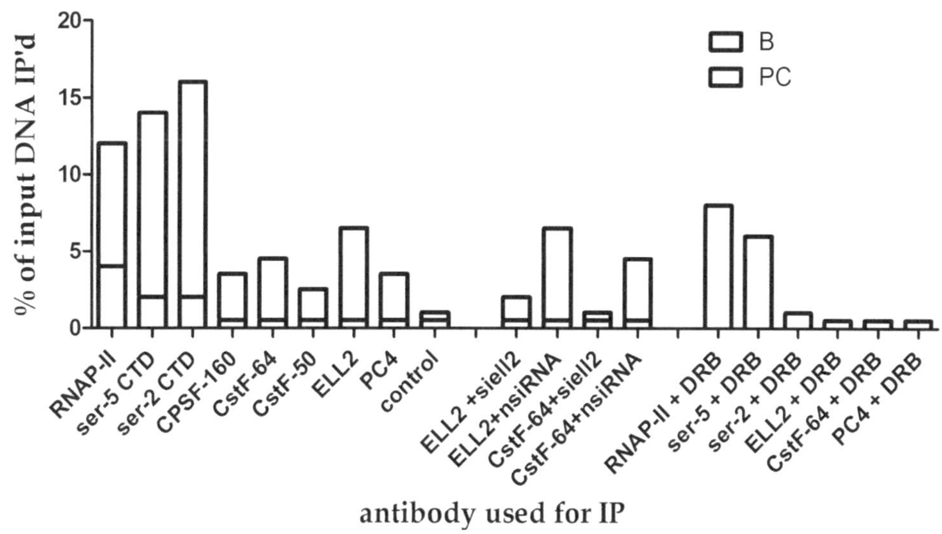

Fig. 3. **Co-activators are differentially loaded onto the IgG2a heavy chain near the promoter.** Chromatin was immune- precipitated with antibodies against the indicated factors. The resulting DNA was amplified in a QPCR with primers for the 5′ end of the Ig gamma 2a H chain transcript, as designated TATA on map of Igh, Figure 2. Grey boxes are the signals from A20 B-cells and white boxes the plasma cell AxJ. Data are simplified and compiled here from two papers: (Shell, Martincic et al. 2007), normal and DRB treatment and siell2 data (Martincic, Alkan et al. 2009). The error bars and statistics showing significance are detailed in those publications and omitted here for clarity.

modifications. The increased CTD phosphorylation, polyadenylation factor, and elongation factor association at the 5′ end in plasma cells vs B-cells are consistent with an RNAP-II on the Ig heavy chain gene in plasma cells that is primed for recognition of the proximal (secretory-specific) poly(A) site. Such polymerases would be expected to produce mRNA, leading to high abundance. The nascent RNAs could be efficiently processed, most likely at the promoter proximal poly(A) site, thereby producing the secreted form of the Igh mRNA and the protein.

In contrast to plasma cells, in the B-cells the polymerase on the Ig heavy chain gene is much less heavily modified with either type of ser-phosphorylation, polyadenylation factors, ELL2 or PC4. These polymerases in B-cells seem more likely to allow the weak donor site for the alternative CH3 to M1 splice to be set up and are not as competent for polyadenylation at the weak sec poly(A) site. Of course the presence of inhibitory factors also plays a role (see below). It appears that the polymerase in B-cells lacking the ser-2 and ser-5 modifications never acquire them in bulk even downstream (Shell, Martincic et al. 2007). Thus they may be dubbed "pauci-polymerases" in so far as they lack the modifications and the factors necessary to efficiently polyadenylate the RNA. This also results in decreased mRNA yield per polymerase pass. This is consistent with recent observations that a strong promoter directs strong association of polyadenylation factors with the polymerase (Nagaike, Logan et al. 2011).

The co-transcriptional processing of nascent RNA can be an inefficient activity even when RNAP-II is transiting the gene. This is evident in the c-H-ras gene where a mutation making a splice stronger significantly up-regulates mature mRNA production and leads to oncogenesis without changing transcription rate (Cohen and Leninson 1988). In the prothrombin gene, increased efficiency of the mRNA 3′ end formation and thus protein production is brought about by mutation near the poly(A) site with no change in transcription rate. The mutation at the poly(A) site causes increased risk for blood clots in people carrying the mutation (Gehring, Frede et al. 2001). So weak *cis* acting signals allow the polymerase to avoid co-transcription processing; this along with pauci-polymerases can also result in low production of mature mRNA.

Changes in the level of rate-limiting, *trans* acting factors, like CstF-64 following lipopolysaccharide stimulation in B-cells (Takagaki, Seipelt et al. 1996) or macrophages (Shell, Hesse et al. 2005) or in the cell cycle (Martincic, Campbell et al. 1998), can also increase mRNA polyadenylation (Getz, Elder et al. 1976). Changes in the level of ELL2, a transcription elongation factor, increase use of the first poly(A) site in the Igh gene (Martincic, Alkan et al. 2009), an important step for plasma cell development. Therefore, the throughput of initiated transcripts to polyadenylated, mature mRNA is limited by a.) *cis* acting elements in the nascent RNA, b.) the availability of *trans* acting polyadenylation factors and c.) the elongation factors and their requisite associations with the polymerase at pause sites.

3.3 Do modifications of the histones regulate alternative processing of Igh RNA?

The appearance of mono-, di-, and tri-methylated forms of histone H3, modified at Lysine 4, Lysine 36 or Lysine 79 (aka $H3K4^{me2/3}$, $H3K36^{me3}$ and $H3K79^{me1,2,3}$) are signals of gene activation (Steger, Lefterova et al. 2008). The K4 mark is associated with the multiple lineage leukemia gene MLL in mammalian cells and yeast SET1 and COMPASS at a number of gene loci (Wang, Lin et al. 2009). MLL interacts with Menin to form a histone methyltransferase for H3K4 (Yokoyama, Lin et al. 2004) which results in the expression of the developmentally important Hoxa7 and -9 genes, hallmarks of MLL induced leukemia (Ayton and Cleary 2003).

The ser-5 modification of the CTD of RNAP-II directs histone modifications especially at H3K4, see Table 2. The H3K36me3 mark has been associated with recruitment of splicing factors to exons (Spies, Nielsen et al. 2009) and it can modulate alternative splicing by recruiting Polypyrimidine Tract Binding (PTB) protein to sub-optimal exons (Luco, Pan et al. 2010). The yeast SET2 enzyme binds to a peptide of CTD phosphorylated at ser-2 and ser-5 with two heptapeptide repeats and three flanking NH_2-terminal residues, whereas a single CTD repeat is insufficient for binding (Vojnic, Simon et al. 2006). The mammalian homolog of SET2 is NSD1 which has been shown to link H3K36methylation and leukemogenesis (Wang, Cai et al. 2007). H3K79 methylations are brought about by Dot1L (Steger, Lefterova et al. 2008); the linkage of Dot1L action to CTD modifications has thus far not been made. Conversion of H3K79 monomethylation into di- and tri-methylation is correlated with the transition from low- to high-level gene transcription. The multi-subunit Dot1 complex (DotCom) includes MLL partners: ENL, AF9/MLLT3, AF17/MLLT6, and AF10/MLLT10 (Mohan, Herz et al. 2010). In another study ENL was shown to associate with Dot1L to methylate K79 (Mueller, Bach et al. 2007); ENL may thus link the super elongation complex (SEC) with H3K79 modifications, see Table 2.

We saw no changes in H3 K9 or K14 acetylation on the Igh by chromatin IP in previous studies although unusual high acetylation was seen near the Igh enhancer region, consistent with its role in gene activation (Shell, Martincic et al. 2007). However, terminal B cell differentiation *in vitro* was induced by the inhibition of histone acetylases (Lee, Bottaro et al. 2003) and knocking out histone deactylase-2 in chicken B cells had an influence on both transcription and alternative processing (Takami, Kikuchi et al. 1999). Studies of other modifications of the histones are clearly warranted and on-going in the Igh locus to understand how these might control alternative processing.

3.4 Polyadenylation of Igh RNA is altered in plasma cells

Most mature eukaryotic mRNAs contain a homopolymer (20-250 nts) of adenosines, the 3′ poly(A) tail, which controls mRNA degradation, mRNA export, and translation efficiency in somatic cells (Sachs and Wahle 1993) and in oocyte maturation (Sheets, Wu et al. 1995). When poly(A) tails were first discovered, hybridization studies revealed some exceptions to the rule, there are unique poly(A) minus mRNAs (Milcarek, Price et al. 1974). A recent look at mRNA expression by deep sequencing has revealed both poly(A)-plus and minus mRNAs but these poly(A)-minus mRNAs are in the minority (Yang, Duff et al. 2011).

Despite these exceptions, polyadenylation is a common means for 3′ end formation; many genes have more than one poly(A) site (Lutz and Moreira 2011). The sequence requirements for poly(A) tail addition are an AAUAAA or a closely related poly(A) **signal**, followed by the **site** where cleavage and poly(A) addition will occur and from 30-50 nts downstream, a GU or U rich **downstream sequence**, illustrated in Figure 4. Minimal protein factors required for the coupled pre-mRNA cleavage and polyadenylation include: cleavage stimulatory factor trimer (CstF 77, 64 & 50); poly(A) polymerase (PAP); cleavage factors (CF) I_m and II_m; nuclear and cleavage and polyadenylation specificity factor complex (CPSF 160, 100, 73 & 30 kDa). CPSF recognizes the AAUAAA signal and CstF recognizes the downstream element. Nuclear poly(A) binding proteins II, involved in transport and cytoplasmic stability, are bound to the newly formed poly(A) tail. CPSF-73 is the presumptive endonuclease for cleavage of the pre-mRNA (Mandel, Kaneko et al. 2006). These factors interact to form a large complex *in vitro* (Moore, Skolnik-David et al. 1988; Stefano and Adams 1988) (Veraldi, Edwalds-Gilbert et al. 2000) and *in vivo* (Shi, Di Giammartino et al. 2009). CPSF interacts with TFIID (transcription factor II D) then RNA polymerase II at the promoter and remains associated with RNAP-II in HeLa cells (Dantonel, Murthy et al. 1997; McCracken, Fong et al. 1997) and on the Igh gene as we have shown (Shell, Martincic et al. 2007)

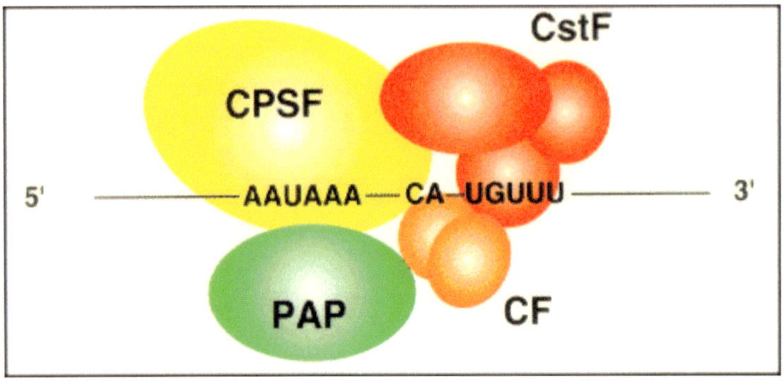

Fig. 4. Minimal factors required for poly(A) tail addition at 3′ end of RNA.

The CstF trimer is required for the cleavage reaction (MacDonald, Wilusz et al. 1994), interacts with CPSF via its 77 kDa subunit, and binds the GU-rich region downstream of the poly(A) site via its 64 kDa subunit (Wilusz and Shenk 1990; Takagaki, MacDonald et al. 1992; Takagaki and Manley 1997). The 50 kDa subunit interacts with BRCA1/BARD1 to modulate polyadenylation during DNA repair (Kleiman and Manley 2001), and with RNAP-II through CTD (McCracken, Fong et al. 1997). The 77 kDa subunit of CstF contains the putative nuclear localization signal for transporting the 50:77:64 trimer into the nucleus (Takagaki and Manley 1994).

3.5 Alterations in trans-acting factors for polyadenylation in B and plasma cells

Nascent RNA cleavage in polyadenylation can be blocked by U1A (Phillips, Pachikara et al. 2004; Ma, Gunderson et al. 2006) or hnRNP F (Veraldi, Arhin et al. 2001); the levels of both of these are high in B-cells and lower in plasma cells (summarized in Table 1) and (Ma, Gunderson et al. 2006) consistent with a loss of their inhibitory function on the poly(A) sites in plasma cells. While hnRNP F might be expected to block any poly(A) site based on its sequence preference for downstream regions (Alkan, Martincic et al. 2006), we found by a micro-array analyses of hnRNP F transfected cells that only some genes were affected, most notable among these were secretory Igh and ELL2, a transcription elongation factor (Martincic, Alkan et al. 2009). The finding that there are U1A binding sites up-stream of the Igh mu secretory poly(A) site indicates a selectivity consistent with the observed increased use of the site when U1A levels fall (Phillips and Virtanen 1997). The data clearly show that a change in the levels of these factors influences the polyadenylation of the Igh secretory site. The smaller number of polyadenylation factors associated with the B cell RNAP-II may not recognize the AAUAAA and downstream regions of the secretory poly(A) site because these two RNPs block access.

Recently, using a knock-down and whole genome array approach, the U1 snRNA itself, not the U1A protein, was shown to protect pre-mRNA from premature cleavage and polyadenylation (Kaida, Berg et al. 2010). This reveals a function for U1 RNA independent of splicing where its interaction with the splice site in the nascent RNA plays a seminal role. In another recent study a fraction of the U1 snRNA, without any of the normal RNP proteins, was found associated with TAF15 aka TAFII-68 (Jobert, Pinzon et al. 2009). This TAF interacts with a distinct population of TFIID so U1 snRNA may play a heretofore unrecognized role in transcription initiation. These unique aspects of U1 snRNA function have not been investigated in B or plasma cells.

The CstF-64 gene (CSTF2) maps to the X chromosome; expression of the protein fluctuates and is rate-limiting for the CstF complex formation (Martincic, Campbell et al. 1998). Knocking out CstF2 in chicken B-cells resulted in changes to viability, Igh transcription, and alternative splicing (Takagaki and Manley 1998). An alternative form of CstF-64 (CSTF2T) was found originally in testes, but then it was also found to be expressed in other tissues including B-cells and plasma cells. The CSTF2T gene maps to an autosome allowing for its transcription in spermatogenesis when the X chromosome is suppressed (Dass, McMahon et al. 2001). CSTF2T protein is induced by LPS in splenocytes just like CSTF2. Deletion of the CSTF2T gene gives rise to spermatogenetic defects but no immunological defects were associated with its loss (Hockert, Martincic et al. 2011). Thus CSTF2T does not play an indispensible part in Igh expression.

3.6 Splicing of Igh RNA is altered in plasma cells

RNA splicing occurs through a concerted series of events facilitated by the U family of small Ribonuclear protein particles (snRNPs) 1, 2, 4, 5, 6 and their associated proteins. Serine arginine (SR) proteins, e.g. SF2/ASF, SRp20, often act as enhancers for splicing while in general heterogenous nuclear ribonucleoproteins (hnRNPs) act as spoilers. The balance between these has been shown to control many genes, reviewed in (House and Lynch 2008). Changes in the levels of the splicing factors in various B cell types (Bruce, Dingle et al. 2003) and during development have been shown to alter splicing patterns (Expert-Bezancon, Sureau et al. 2004). For, example, SRp20 plays an important role in alternative splicing of the ED1 exon (de la Mata and Kornblihtt 2006). The finding that the levels of SRp20 increase in plasma cells is intriguing (Table 1). How SRp20 is influencing the balance between splicing and polyadenylation is not known. It is tempting to speculate that it blocks use of the weak splice site in the secretory exon in plasma cells.

RNA processing events and transcription are tightly linked (Proudfoot, Furger et al. 2002). The recruitment of different factors to control splice site selection occurs on the carboxyl-terminal domain (CTD) of RNAP-II (McCracken, Fong et al. 1997). Elongation rates were shown to modulate alternative splicing with high processivity of the polymerase correlating with exon skipping, reviewed in (Kornblihtt 2006). A key role for pTEFb was found for coupling transcription elongation with alternative splicing (Barboric, Lenasi et al. 2009). But chromatin modifications also seem to be important. For example, H3K36me3 marks are associated with recruitment of splicing factors to exons (Spies, Nielsen et al. 2009). The histone tail-binding protein MORF-related gene 15 (MRG15), a component of the retinoblastoma binding protein 2 (RBP2)/H3-K4 demethylase complex, recruits Polypyrimidine Tract Binding protein to sub-optimal exons (Luco, Pan et al. 2010). The mammalian ortholog of the SWI/SNF (SWItch/Sucrose NonFermentable) yeast nucleosome remodeling complex has been shown to play a role in CD44 alternative splicing (Batsche,

Yaniv et al. 2006). In addition, H3K9 hyperacetylation outside the promoter stimulates alternative splicing (Schor, Rascovan et al. 2009).
Several models for coupling alternative splicing to elongation or chromatin have been considered recently. The modulation of elongation rates to splicing has been advocated (de la Mata, Lafaille et al. 2010). Meanwhile nucleosome positioning has been discussed as a regulator (Tilgner, Nikolaou et al. 2009). And chromatin as a scaffold for pre-mRNA splicing regulation has been discussed (Allemand, Batsché et al. 2008). While there is a link between transcription elongation and RNA splicing, the details of these connections are still emerging and chromatin modifications may play a large role as well. Our data clearly indicate a role for transcription elongation factor ELL2 in modulating alternative splicing (see below) but much more needs to be done to understand how this is accomplished.

4. RNAP-II elongation is altered in Igh gene regulated RNA processing

4.1 Elongation regulation is crucial

Photo-bleaching of fluorescent RNA polymerase II in living cells reveals that transcription elongation is much faster than expected but the polymerases enters a paused state for unexpectedly long times (Darzacq, Sahav-Tal et al. 2007). Genome wide studies indicated that a number of developmentally important genes in *Drosophila* embryos that were not yet being actively transcribed but are scheduled to be expressed in subsequent stages have a paused polymerase at the 5′ end (Zeitlinger, Stark et al. 2007).
The dysregulation of elongation and subsequent aberrant gene expression have been strongly associated with the genesis of several cancers. The von Hippel-Lindau tumor suppressor gene (VHL) predisposes individuals to a variety of tumors by inhibiting elongin SIII, a normal component of the elongation machinery (Duan, Pause et al. 1995). The tumor suppressor Cdc73, a component of the mPAF elongation complex, is inactivated by mutation in hereditary and sporadic parathyroid tumors and alters poly(A) site choice (Rozenblatt-Rosen, Nagaike et al. 2009).
In multiple lineage leukemia (MLL), which has provided an important window to the role of elongation and chromatin modification (Shilatifard 1998) and (Lin, Smith et al. 2010; Mohan, Herz et al. 2010), fusions occur with different elongation factors in different tumors to bring MLL protein in close association with the start of target genes, like the hox genes, and thereby inappropriately activate them (Meyer, Kowarz et al. 2009). The regulation of pausing and elongation are therefore emerging as important steps in gene regulation.

4.2 ELL genes in general transcription elongation

ELL1 (Eleven-nineteen Lysine-rich Leukemia gene 1) was discovered as a translocation partner with the MLL gene in individuals with acute leukemia (Thirman, Levitan et al. 1994). The closely related family member ELL2, isolated by homology with ELL1, can also stimulate RNAP-II elongation *in vitro* (Shilatifard, Lane et al. 1996), (Shilatifard, Duan et al. 1997), and (Miller, Williams et al. 2000). ELL3 is primarily expressed in testis and tumor cells; it also increases the catalytic rate of transcription elongation *in vitro* (Miller, Williams et al. 2000).
The mRNAs for the ELL1 and 2 are widely expressed but vary from tissue to tissue, suggesting they may serve a regulatory role (Shilatifard, Duan et al. 1997). Human ELL1 protein is 621 amino-acids long while ELL2 is 640, see Figure 5 for ELL2. They are very similar from aa 1-345. This region is responsible for elongation enhancement. The segments

of ELL2 from aa 168-180 and from 239 to 250 were shown to interact with mediator in a proteomic screen which has not yet been verified by functional assays (Sato, Tomomori-Sato et al. 2004). ELL1 and 2 differ from aa ~352-443 and 473-516, amino acids that map primarily to the later ~75% of exon 8. The 352-516 region differences may explain some of the unique associations of ELL1 versus ELL2. This region is rich in hydrophobic amino acids like proline and leucine but also contains hydrophilic charged residues like lysine and glutamate. No known protein motif has been identified in this domain. The mid-portion of ELL has been determined to be the region that is required for its association with heat shock puffs in *Drosophila* (Gerber, Shilatifard et al. 2005).

From aa 520 to the carboxyl-end ELL1 and 2 are very similar. The C-terminal domain is conserved in all the members of the ELL-family including Drosophila; it shares homology with occludin, an integral plasma membrane protein located in tight junctions. The functional significance of the homology is unknown but this C-terminal domain is required for viability in Drosophila (Eissenberg, Ma et al. 2002; Gerber, Shilatifard et al. 2005). The C-terminal domain of ELL is sufficient for immortalization of myeloid progenitors most likely through its interactions with p53, although the MLL:ELL fusion is more efficient than ELL alone (Wiederschain, Kawai et al. 2003).

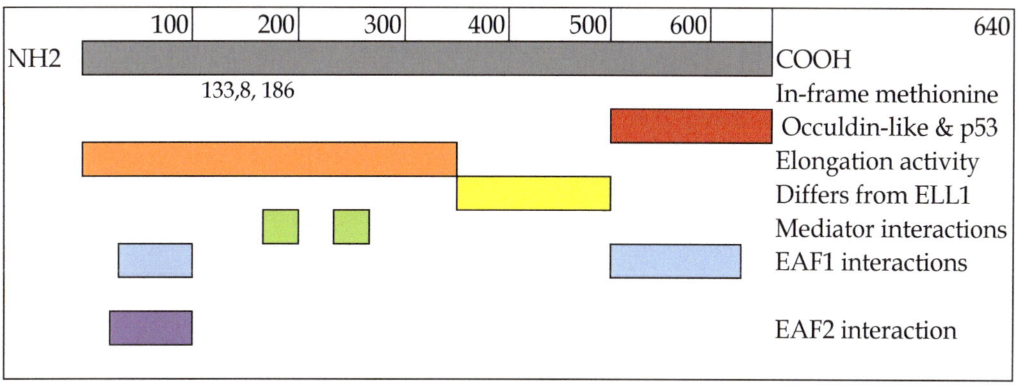

Fig. 5. Map of ELL2 indicating important regions discussed in text.

In addition, ELL1 was found to bind to the promoter and to have direct transcriptional activity on the thrombospodin-1 gene in mammalian cells (Zhou, Feng et al. 2009). The DNA binding domain maps to the aa 1-45. Studies using zebrafish, confirmed that ELL regulates TSP-1 mRNA expression *in vivo*; the conserved C-domain found in MLL fusions was the region involved in this activation (Zhou, Feng et al. 2009). This is the first report of ELL acting without binding to RNAP-II.

4.3 EAF genes in transcription elongation

EAF1 and EAF2 (ELL associated factors 1 and 2) were discovered via two-hybrid and co-IP studies to be associated with ELL. The association of EAF1 was mapped to amino acids 28-117 and 508-621 of ELL1 while the EAF2 associations mapped to aa 23 to 90 of ELL1 (Luo, Lavau et al. 2001; Simone, Luo et al. 2003), see Figure 5. Both EAF1 and 2 are required for viability in Drosophila (Liu, Hu et al. 2009). EAF2/U19/FESTA is associated with another elongation factor, SII/TCEA/TFIIS. The eaf2-/- mice are viable but form tumors in the spleen and prostate later in life (Xiao, Zhang et al. 2008). Therefore, not having EAF2 is not fatal but sufficient to produce a back-up at the mature B-cell stage. Investigation of the production of secreted Igh in the eaf2-/- mice would be an important problem.

4.4 pTEFb in transcription elongation

Cyclin T1 or T2 and cdk9, a cyclin dependent kinase, form the core of pTEFb, which has been implicated in many studies of gene regulation through alleviation of RNAP-II pausing (He, Pezda et al. 2006). The c-myc gene was among the earliest genes studied that displays a strong pause site, which can either be alleviated or cause transcription termination leading to aborted mRNA production (Roberts and Bentley 1992). Recent studies have shown that myc requires pTEFb, the positive transcription elongation factor, to relieve the pause and empower the polymerase to make mature mRNA, or in other words, increase thoughput (Rahl, Lin et al. 2010). The heat shock genes were recognized as having a paused polymerase with a requirement for pTEFb to drive elongation (Lis, Mason et al. 2000). The factor pTEFb has been shown to be required for the expression or repression of several immunologically important genes including AIRE (Oven, Brdickova et al. 2007), p53 (Gomes, Bjerke et al. 2006), runx in double positive T cells (Jiang and Peterlin 2008) and primary response genes in macrophages following Toll-Like-Receptor signaling (Hargreaves, Horng et al. 2009). Thus an examination of the pTEFb factor is important for understanding pausing and subsequent elongation.

Inactive pTEFb is associated with the small nuclear 7SK snRNA and HEXIM 1 or 2 plus other proteins. HEXIM is induced by a hexamethylene bis-acetamide and has no introns. Its levels vary with developmental stage in a number of studies. HEXIM molecules can associate as homo- or hetero-dimers, through their carboxyl-terminal tails (Dulac, Michels et al. 2005). Multiple complexes of HEXIM dimers with their associated pTEFb bind to 7SK with a conformation change in 7SK structure (Krueger, Varzavand et al. 2010); cdk9 is thus inhibited in its enzymatic ability to phosphorylate substrates. The inactive form of pTEFb is released from HEXIM and binds other factors to become activated. The equilibrium between active and inactive forms shifts based on the amount of HEXIM expressed, linking the pTEFb equilibrium to the intracellular transcriptional demands, proliferation, and differentiated states of cells (He, Pezda et al. 2006). When pTEFb is released from the inactive state it can be brought to the DNA: RNA polymerase complex by Brd4 through recognition of acetylated chromatin structures (Vollmuth, Blankenfeldt et al. 2009) or to virus transcription by specialized mechanisms.

The DRB sensitive factor DSIF (composed of Spt1 and Spt5(h) aka p160) and a multi-subunit negative elongation factor (NELF) act together to arrest RNAP-II shortly after initiation. The recruitment of the kinase activity of cdk9 in pTEFb to the polymerase phosphorylates not only the ser-2 of the CTD of RNAP-II, linking to H3K36 modifications (see Table 2), but also the C-terminal region of the Spt5h subunit of DSIF. This releases NELF from the complex and converts DSIF into a positively acting elongation factor. DSIF then cooperates with Tat-SF1 and the mPAF complex to super-charge elongation. The on-going ser-2 phosphorylation of the CTD of RNAP-II is associated with histone H2B mono-ubitination of K 120. The FACT complex is then recruited to help unwind nucleosomes (Barboric, Lenasi et al. 2009).

Mammalian polymerase associated factor complex (mPAF) functions in transcription after mediator recruits RNAP-II; mPAF helps recruit the histone methylases and possibly RNA processing factors to the RNAP-II based on CTD phosphorylation. PAF binds the polyadenylation factors at the promoter and transfers them to the elongating polymerase. The mPAF subunit parafibromin alters poly(A) site choice by association with CPSF/CstF (Rozenblatt-Rosen, Nagaike et al. 2009; Shi, Di Giammartino et al. 2009) and alterations in parafibromin cause tumors. Thus it is clear that pTEFb plays a pivotal role in elongation, polyadenylation thru mPAF recruitment, and splicing through the H3K36 modifications.

4.5 The associations of pTEFb and ELL2 to form the super elongation complex

Two recent papers have shown that pTEFb can be found in distinct complexes based on cell type and HIV status. There are numerous shared proteins between these complexes see Table 3, with potential fusion partners of the MLL gene in each complex. A super elongation complex (SEC) was demonstrated in 293, a human embryonic kidney derived cell line generated by adenovirus DNA transformation; the 293 line shares many properties with neuronal cells (Shaw, Morse et al.). The SEC was isolated (Lin, Smith et al. 2010) using antibody-mediated purification of epitope-tagged MLL-ELL1, MLL-ENL, MLL-AFF1 or MLL-AF9 transfected into the cells, with subsequent analysis of the immune-precipitate by mass spectrometry. The complexes all contained: cdk9, cyclin T1, T2a and b; AFF1, AFF4, AF9, ENL, and an ELL gene product, 1, 2 or 3. If the AFF4 was used for the pull-down EAF1 and all three ELLs were present. If epitope-tagged ELL1 or ELL2 was used for the pull-down the other was found in the complex, perhaps implying mixed dimers, while if ELL3 was used for the pull-down ELL1 but not ELL2 was found. With antibodies to tagged ELL1, no EAF was found while if ELL2 or ELL3 was used EAF1 and 2 were co-immuno-precipitated in the complex. This variety indicates that there may be several different complexes based on which ELL is expressed in the cells. What emerges is that the AFF4 is crucial for the formation of the SEC and recruitment to the HSP70 both at the promoter and into the body of the gene during transcription (Lin, Smith et al. 2010). Those studies did not address the recruitment of the pTEFb in the SEC from the 7SK:hexim complexes. This is an area that will be of interest in the future. Our ChIP experiments, outlined in Figure 3,

Major MLL fusion partners (Meyer, Kowarz et al. 2009)	**Super elongation complex components** (Lin, Smith et al. 2010)	**DotCom components** (Mohan, Herz et al. 2010)	**TAR:TAT interacting complex** (He, Liu et al. 2010)	**Up-regulated in plasma cells** (Martincic, Alkan et al. 2009)
AFF1/AFF4	*AFF4*	-	*AFF4*	*AFF1*
ELL1	***ELL1, 2 or 3***	**-**	***ELL2***	***ELL2***
EPS15/AF1P	-	-	*AFF1*	
MLLT1/ENL	*ENL*	*ENL*	*ENL*	*ENL*
MLLT3/AF9	*AF9*	*AF9*	*AF9*	
MLLT4/AF6	-	-	-	
MLLT6/AF17	*AF17*	*AF17*	-	
MLLT10/AF10	*AF10*	*AF10*	-	
SEPT6	-		-	
	EAF1 or 1+2		*EAF2*	*EAF2*
	Cdk9		*Cdk9*	*Cdk9*
	Cyclin T		*Cyclin T*	*Cyclin T*
				PC4/ sub1 Supt5h/ suppressor of Ty5

Table 3. Potential transcription elongation factors implicated in each process or complex.

showed that DRB treatment to inactivate pTEFb and ser-2 phosphorylation of the CTD eliminated the binding of ELL2 and CstF-64 to the TATA region of Igh. In the light of the discovery of the SEC this indicates that pTEFb and ELL2 and all of the SEC components may be associated in plasma cells as they are in 293 cells.

In HIV infection of T cells, the rate limiting step for transcription is RNA polymerase pausing on viral genes near the 5′ end of all viral transcripts in the Long Terminal Repeat (Peterlin and Price 2006). The pause in transcription is relieved by the action of the HIV-1 Tat protein that recruits the host pTEFb to the TAR element in the viral RNA. TAR is a stem-loop structure near the 5′ end of the LTR that resembles the 7SK RNA and may thus serve as a binding site for pTEFb recruitment. Epitope tagged factors cdk9-F and inducible expression of Tat-HA were used for sequential affinity purifications of proteins (He, Liu et al. 2010) and (Sobhian, Laguette et al. 2010). Associated with pTEFb and Tat were AFF4, ENL, AF9, and ELL2, summarized in Table 3. These complexes are similar to the SEC but differ as well. In the absence of Tat, AFF4 can mediate the ELL2 to pTEFb interaction but less efficiently than with Tat present. This is consistent with the SEC studies where AFF4 seems to be the core of the complex. AFF17 and 10 were not found in the Tat mediated complex and ELL1 was missing; AFF17 and 10 may serve the role that Tat does in holding the SEC together. ELL2 may be more likely to associate when Tat is present than when AFF17 or 10 are part of the complex. The over-expression of Tat or AFF4 seem to use a common mechanism to stabilize ELL2 which is mediated by the cdk9 kinase activity of pTEFb and the sequestration of ELL2 in the complex to block proteolysis. Whether ELL2 is a substrate for pTEFb phosphorylation has not yet been determined but ELL2 shows a mobility shift in the experiments.

Another interesting observation was that the ELL2:pTEFb complexes were associated with a number of cellular promoters, in the absence of TAT:TAR (He, Liu et al. 2010). This implies that the complex is able to enhance the regulation of elongation on many promoters. This has implications for the role of ELL2 in regulating plasma cell genes besides Igh, for example, it could enhance the expression of IRF-4 and blimp-1, thus solidifying their expression and the plasma cell phenotype.

5. Role of ELL2 in Igh expression and alternative RNA processing

5.1 ELL2 is induced and binds to the Igh TATA region in plasma cells

The mRNA for ELL2 has been shown to be induced at least 4 to 6-fold in plasma cells when compared to B-cells by micro-array analyses by several labs (Underhill, George et al. 2003) and (Turner, Mack et al. 1994; Lin, Wong et al. 1997). We showed that both a 59 kDa cleavage product of full length ELL2 protein and a shorter, internal Methionine (M186) initiated 58kDa form of ELL2 were increased in plasma cells and after stimulation of splenic B-cells to Igh secretion (Martincic, Alkan et al. 2009). Taken together these data suggest an important role for ELL2 in Igh chain expression.

The mRNA and protein for ELL2 increase when Ig sec mRNA production increases and ELL2 is decreased with over-express hnRNP F; over-expression of hnRNP F decreases production of Igh sec mRNA (Martincic, Alkan et al. 2009). By chromatin immunoprecipitations, ELL2 is associated with the endogenous Ig mu heavy chain gene in primary mouse splenic B cells and with the gamma Igh in cultured mouse B and plasma cells. An siRNA to ELL2 is able to diminish Ig secretory mRNA production not only of Ig gamma in cultured plasma cells, but also of Ig mu in primary splenic B cells. That same siRNA to ELL2 is able to inhibit the binding of not only itself but also of CstF-64, a factor in the poly(A) addition reaction, to the promoter of an Igh gene transfected into J558L plasma cells which lack their own Ig gene (summarized in Figure 3).

Increased phosphorylation of both ser-5 and ser-2 on the CTD of RNAP-II and loading of polyadenylation factors and ELL2 onto the polymerase at the promoter in plasma cells vs B-cells (see Figure 3) contribute to regulation of production of Igh mRNA (Shell, Martincic et al. 2007). RNAP-II is therefore more competent to deliver the factors to the first poly(A) site encountered, the sec-poly(A) site in plasma cells. Hence, in the absence of the competing factors that would be both negative for the sec poly(A) site and positive for splicing, and with higher local concentrations of CstF and CPSF, the polyadenylation reaction could be favored over splicing by mass-action. How do the polyadenylation factors load better in plasma cells? We hypothesize that the polyadenylation factor loading onto RNAP-II is directed at least in part by ELL2 in its association with pTEFb and subsequent mPAF interactions.

5.2 ELL2, but not ELL1 or PC4, influences the sec poly (A) site choice in Igh reporters

We had previously cloned the ~11 kb IgGb heavy chain gene with an intact Ig heavy chain promoter, introns and enhancer between VDJ and CH1; production of B- or plasma cell specific Igh sec vs membrane forms of mRNA was shown to be dependent on the cell-type with this reporter (Kobrin, Milcarek et al. 1986). The Igh gene was co-transfected into A20 B-cells along with an empty expression vector or full length cDNAs for ELL2, ELL1, CstF-64 or PC4 cloned into that vector. We also assessed the effect of NH2 terminal, COOH terminal portions of ELL2 and a mutant in which the M 133, 138, 186 were changed to Ileu to prevent internal translational initiation. The ratio of sec (polyadenylated at first site): mb (splicing to M1) heavy chain mRNA species produced in these cells after 48 hours was quantified by QPCR following RT using the primers specific for sec p(A) site use or splicing. The data are summarized in Figure 6, below. Equal efficiency of transfection by the ELL1 & 2, CstF-64 and PC4 plasmids was assessed by RT-QPCR of their mRNAs using primers unique for the transfected products.

Considering the sec:mb mRNA ratio produced by the IgG2b heavy chain reporter in the B-cells as 1, we saw, in the data summarized in Figure 6, an increase in secretory specific mRNA production of approximately 4.5-fold when A20 B cells were transfected with mRNA for wild-type ELL2. This stimulation of secretory mRNA is more efficient with ELL2 than co-transfection with CstF-64, shown previously to drive first site poly(A) selection in chicken DT-40 cells (Takagaki, Seipelt et al. 1996). A dominant negative mutation of CstF-64 (d/n), which can assemble into the CstF complex but lacks the essential final 282 a.a.s at the COOH domain, suppressed sec poly (A) site use, as we predicted. Co-transfection of the Igh reporter and shRNA plasmid targeted to ELL2 expression (iELL2) reduced production of the Igh secretory form while a nonsense shRNA (nsiRNA) had no effect.

When cells were transfected with a plasmid carrying engineered ELL2 with Met 133, 138 and 186 to Ileu mutations, (see Figure 5 for location of the in-frame methionines) the production of Ig secretory mRNA was still stimulated relative to empty vector, about 4-fold. These cells would presumably be making primarily full length ELL2 protein and the cleaved 59 kDa form but not the 58 kDa internally initiated form. Using a clone with a segment of ELL2 corresponding to only the amino-terminal (NH2) or the 58 kDa protein (COOH ELL2), we observed virtually no stimulation in the production of the secretory specific Ig heavy chain mRNA over that with empty vector in B-cells. Taken together the data indicate that

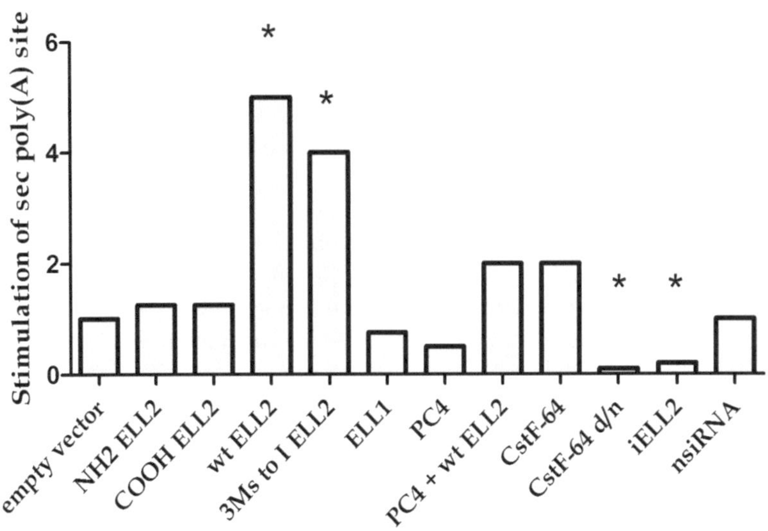

Fig. 6. ELL2 stimulates sec mRNA production. A reporter containing the intact Igh locus with promoter and enhancer and normal sec poly(A) site in competition with M1 splice (see Figure 2) was transfected into A20 B-cells along with the indicated expression vector (pEF4) containing either no insert (empty vector), portions of ELL2 , the full wt. ELL2, an ELL2 where the methionine at M 133, 138 and 185 was substituted with Isoleucine so they could not internally initiate, ELL1, PC4, CstF-64, a dominant negative (d/n) form of CstF-64 that can inhibit action of the CstF trimer, or with a vector containing siELL2 or non-specific siRNA. The output of poly(A)+ mRNA either secretory or mb specific was assessed by QPCR using probes outlined in Figure 2. The asterisk * indicates P=<0.05 indicating a different from the empty vector as a control using ANOVA and a Tukey's post-test. Data adapted and simplified from (Martincic, Alkan et al. 2009).

the wild type, full length form of ELL2 is the most efficient at stimulating secretory-specific mRNA production from the Igh reporter. We speculate that the increased production of full length ELL2 results in rapid turnover into the 59/58kDa forms after having had its effect on Igh poly(A) splicing choice. Some of the ELL2 could be stabilized in the complex with pTEFb as it is in the TAT:TAR complex during HIV infection.
Meanwhile, full length ELL1 was unable to stimulate secretory specific mRNA production, a surprising result in light of the similarities of the sequences of the two proteins and their role at enhancing elongation. With PC4, a co-transcriptional factor with multiple activities (Calvo and Manley 2005) and (Garcia, Rosonina et al. 2010), there was also no stimulation of sec-specific mRNA production, even though we showed that PC4 bound to the Igh promoter in plasma cells.

5.3 ELL2 influences splicing of alternative exons with several promoters

To assess the effects of elongation factors on splicing we used transient transfections with the alternative splicing constructs (Kornblihtt, De La Mata et al. 2004) with the ED1 exon driven by the alpha-globin promoter. This reporter has been used extensively to study the role of elongation on splicing. First we used the alpha-globin promoter to drive transcription and saw an effect of ELL2 on splicing (see Table 4). Then we cloned in the J558 Igh promoter and enhancer to replace the alpha-globin promoter in the reporter to control for potential promoter effects. We used RT QPCR to assess ED exon inclusion or skipping in A20 B-cells. As summarized in Table 4, we saw significant increases in skipping with ELL2 ($P<0.001$) vs the vector control. ELL1 had a 2 to 4 fold effect on skipping (with $P<0.05$). The COOH portion of ELL2 (aka 58 kDa ELL2, amino acids 186-640) was effective at the splicing choice and this may reflect a role for it in the plasma cell. We saw a greater effect with the NH2 terminal end (aa 1-285) than the whole ELL2 molecule on the alpha-globin-promoter driven splicing reporters but not the Ig promoter constructs. This reveals differences in the two reactions and could indicate a role for interactions of the promoter, other factors, or the RNAP-II with portions of ELL2.

	Fold increase over control			
	ELL2 (aa 1-640)	ELL2 NH2 (aa 1-285)	ELL2 COOH (aa 186-640)	ELL1
Igh sec poly(A) site> splicing (Igh promoter)	4.5	-	-	-
Exon skipping with Igh promoter	3	-	3	3
Exon skipping with alpha-globin promoter	3	6	4	2
Proximal poly(A) site choice (400 nts bw sites)	-	-	-	-
Proximal poly(A) site choice 1 kb spacing	3	-	4.5	Not done

Table 4. Summary of transfection experiments with ELLs

Meanwhile we saw no effects on poly(A) choice with ELL2 or ELL1 in B cells where tandem poly(A) sites were only about 400 nts apart in the reporter (Table 4). In the Igh gene the two poly(A) sites (sec vs mb) are ~3kb apart. When the sites were moved >1kb apart in our polyadenylation only vector, full length ELL2 stimulated proximal poly(A) site use. Interestingly the fraction of ELL2 from aa 186 to 640 amino-acids was better than the full length molecule. ELL1 was not tested in this assay but should be for completeness. Thus various portions of the ELL2 have different activities. It will be important to determine which of the components of the SEC or TAT:TAR complex interact directly with which portions of ELL2. Yeast two-hybrid studies with cloned portions of the ELL2 molecule are in progress to determine this. The region corresponding to the occludin-like and p53 interacting domain shows trans-activation by itself, indicating that it interacts with the basal transcription machinery in yeast.

6. Insights from viral systems

Other model systems for poly(A) site use include virus infection. In adenovirus distal poly(A) sites in the major late transcript are favored later in infection (DeZazzo, Falck-Pedersen et al. 1991); is this because the levels of polyadenylation factors and elongation factors fall? This has not been explored. It would be interesting to examine the levels of the subunits of the SEC both in the differentiated cells and late in viral infection. The prediction would be that they decline leading to pauci-polymerases with little ability to polyadenylate efficiently. Perhaps a similar situation pertains late in development of a particular tissue, a kind of elongation exhaustion.

The ICP4 gene of Herpes Simplex Virus Type 1 (HSV-1) targets TFIID, a general transcription factor bound at the promoter (Grondin and DeLuca 2000) to high-jack transcription towards viral genes. ICP4 forms complexes with TFIID and mediator (Lester and DeLuca 2011). The prediction would be that the presumed association of the polyadenylation factors with TFIID would allow the HSV genes to associate with mPAF and the elongation factors more efficiently. In addition another HSV gene, ICP27, mediates the inhibition of cellular splicing early in infection, whereas, later it helps to recruit cellular RNA polymerase II to viral replication sites and to facilitate viral RNA export (Sandri-Goldin 2008). Early on, ICP27 specifically mediates the reduction of phosphorylation of cellular SR proteins and thereby changes their subcellular location; this favors viral mRNA production (Sciabica, Dai et al. 2003). Phosphorylation of SR proteins has been shown to influence RNA binding and is variable based on physiological changes (Ghosh, Adams et al. 2011). What if any changes may occur in the phosphorylation of SR proteins during B cell maturation has not been explored.

An earlier discussion of the HIV-1 TAT:TAR interaction with components of the SEC shows how viruses can help us clearly get at molecular events in elongation. In HIV-1 the long terminal repeat RNA contains not only the TAR stem loop, for TAT association, but also a poly(A) site followed by a major splice donor. This arrangement of sites is repeated at the 3′ end of the virus where the poly(A) site functions. The promoter proximal poly(A) site is occluded by the presence of the major splice donor (Ashe, Griffin et al. 1995) and the U1 RNA binding there at the splice donor plays a role in the occlusion (Ashe, Furger et al. 2000). In addition there is a gene loop structure that is found between the 5'LTR promoter and 3'LTR poly (A) signal. An inhibitor of pTEFb (flavopiridol) blocks 5' to 3'LTR juxtaposition, indicating that this structure is maintained during transcription. Activation of the 5'LTR poly (A) signal or inactivation of the 3'LTR poly (A) signal abolishes gene loop formation. Thus transcription, elongation factors, and pre-mRNA processing are essential for gene loop formation (Perkins, Lusic et al. 2008). The prediction is that these structures represent a defining feature of regulation for the virus. It has been suggested that the transcription factory for cellular genes stays put while the DNA and RNA thread through. The role of elongation factors in formation of this structure is unknown.

7.1 Model for regulated alternative RNA processing in the Igh gene

In Figure 7 a model for what we know about Igh alternative mRNA processing is presented. In B-cells, U1A (Milcarek, Martincic et al. 2003), hnRNP F (Veraldi, Arhin et al. 2001), and Serine-Arginine-rich (SR) proteins like ASF/SF2 (Bruce, Dingle et al. 2003) are expressed in relatively higher concentrations than in plasma cells. The CTD of RNAP-II on the Igh gene is relatively under-phosphorylated; the polyadenylation factors CPSF and CstF and ELL2 are not strongly associated (Shell, Martincic et al. 2007) with the polymerase. The question mark indicates that we do not know if enhancing SR protein(s) like SF2/ASF for the 5′ splice to the M1 exon is/are associated with the RNAP-II. When the secretory-specific poly(A) site is transcribed there are few polyadenylation factors on RNAP-II to recognize it (thus it is a pauci-polymerase). In B-cells splicing between the 5′ splice site in the terminal (CH3 in gamma, CH4 in mu) exon, occurs presumably as the default pathway. This leads to the production primarily but not exclusively of the membrane-specific form of the Igh mRNA and protein at a low level. (Some sec mRNA is made at a low level.)

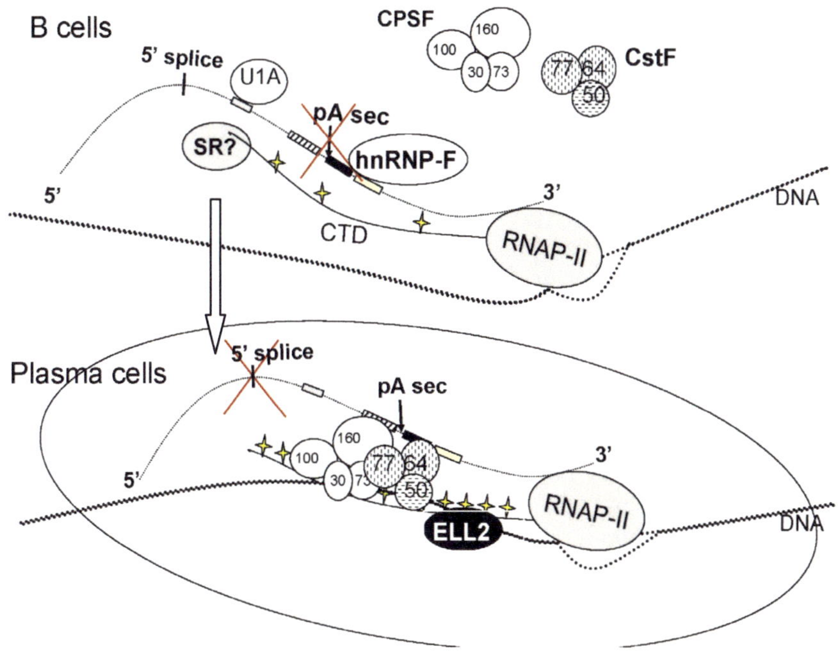

Fig. 7. Model for the use of the splice site to M1 in B cells and the sec poly(A) site in plasma cells, mediated by elongation factors like ELL2, part of the SEC.

In plasma cells the RNAP-II is more heavily phosphorylated early on, perhaps by cyclin C and cdk8, perhaps through the action of NF-kB, and RNAP-II is associated with the polyadenylation factors and ELL2 via the associated pTEFb kinase activity. Polyadenylation factors are also associated with the polymerase, perhaps through the action of mPAF. When the RNAP-II reaches the sec poly(A) site the factors act upon the pre-mRNA and trigger production primarily but not exclusively of the sec-specific mRNA. This is an efficient process and mRNA yield per polymerase pass is much higher. The splice to M1 cannot then occur on the cleaved RNA; the CH3 exon splice to M1 is thus "undefined" by either an active or passive mechanism.

7.2 Questions remaining

Since the secretory poly(A) site occurs first in the Igh transcript, how is membrane-specific Igh mRNA ever made? We know that the levels of U1 snRNP splice factor and Serine Arginine (SR) exon enhancing factors are higher in B-cells than in plasma cells. This could facilitate stronger 5′ splice site recognition. In B-cells ELL2 levels are lower and the RNAP-II is quite deficient in polyadenylation factors. U1A and hnRNP F block access to the poly(A) site as well (Phillips, Pachikara et al. 2004; Ma, Gunderson et al. 2006) & (Veraldi, Arhin et al. 2001). The sec-poly(A) site is therefore weakest in B-cells and used less than half the time. As a result, some RNAP-IIs ignore it and proceed downstream the 3 kb to the membrane poly(A) site. The long intron (~3 kb) allows the setting up of the weak 5′ splice site in CH3 with its associated enhancing factors on the pre-mRNA. Meanwhile the RNAP-II may have acquired polyadenylation factors in the IVS between CH3 and M1, 'on the fly' as it were, as is seen for the c-myc and GAPDH genes (Glover-Cutter, Kim et al. 2008). Acquisition of polyadenylation factors by the polymerase 'on the fly' may be a less efficient process and could account for the overall reduced amount of processed Igh transcript seen in B-cells. This may explain the pause seen in some studies after the secretory poly(A) site in both B cells and plasma cells (Peterson, Bertolino et al. 2002), and listed in Table 1. In the case of B cells perhaps the polyadenylation factors are added to RNAP-II at the pause, although at a sufficiently low level so that we were not able to see them in our chromatin IP studies. In plasma cells the polymerase may pause to allow time for the polyadenylation reaction to occur. *In vitro* a coupling between splice sites and poly(A) sites has been seen which may slow the polymerase down (Rigo and Martinson 2008) and this may explain the pause. The poly(A) site at the last membrane-encoding exon is known to be a strong default site but the RNAP-II must be competent for processing the RNA when it reaches it. Some transcripts probably never get processed at all and turn-over rapidly in the nucleus.

Is the skipping of the 5′ splice site in CH3 an active or passive process and are SR proteins involved? The increase of SRp20 levels in plasma cells suggests that the splicing inhibitory process of this SR protein may play a significant role. It is not known if it travels with the RNAP-II complex in plasma cells or associates with the nascent RNA. This remains an interesting and open question.

What role does histone modification play in directing polyadenylation? The increase in ser-5 and ser-2 near the Igh promoter should be accompanied by increases in H3 K4, K36 and perhaps K79 methylations. This is another open question in the regulation of the alternative processing of Igh RNA.

An additional question is what is the role of ELL2 vs ELL1 in the splicing vs polyadenylation choice. Both ELL2 and ELL1 direct exon skipping with an alpha-globin or the Igh promoter (Table 4). When we assessed the ability of the "COOH" portion of ELL2 (aa 186-640) in the Igh reporter assay it had minimal effect on first poly(A) site use. However that protein was lacking the first 186 amino-acids encompassing one region thought to interact with the mediator complex (aa168-186) as well as the EAF2 interaction region (aa 6-80). Therefore we hypothesize that when ELL2 was enhancing the choice of the sec poly(A) site it might have been acting as a bridge between several factors. This is in keeping with two regions of ELL2 interacting with either different mediator subunits or EAF1 . Hence maintaining proper spacing may be key. It will be interesting to determine what proteins uniquely interact with ELL1 versus ELL2. Perhaps they are AF17 and AF10, see Table 3.

A major issue for plasma cell development is whether ELL2 drives the expression of other genes besides Igh. In the TAT:TAR studies ELL2 was found on several promoters by chromatin IP. Our preliminary data support a more broad distribution of ELL2 on plasma cell genes. If ELL2 acts independently of the Igh promoter it may assist the expression of IRF4 and blimp-1, thus providing a feed-forward loop for its own expression. More IRF4 would lead to more ELL2 which would lead to more IRF4 and so on. Global genome wide mapping of ELL2 binding would help to reveal its targets. Knocking ELL2 out in a conditional way so the animals survived would also help show what it was responsible for activating in specific cell lineages. These are separate but complementary questions.

8. Conclusions

The Igh locus has been a useful model in an important biological system; we have much more to learn from it. The experiments done thus far on the role of elongation in directing poly (A) site use and choice provide us with worth-while glimpses of how RNAP-II functions with a myriad of other factors to produce large amounts of mature mRNA. The interactions of these complexes with the specific modifications of the CTD of RNAP-II may only be able to be approached by *in vitro* methodologies as was done for the interactions of SET2 with phosphorylated CTD (Vojnic, Simon et al. 2006). The role of individual factors like ELL2 may have some redundancy with other elongation factors but the observation that portions of ELL1 and 2 differ in primary sequence permit us to consider that each factor may play a unique role in gene expression. The additive effect of all the factors in a single complex (SEC) implies they are all needed. The immune system is particularly suited to the study of conditional knock-outs targeted specifically at B-cell or T-cells. Knocking out ELL2 specifically in the B-cell lineage should provide valuable insights into its role in elongation and Igh mRNA processing. Once we fully understand how polyadenylation is linked to transcription we may then be able to more easily see how the competition between splicing and polyadenylation can be accomplished.

9. Acknowledgements

I extend my sincere thanks to all my trainees who participated in the research presented here and to many colleagues who have honed my thinking on this topic. I apologize to those whose publications I was not able to discuss or cite due to space limitations. This work was support by grant # MCB-0842725 from the National Science Foundation.

10. References

Akhtar, M. S., M. Heidemann, et al. (2009). "TFIIH Kinase Places Bivalent Marks on the Carboxy-Terminal Domain of RNA Polymerase II." Mol Cell 34(3): 387-393.

Alkan, S. A., K. Martincic, et al. (2006). "The hnRNPs F and H2 bind to similar sequences to influence gene expression." Biochem. J. 393: 361-371.

Allemand, E., E. Batsché, et al. (2008). "Splicing, transcription, and chromatin: a ménage à trois." Current Opinion in Genetics & Development 18(2): 145-151.

Amir-Zilberstein, L., E. Ainbinder, et al. (2007). "Differential Regulation of NF-{kappa}B by Elongation Factors Is Determined by Core Promoter Type." Mol Cell Biol 27(14): 5246-5259.

Ashe, M. P., A. Furger, et al. (2000). "Stem-loop of the U1 snRNP plays a critical role in the suppression of HIV-1 polyadenylation." RNA 6: 170-177.

Ashe, M. P., P. Griffin, et al. (1995). "Poly(A) site selection in the HIV-1 provirus: inhibition of promoter-proximal polyadenylation by the downstream major splice donor site." Genes Dev 9: 3008-3025.

Ayton, P. M. and M. L. Cleary (2003). "Transformation of myeloid progenitors by MLL oncoproteins is dependent on Hoxa7 and Hoxa9." Genes Dev. 17: 2298-2307.

Barboric, M., T. Lenasi, et al. (2009). "7SK snRNP/pTEFb couples transcription elongation with alternative splicing and is essential for vertebrate development." Proc Natl Acad Sci, USA 106: 7798-7803.

Batsche, E., M. Yaniv, et al. (2006). "The human SWI/SNF subunit Brm is a regulator of alternative splicing." Nat. Struct. Mol. Biol. 13: 973-980.

Borghesi, L. and C. Milcarek (2006). "From B cell to plasma cell: regulation of V(D)J recombination and antibody secretion " Immunological Research 36((1-3)): 27-32.

Bruce, S. R., R. W. C. Dingle, et al. (2003). "B-cell and plasma-cell splicing differences: A potential role in regulated immunoglobulin RNA processing." RNA 9(10): 1264-1273.

Calkhoven, C. F., C. Muller, et al. (2000). "Translational control of C/EBPalpha and C/EBPbeta isoform expression." Genes Dev 14(15): 1920-1932.

Calvo, C. and J. L. Manley (2005). "The transcriptional coactivator PC4/sub1 has multiple functions in RNA polymerase II transcription." The EMBO Journal 24: 1009-1020.

Chen, X., W. Liu, et al. (1997). "Impaired generation of bone marrow B lymphocytes in mice deficient in C/EBPbeta." Blood 90(1): 156-164.

Cohen, J. B. and A. D. Leninson (1988). "A point mutation in the last intron responsible for increased expression and transforming activity of the c-Ha-ras oncogene." Nature 334: 119-124.

Cramer, P., J. F. Caceres, et al. (1999). "Coupling of transcription with alternative splicing: RNA polII promoters modulate SF2/ASF and 9G8 effects on an exonic splicing enhancer." Mol Cell 4: 251-258.

Dantonel, J.-C., K. Murthy, et al. (1997). "Transcription factor TFIID recruits factor CPSF for formation of 3' end of mRNA." Nature 389: 399-402.

Darzacq, X., Y. Sahav-Tal, et al. (2007). "In vivo dynamics of RNA polymerase II transcription." Nature Struct & Mol Biol 14: 796-806.

Dass, B., W. McMahon, et al. (2001). "The gene for a variant form of the polyadenylation protein CstF-64 is on chromosome 19 and is expressed in pachytene spermatocyctes in mice." J Biol Chem 11: 8044-8050.

de la Mata, M. and A. R. Kornblihtt (2006). "RNA polymerase II C-terminal domain mediates regulation of alternative splicing by SRp20." Nature Struct & Mol Biol 13(11): 973-980.

de la Mata, M., C. Lafaille, et al. (2010). "First come, first served revisited: factors affecting the same alternative splicing event have different effects on the relative rates of intron removal." RNA 16: 904-912.

DeZazzo, J., E. Falck-Pedersen, et al. (1991). "Sequences regulating temporal polyA site switching in the Adenovirus major late transcription unit." Mol Cell Biol 11: 5977-5984.

Dikstein, R., S. Zhou, et al. (1996). "Human TAFII105 is a cell type-specific TFIID subunit related to hTAFII130." Cell 87: 137-146.

Duan, D. R., A. Pause, et al. (1995). "Inhibition of transcription elongation by the VHL tumor suppressor protein." Science 269(5229): 1402-1406.

Dulac, C., A. A. Michels, et al. (2005). "Transcription-dependent Association of Multiple Positive Transcription Elongation Factor Units to a HEXIM Multimer." J Biol Chem 280(34): 30619-30629.

Edwalds-Gilbert, G. and C. Milcarek (1995). "The binding of a subunit of the general polyadenylation factor cleavage polyadenylation specificity factor (CPSF) to polyadenylation sites changes during B cell development." Nucleic Acids Symposium Series 33: 229-233.

Edwalds-Gilbert, G. and C. Milcarek (1995). "Regulation of poly(A) site use during mouse B-cell development involves a change in the binding of a general polyadenylation factor in a B-cell stage-specific manner." Mol Cell Biol 15: 6420-6429.

Edwalds-Gilbert, G., K. Veraldi, et al. (1997). "Alternative poly(A) site selection in complex transcription units: means to an end?" Nucleic Acids Res 25: 2547-2561.

Eissenberg, J. C., J. Ma, et al. (2002). "dELL is an essential RNA polymerase II elongation factor with a general role in development." Proc. Natl. Acad. Sci., USA 99(15): 9894-9899.

Emslie, D., K. D'Costa, et al. (2008). "Oct2 enhances antibody-secreting cell differentiation through regulation of IL-5 receptor {alpha} chain expression on activated B cells." J. Exp. Med. 205(2): 409-421.

Expert-Bezancon, A., A. Sureau, et al. (2004). "HnRNP A1 and SR proteins, ASF/SF2 and SC35 have antagonistic functions in splicing of beta -tropomyosin exon 6B." J. Biol. Chem.: M405377200.

Fields, E. R., B. J. Seufzer, et al. (2000). "A switch in distinct IkBalpha degradation mechanisms mediates constitutive NF-kB activation in mature B cells." J. Immunol 164: 4762-4767.

Flaspohler, J. A., D. Boczkowski, et al. (1995). "The 3'-untranslated region of membrane exon 2 from the gamma 2a immunoglobulin gene contributes to efficient transcription termination." J Biol Chem 270: 11903-11911.

Flaspohler, J. A. and C. Milcarek (1992). " Use of in vitro-transcribed RNAs as immobilized targets during RNA:RNA hybridization." BioTechniques 13(1): 68-72.

Flaspohler, J. A. and C. Milcarek. (1990). "Myelomas and lymphomas expressing the IgG2a H chain gene have similar transcription termination regions." Journal of Immunology 144: 2802-2810.

Freiman, R. N., S. R. Albright, et al. (2002). "Redundant role of tissue-selective TAFII105 in B lymphocytes." Mol Cell Biol 22(18): 6564-6572.

Garcia, A., E. Rosonina, et al. (2010). "Sub1 Globally Regulates RNA Polymerase II C-Terminal Domain Phosphorylation." Mol. Cell. Biol. 30(21): 5180-5193.

Gehring, N. H., U. Frede, et al. (2001). "Increased efficiency of mRNA 3' end formation: a new genetic mechanism contributing to heriditary thrombophilia." Nature Genet 28: 389-392.

Gendra, E., D. F. Colgan, et al. (2007). "A Sequence Motif in the Simian Virus 40 (SV40) Early Core Promoter Affects Alternative Splicing of Transcribed mRNA." J. Biol. Chem. 282(16): 11648-11657.

Gerber, M. A., A. Shilatifard, et al. (2005). "Mutational Analysis of an RNA Polymerase II Elongation Factor in Drosophila melanogaster." Mol. Cell. Biol. 25(17): 7803-7811.

Getz, M. J., P. K. Elder, et al. (1976). "Effect of cell proliferation on levels and diversity of poly(A)-containing mRNA." Cell 7: 255.

Ghosh, G., J. A. Adams, et al. (2011). "Phosphorylation mechanism and structure of serine-arginine protein kinases." FEBS Journal 278: 587-597.

Glover-Cutter, K., S. Kim, et al. (2008). "RNA polymerase II pauses and associates with pre-mRNA processing factors at both ends of genes." Nat. Struct. Mol. Biol. 15: 71-78.

Glover-Cutter, K., S. Larochelle, et al. (2009). "TFIIH-Associated Cdk7 Kinase Functions in Phosphorylation of C-Terminal Domain Ser7 Residues, Promoter-Proximal Pausing, and Termination by RNA Polymerase II." Mol. Cell. Biol. 29(20): 5455-5464.

Gomes, N. P., G. Bjerke, et al. (2006). "Gene-specific requirement for p-TEFb activity and RNA polymerase II phosphorylation within the p53 transcriptional program." Genes Dev. 20(5): 601-612.

Grondin, B. and N. DeLuca (2000). "Herpes Simplex Virus Type 1 ICP4 Promotes Transcription Preinitiation Complex Formation by Enhancing the Binding of TFIID to DNA." J. Virol. 74(24): 11504-11510.

Hargreaves, D. C., T. Horng, et al. (2009). "Control of inducible gene expression by signal-dependent transcriptional elongation." Cell 138: 129-145.

He, N., M. Liu, et al. (2010). "HIV-1 Tat and Host AFF4 Recruit Two Transcription Elongation Factors into a Bifunctional Complex for Coordinated Activation of HIV-1 Transcription." Molecular Cell 38(3): 428-438.

He, N., A. C. Pezda, et al. (2006). "Modulation of a P-TEFb Functional Equilibrium for the Global Control of Cell Growth and Differentiation." Mol. Cell. Biol. 26(19): 7068-7076.

Hinz, M., D. Krappmann, et al. (1999). "NF-kB function in growth control: regulation of cyclin D1 expression and Go/G1-to-S-phase transition." Mol Cell Biol 19: 2690-2698.

Hockert, K. J., K. Martincic, et al. (2011). "Spermatogenetic But Not Immunological Defects in Mice Lacking the &[tau]CstF-64 Polyadenylation Protein." Journal Reproductive Immunology 89: 26-37.

Horowitz, B., P. Zalazowski, et al. (1999). "The p65 subunit of NF-kB is redundant with p50 during B cell proliferative responses, and is required for germline CH transcription and class switching to IgG3." J. Immunol 162: 1941-1946.

House, A. E. and K. W. Lynch (2008). "Regulation of Alternative Splicing: More than Just the ABCs." J. Biol. Chem. 283(3): 1217-1221.

Ji, Z., J. Y. Lee, et al. (2009). "Progressive lengthening of 3' untranslated regions of mRNAs by alternative polyadenylation during mouse embryonic development." Proc Natl Acad Sci., USA 106(17): 7028-7033.

Ji, Z. and B. Tian (2009). "Reprogramming of 3'UTR Untranslated Regions of mRNAs by Alternative Polyadenylation in Generation of Pluripotent Stem Cells from Different Cell Types." PLoS ONE 4(12): e8419.

Jiang, H. and B. M. Peterlin (2008). "Differential Chromatin Looping Regulates CD4 Expression in Immature Thymocytes." Mol. Cell. Biol. 28(3): 907-912.

Jobert, L., N. Pinzon, et al. (2009). "Human U1 snRNA forms a new chromatin-associated snRNP with TAF15." EMBO Rep 10(5): 494-500.

Johnston, C. M., A. L. Wood, et al. (2006). "Complete Sequence Assembly and Characterization of the C57BL/6 Mouse Ig Heavy Chain V Region." J Immunol 176(7): 4221-4234.

Kaida, D., M. G. Berg, et al. (2010). "U1 snRNP protects pre-mRNAs from premature cleavage and polyadenylation." Nature 468(7324): 664-668.

Kelly, D. E. and R. P. Perry (1986). "Transcriptional and post-transcriptional control of Ig mRNA production during B lymphocyte development." Nucleic Acids Research 14: 5431-5441.

Kim, U., R. Siegel, et al. (2003). "Identification of transcription coactivator OCA-B-dependent genes involved in antigen-dependent B cell differentiation by cDNA array analyses." Proc Natl Acad Sci, USA 100: 8868-8873.

Kleiman, F. and J. Manley (2001). "The BARD1-CstF50 interaction links mRNA 3' end formation to DNA damage and tumor suppression." Cell 104: 743-753.

Kobrin, B. J., C. Milcarek, et al. (1986). "Sequences near the 3' secretion-specific polyadenylation site influence levels of secretion-specific and membrane-specific IgG2b mRNA in myeloma cells." Mol Cell Biol 6: 1687-1697.

Kornblihtt, A. R. (2006). "Chromatin, transcription elongation and alternative splicing." Nat. Struct. Mol. Biol. 13: 5-7.

Kornblihtt, A. R., M. De La Mata, et al. (2004). "Multiple links between transcription and splicing." RNA 10(10): 1489-1498.

Krueger, B. J., K. Varzavand, et al. (2010). "The Mechanism of Release of P-TEFb and HEXIM1 from the 7SK snRNP by Viral and Cellular Activators Includes a Conformational Change in 7SK." PLoS ONE 5(8): e12335.

Kuo, T. C. and K. L. Calame (2004). "B Lymphocyte-Induced Maturation Protein (Blimp)-1, IFN Regulatory Factor (IRF)-1, and IRF-2 Can Bind to the Same Regulatory Sites." J Immunol 173(9): 5556-5563.

Lassman, C. R., S. Matis, et al. (1992). "Plasma cell-regulated polyadenylation at the Ig gamma 2b secretion-specific poly(A) site." J Immunol 148(4): 1251-1260.

Lassman, C. R. and C. Milcarek (1992). " Regulated expression of the mouse γ2b Ig H chain gene is influenced by polyA site order and strength." J Immunol 148(8): 2578-2585.

Lee, S. C., A. Bottaro, et al. (2003). "Activation of terminal B cell differentiation by inhibition of histone deacetylation." Mol Immunol 39(15): 923-932.

Lekstrom-Himes, J. and K. G. Xanthopoulos (1999). "CCAAT/enhancer binding protein epsilon is critical for effective neutrophil-mediated response to inflammatory challenge." Blood 93(9): 3096-3105.

Lester, J. T. and N. A. DeLuca (2011). "Herpes Simplex Virus Type 1 (HSV-1) ICP4 forms complexes with TFIID and Mediator in Virus Infected Cells." J. Virol.: in press.

Lewis, B. A. and D. Reinberg (2003). "The mediator coactivator complex: functional and physical roles in transcription regualtion." J. Cell Science 116: 3667-3675.

Lin, C., E. R. Smith, et al. (2010). "AFF4, a Component of the ELL/P-TEFb Elongation Complex and a Shared Subunit of MLL Chimeras, Can Link Transcription Elongation to Leukemia." Molecular Cell 37(3): 429-437.

Lin, Y., K. Wong, et al. (1997). "Blimp-1, an inducer of terminal B-cell differentiation, represses c-Myc transcription." Science 276: 596-599.

Lis, J. T., P. Mason, et al. (2000). "P-TEFb kinase recruitment and function at heat shock loci." Genes Dev. 14(7): 792-803.

Liu, J.-X., B. Hu, et al. (2009). "Zebrafish eaf1 and eaf2/u19 mediate effective convergence and extension movements through the maintenance of wnt11 and wnt5 expression." J. Biol. Chem.: M109.009654.

Lu, R. (2008). "Interferon regulatory factor 4 and 8 in B-cell development." Trends in Immunology 29(10): 487-492.

Luco, R. F., Q. Pan, et al. (2010). "Regulation of Alternative Splicing by Histone Modifications." Science 327(5968): 996-1000.

Luo, R. T., C. Lavau, et al. (2001). "The Elongation Domain of ELL Is Dispensable but Its ELL-Associated Factor 1 Interaction Domain Is Essential for MLL-ELL-Induced Leukemogenesis." Mol. Cell. Biol. 21(16): 5678-5687.

Lutz, C. S. and A. Moreira (2011). "Alternative mRNA polyadenylation in eukaryotes: an effective regulator of gene expression." WIRES RNA 2: 23-31.

Ma, J., S. I. Gunderson, et al. (2006). "Non-snRNP U1A levels decrease during mammalian B-cell differentiation and release the IgM secretory poly(A) site from repression." RNA 12(1): 122-132.

MacDonald, C., J. Wilusz, et al. (1994). "The 64 kDa subunit of the CstF polyadenylation factor binds to pre-mRNAs downstream of cleavage site and influences cleavage site location." Mol Cell Biol 14: 6647-6654.

Mandel, C. R., s. Kaneko, et al. (2006). "Polyadenylation factor CPSF-73 is the pre-mRNA 3'-end processing endonuclease." Nature 444: 953-956.

Martincic, K., S. A. Alkan, et al. (2009). "Transcription elongation factor ELL2 directs immunoglobulin secretion in plasma cells by stimulating altered RNA processing." Nat Immunol 10(10): 1102-1109.

Martincic, K., R. Campbell, et al. (1998). "Increase in the 64-kDa subunit of the polyadenylation/cleavage stimulatory factor during the G_0 to S phase transition." Proc Natl Acad Sci USA 95(19): 11095-11100.

Martins, G. and K. Calame (2008). Regulation and Functions of Blimp-1 in T and B Lymphocytes. Ann Rev Immunology. P. Littman. Palo Alto, CA, Annual Reviews. 26: 133-169.

Matis, S. A., K. Martincic, et al. (1996). "B-lineage regulated polyadenylation occurs on weak poly(A) sites regardless of sequence composition at the cleavage and downstream regions." Nucleic Acids Research 24: 4684-4692.

McCracken, S., N. Fong, et al. (1997). "The C-terminal domain of RNA polymerase II couples mRNA processing to transcription." Nature 385: 357-361.

Meyer, C., E. Kowarz, et al. (2009). "New insights to the MLL recombinome of acute leukemias." Leukemia.

Milcarek, C. and B. Hall (1985). "Cell-specific expression of secreted versus membrane forms of immunoglobulin gamma 2b mRNA involves selective use of alternate polyadenylation sites." Mol. Cell. Biol. 5(10): 2514-2520.

Milcarek, C., M. Hartman, et al. (1996). "Changes in abundance of IgG 2a mRNA in the nucleus and cytoplasm of a murine B-lymphoma before and after fusion to a myeloma cell." Mol Immunol 33(7-8): 691-701.

Milcarek, C., K. Martincic, et al. (2003). "The snRNP-associated U1A levels change following IL-6 stimulation of human B-cells." Mol Immunol 39: 809-814.

Milcarek, C., R. Price, et al. (1974). "The metabolism of a poly(A) minus mRNA fraction in HeLa cells." Cell 3: 1-10.

Miller, T., K. Williams, et al. (2000). "Identification, cloning, expression, and biochemical characterization of the testis-specific RNA polymerase II elongation factor ELL3." J. Biol. Chem. 275: 32052-32056.

Mohan, M., H.-M. Herz, et al. (2010). "Linking H3K79 trimethylation to Wnt signaling through a novel Dot1-containing complex (DotCom)." Genes & Development 24(6): 574-589.

Moore, C. L., H. Skolnik-David, et al. (1988). "Sedimentation analysis of polyadenylation specific complexes." Mol Cell Biol 8: 226-233.

Mueller, D., C. Bach, et al. (2007). "A role for the MLL fusion partner ENL in transcriptional elongation and chromatin modification." Blood 110(13): 4445-4454.

Muñoz, M. J., M. de la Mata, et al. (2010). "The carboxy terminal domain of RNA polymerase II and alternative splicing." Trends in Biochemical Sciences 35(9): 497-504.

Nagaike, T., C. Logan, et al. (2011). "Transcriptional Activators Enhance Polyadenylation of mRNA Precursors." Molecular Cell 41(4): 409-418.

Nechaev, S. and K. Adelman (2011). "Pol II waiting in the starting gates: Regulating the transition from transcription initiation into productive elongation." Biochimica et Biophysica Acta (BBA) - Gene Regulatory Mechanisms 1809(1): 34-45.

Oven, I., N. Brdickova, et al. (2007). "AIRE Recruits P-TEFb for Transcriptional Elongation of Target Genes in Medullary Thymic Epithelial Cells." Mol. Cell. Biol. 27(24): 8815-8823.

Pal, R., M. Janz, et al. (2009). "C/EBP{beta} regulates transcription factors critical for proliferation and survival of multiple myeloma cells." Blood 114(18): 3890-3898.

Perales, R. and D. Bentley (2009). ""Cotranscriptionality": The Transcription Elongation Complex as a Nexus for Nuclear Transactions." Mol Cell 36(2): 178-191.

Perkins, K., M. Lusic, et al. (2008). "Transcription-Dependent Gene Looping of the HIV-1 Provirus Is Dictated by Recognition of Pre-mRNA Processing Signals." Mol Cell 29: 56-68.

Peterlin, B. M. and D. H. Price (2006). "Controlling the Elongation Phase of Transcription with P-TEFb." Mol Cell 23(3): 297-305.

Peterson, M. L. (2007). "Mechanisms controlling production of membrane and secreted immunoglobulin during B cell development." Immunol Res 37(1): 33-48.

Peterson, M. L., S. Bertolino, et al. (2002). "An RNA Polymerase Pause Site Is Associated with the Immunoglobulin {micro}s Poly(A) Site." Mol. Cell. Biol. 22(15): 5606-5615.

Peterson, M. L. and R. P. Perry (1986). "Regulated production of mu-m and mu-s mRNA requires linkage." Proc Natl Acad Sci, USA 83: 8883-8887.

Peterson, M. L. and R. P. Perry (1989). "The regulated production of mu-m and mu-s mRNA is dependent on the relative efficiencies of mu-s poly(A) site usage and the Cmu4 to M1 splice." Mol. Cell. Biol. 9: 726-738.

Phillips, C., N. Pachikara, et al. (2004). "U1A Inhibits Cleavage at the Immunoglobulin M Heavy-Chain Secretory Poly(A) Site by Binding between the Two Downstream GU-Rich Regions." Mol. Cell. Biol. 24(14): 6162-6171.

Phillips, C. and A. Virtanen (1997). "The murine IgM secretory poly(A) site contains dual upstream and downstream elements which affect polyadenylation." Nucleic Acids Research 25: 2344-2351.

Pirngruber, J., A. Schhebet, et al. (2009). "Insights into the function of the human pTEFb component cdk9 in the regulation of chromatin modifications and co-transcriptional mRNA processing." Cell Cyle 8: 3636-3642.

Poli, V. (1998). "The role of C/EBP isoforms in the control of inflammatory and native immunity functions." J Biol Chem 273(45): 29279-29282.

Proudfoot, N. J., A. Furger, et al. (2002). "Integrating mRNA processing with transcription." Cell 108: 501-512.

Qin, X. F., A. Reichlin, et al. (1998). "OCA-B integrates B cell antigen receptor-, CD40L- and IL4-mediated signals for the germinal center pathway of B cell development." EMBO J. 17: 5066-5075.

Rahl, P. B., C. Y. Lin, et al. (2010). "c-Myc Regulates Transcriptional Pause Release." Cell 141(3): 432-445.

Rigo, F. and H. G. Martinson (2008). "Functional Coupling of Last-Intron Splicing and 3'-End Processing to Transcription In Vitro: the Poly(A) Signal Couples to Splicing before Committing to Cleavage." Mol. Cell. Biol. 28(2): 849-862.

Roberts, S. and D. L. Bentley (1992). "Distinct modes of transcription read through or terminate at the c-myc attenuator." EMBO J. 11: 1085-1093.

Rozenblatt-Rosen, O., T. Nagaike, et al. (2009). "The tumor suppressor Cdc73 functionally associates with CPSF and CstF mRNA processing factors." Proc. Natl. Acad. Sci., USA 106(3): 755-760.

Sachs, A. and E. Wahle (1993). "Poly(A) tail metabolism and function in eucaryotes." J Biol Chem 268(31): 22955-22958.

Sandri-Goldin, R. (2008). "The many roles of the regulatory protein ICP27 during herpes simplex virus infection." Front. Biosci. 13: 5241-5256.

Sato, S., C. Tomomori-Sato, et al. (2004). "A Set of Consensus Mammalian Mediator Subunits Identified by Multidimensional Protein Identification Technology." Mol Cell 14(5): 685-691.

Schor, I. E., N. Rascovan, et al. (2009). "Neuronal cell depolarization induces intragenic chromatin modifications affecting NCAM alternative splicing." Proc. Natl. Acad. Sci., U.S.A. 106: 4325-4330.

Sciabica, K. S., Q. J. Dai, et al. (2003). "ICP27 interacts with SRPK1 to mediate HSV splicing inhibition by altering SR protein phosphorylation." EMBO J 22(7): 1608-1619.

Sciammas, R., A. L. Shaffer, et al. (2006). "Graded Expression of Interferon Regulatory Factor-4 Coordinates Isotype Switching with Plasma Cell Differentiation." Immunity 25(2): 225-236.

Screpanti, I., L. Romani, et al. (1995). "Lymphoproliferative disorder and imbalanced T-helper response in C/EBP beta-deficient mice." Embo J 14(9): 1932-1941.

Selth, L. A., S. Sigurdsson, et al. (2010). "Transcript Elongation by RNA Polymerase II." Ann Rev Biochem 79(1): 271-293.

Shaffer, A., X. Yu, et al. (2000). "BCL-6 represses genes that function in lymphocyte differentiation, inflammation and cell cycle control." Immunity 13(2): 199-212.

Shaffer, A. L., N. C. T. Emre, et al. (2008). "IRF4 addiction in multiple myeloma." Nature 454: 226-231.

Shaffer, A. L., M. Shapiro-Shelef, et al. (2004). "XBP1, Downstream of Blimp-1, Expands the Secretory Apparatus and Other Organelles, and Increases Protein Synthesis in Plasma Cell Differentiation." Immunity 21: 81-93.

Shaw, G., S. Morse, et al. "Preferential transformation of human neuronal cells by human adenoviruses and the origin of HEK 293 cells." The FASEB Journal.

Sheets, M. D., M. Wu, et al. (1995). "Polyadenylation of c-mos mRNA as a control point in Xenopus meiotic maturation." Nature 374: 511-516.

Shell, S. A., C. Hesse, et al. (2005). "Elevated Levels of the 64-kDa Cleavage Stimulatory Factor (CstF-64) in Lipopolysaccharide-stimulated Macrophages Influence Gene Expression and Induce Alternative Poly(A) Site Selection." J. Biol. Chem. 280(48): 39950-39961.

Shell, S. A., K. Martincic, et al. (2007). "Increased phosphorylation of the carboxyl terminal domain of RNA polymerase II and loading of polyadenylation and co-transcriptional factors contribute to regulation of the Ig heavy chain mRNA in plasma cells." J. Immunol. 179: 7663-7673.

Shi, Y., D. C. Di Giammartino, et al. (2009). "Molecular Architecture of the Human Pre-mRNA 3' Processing Complex." Mol Cell 33(3): 365-376.

Shilatifard, A. (1998). "Factors regulating the transcriptional elongation activity of RNA polymerase II." FASEB J. 12: 1437-1446.

Shilatifard, A., D. R. Duan, et al. (1997). "ELL2, a new member of an ELL family of RNA polymerase II elongation factors." Proc. Natl. Acad. Sci. USA 94: 3639-3643.

Shilatifard, A., W. S. Lane, et al. (1996). "An RNA polymerase II elongation factor encoded by the human ELL gene." Science 271: 1873-1876.

Simone, F., R. T. Luo, et al. (2003). "ELL-associated factor 2 (EAF2), a functional homolog of EAF1 with alternative ELL binding properties." Blood 101(6): 2355-2362.

Sobhian, B., Laguette, N., Yatim, A., Nakamura, M., Levy, Y., Kiernan, R., and Benkirane, M. (2010) *Molecular Cell* 38, 439-451Spies, N., C. B. Nielsen, et al. (2009). "Biased Chromatin Signatures around Polyadenylation Sites and Exons." Mol Cell 36(2): 245-254.

Stefano, J. and D. Adams (1988). "Assembly of a polyadenylation-specific 25S ribonucleoprotein complex in vitro." Mol Cell Biol 8(5): 2052-2062.

Steger, D. J., M. I. Lefterova, et al. (2008). "DOT1L/KMT4 Recruitment and H3K79 Methylation Are Ubiquitously Coupled with Gene Transcription in Mammalian Cells." Mol. Cell. Biol. 28(8): 2825-2839.

Taatjes, D. J., M. T. Marr, et al. (2004). "Regulatory diversity among metazoan co-activator complexes." Nature Reviews 5: 403-410.

Takagaki, Y., C. MacDonald, et al. (1992). "The human 64- kDa polyadenylation factor contains a ribonucleoprotein-type RNA binding domain and unusual auxilary motifs." Proc Natl Acad Sci USA 89: 1403-1407.

Takagaki, Y. and J. Manley (1994). "A polyadenylation factor subunit is the human homologue of the *Drosophila suppressor of forked* protein." Nature 372: 471-474.

Takagaki, Y. and J. Manley (1998). "Levels of polyadenylation factor CstF-64 control IgM heavy chain mRNA accumulation and other events associated with B cell differentiation." Mol. Cell 2: 761-771.

Takagaki, Y. and J. L. Manley (1997). "RNA recognition by the human polyadenylation factor CstF." Mol Cell Biol 17: 3907-3914.

Takagaki, Y., R. Seipelt, et al. (1996). "The polyadenylation factor CstF-64 regulates alternative processing of IgM heavy chain pre-mRNA during B-cell differentiation." Cell 87: 941-952.

Takami, Y., H. Kikuchi, et al. (1999). "Chicken histone deacetylase-2 controls the amount of the IgM H-chain at the steps of both transcription of its gene and alternative processing of its pre-mRNA in the DT40 cell line." J Biol Chem 34: 23977-23990.

Tanaka, T., S. Akira, et al. (1995). "Targeted disruption of the NF-IL6 gene discloses its essential role in bacteria killing and tumor cytotoxicity by macrophages." Cell 80(2): 353-361.

Teitell, M. A. (2003). "OCA-B regulation of B-cell development and function." Trends in Immunology 24(10): 546-553.

Thirman, M. J., D. A. Levitan, et al. (1994). "Cloning of ELL, a gene that fuses to MLL in a t(11:19)(q23:p13.1) in acute myeloid leukemia." Proc. Natl. Acad. Sci. USA 91: 12110-12114.

Tian, B., J. Hu, et al. (2005). "A large-scale analysis of mRNA polyadenylation of human and mouse genes." Nucl. Acids Res. 33(1): 201-212.

Tian, B., Z. Pan, et al. (2007). "Widespread mRNA polyadenylation events in introns indicate dynamic interplay between polyadenylation and splicing." Genome Res. 17(2): 156-165.

Tietjen, J. R., D. W. Zhang, et al. (2010). "Chemical-genomic dissection of the CTD code." Nat Struct Mol Biol 17(99): 1154-1161.

Tilgner, H., C. Nikolaou, et al. (2009). "Nucleosome positioning as a determinant of exon recognition." Nat Struct Mol Biol 16(9): 996-1001.

Turner, C., D. Mack, et al. (1994). "Blimp-1, a novel zinc finger-containing protein that can drive the maturation of B lymphocytes into immunoglobulin-secreting cells." Cell 77: 297-306.

Underhill, G. H., D. George, et al. (2003). "Gene expression profiling reveals a highly specialized genetic program of plasma cells." Blood 101(10): 4013-4021.

Veraldi, K., G. Edwalds-Gilbert, et al. (2000). "Isolation and characterization of polyadenylation complexes assembled *in vitro*." RNA 6: 768-777.

Veraldi, K. L., G. K. Arhin, et al. (2001). "hnRNP F influences binding of a 64-kilodalton subunit of cleavage stimulation factor to mRNA precursors in mouse B-cells." Mol. Cell. Biol. 21: 1228-1238.

Vojnic, E., B. Simon, et al. (2006). "Structure and Carboxyl-terminal Domain (CTD) Binding of the Set2 SRI Domain That Couples Histone H3 Lys36 Methylation to Transcription." J Biol Chem 281(1): 13-15.

Vollmuth, F., W. Blankenfeldt, et al. (2009). "Structures of the dual bromodomains of the P-TEFb activating protein Brd4 at atomic resolution." J Biol Chem: -.

Wang, G. G., L. Cai, et al. (2007). "NUP98-NSD1 links H3K36 methylation to Hox-A gene activation and leukaemogenesis." Nat Cell Biol 9(7): 804-812.

Wang, P., C. Lin, et al. (2009). "Global Analysis of H3K4 Methylation Defines MLL Family Member Targets and Points to a Role for MLL1-Mediated H3K4 Methylation in the Regulation of Transcriptional Initiation by RNA Polymerase II." Mol. Cell. Biol. 29(22): 6074-6085.

Wiederschain, D., H. Kawai, et al. (2003). "Molecular Basis of p53 Functional Inactivation by the Leukemic Protein MLL-ELL." Mol. Cell. Biol. 23(12): 4230-4246.

Wilusz, J. and T. Shenk (1990). "A uridylate tract mediates efficient hnRNP C protein-RNA crosslinking and functionally substitutes for the downstream element of the polyadenylation signal." Mol Cell Biol 10: 6397-6407.

Wolstein, O., A. Silkov, et al. (2000). "Specific interaction of TAFII105 with OCA-B is involved in activation of octamer-dependent transcription." J Biol Chem 275(22): 16459-16465.

Xiao, W., O. Zhang, et al. (2008). "U19/Eaf2 knockout causes lung adenocarcinoma, B-cell lymphoma, hepatocellular carcinoma and prostatic intraepithelial neoplasia." Oncogene 6: 1536-1544.

Xu, Y.-X. and J. L. Manley (2007). "Pin1 modulates RNA polymerase II activity during the transcription cycle." Genes & Development 21(22): 2950-2962.

Yamaguchi, Y., T. Wada, et al. (1998). "Interplay between positive and negative elongation factors: drawing a new view of DRB." Genes to Cells 3: 9-15.

Yang, L., M. Duff, et al. (2011). "Genomewide characterization of non-polyadenylated RNAs." Genome Biology 12(2): R16.

Yokoyama, A., M. Lin, et al. (2004). "A Higher-Order Complex Containing AF4 and ENL Family Proteins with P-TEFb Facilitates Oncogenic and Physiologic MLL-Dependent Transcription." Cancer Cell 17(2): 198-212.

Zeitlinger, J., A. Stark, et al. (2007). "RNA polymerase stalling at developmental control genes in the Drosophila melanogaster embryo." Nat Genet 39(12): 1512-1516.

Zhao, J., L. Hyman, et al. (1999). "Formation of mRNA 3' ends in eukaryotes: mechanism, regulation, and interrelationships with other steps in mRNA synthesis." Microbiol Mol Biol Rev 63(2): 405-445.

Zhou, J., X. Feng, et al. (2009). "Elongation Factor ELL (Eleven-Nineteen Lysine-rich Leukemia) Acts as a Transcription Factor for Direct Thrombospondin-1 Regulation." J. Biol. Chem. 284(28): 19142-19152.

3

The Worlds of Splicing and Chromatin Collide

J. Adam Hall and Philippe T. Georgel
Byrd Biotechnology Science Center
Department of Biological Sciences, Marshall University
USA

1. Introduction

A. Integration of transcription and splicing

1. Chromatin, transcription, and splicing.

Both transcription and splicing take place in a nuclear environment which, at face value, may seem refractory to the efficiency afforded by the coupling of both processes. This environment, chromatin, was once viewed as only a passive packaging system for genetic material, with very little contribution to the variety of nuclear activities occurring within and around it. However, overwhelming evidence now points to the chromatin environment as being highly dynamic, and an active player in nuclear activities. Residues on all four histone N-termini (also known as tails) have been shown to be post-translationally modified in a variety of ways. Many of these modifications have been found to be recognized by factors involved in the regulation of gene expression and are associated with particular activating or repressive states, leading to the proposal of a "histone code" that directs (contributes to) the activity of gene regulatory factors ([1]). In addition to compositional changes, chromatin structure has also been proven to be dynamic. Specific enzymes have been characterized to utilize the energy from ATP hydrolysis to physically disrupt histone-DNA contacts, "remodeling" chromatin and altering the accessibility of DNA ([2]). These chromatin remodelers can slide nucleosomes along the DNA template, and even remove individual or subset of histones or entire nucleosomes at a particular genetic locus. In addition to changes in nucleosome (histone octamer plus 146 base-pairs of DNA) density at the primary level, chromatin structure can also be altered at a secondary level, exhibiting the ability to form compacted (and de-compacted) structures. Overall, the role of chromatin and factors acting upon it in the regulation of transcription (generally referred to as *epigenetics*) has become a well-studied topic, and a much better understanding of gene regulation has lead to many important breakthroughs in the fields of cellular differentiation, development, and disease. Because of the popularity of epigenetics and the knowledge that transcription and splicing are not mutually-exclusive, the role of chromatin in splicing is becoming an important area of research foci as well.

2. Co-transcriptionality.

Nuclear processes that involve the generation and manipulation of messenger RNA (mRNA) occur within remarkable spatial and temporal proximity. These processes include transcription, 5′ capping, splicing, and polyadenylation. Two of these mechanisms, transcription and splicing, are utilized by the cell to create phenotypic variation from otherwise identical genotypes. Both complex and elegant, these two nuclear events provide an explanation as to how organisms with relatively identical genetic information can differ severely in appearance and behavior. All aspects of transcription (initiation, elongation, termination, activation, repression, etc.) have been the subject of intense research focus since the first articulation of the central dogma of molecular biology: *DNA>RNA>protein* ([3]). The molecular mechanisms of RNA splicing have been increasingly investigated throughout the past few decades, with its importance highlighted by the fact that more than 90% of all human genes undergo alternative splicing ([4,5]). Although each transcription and splicing processes were initially studied and characterized as being mutually exclusive, mounting evidence has proven them to occur simultaneously and in concert, maximizing the efficiency and fidelity of mature transcript synthesis. The first evidence for the coupling of transcription and splicing, or "co-transcriptionality", came almost 25 years ago, as electron microscopy on transcripts from *Drosophila* embryos revealed co-transcriptional splicing ([6]). Shortly after, on a more specific basis, the human gene *dystrophin* was described as being co-transcriptionally spliced ([7]). Underscoring the need for efficiency in transcript synthesis and processing, this 2400 kb gene takes up to 16 hours to be transcribed. As the distinct factors and mechanisms involved in both processes have been comprehensively elucidated, a rather clear picture as to how the cell integrates transcription and splicing has begun to emerge. In fact, two models have recently been proposed to explain this "coupling" process: kinetic and recruitment ([8]). The kinetic coupling model proposes that the rate of transcription elongation by RNA polymerase II (RNA pol II), the enzyme responsible for transcription catalysis, directly modulates splicing decisions. Recruitment coupling revolves around the association and interaction of transcription factors with the splicing machinery. These models are not mutually exclusive, and focus on two critical nuclear elements which will be fully explored in this chapter: the C-terminal domain of pol II and the chromatin environment in which both transcription and splicing take place.

3. Transcription and the RNA pol II CTD.

RNA polymerase II catalyzes the transcription of eukaryotic genes and is distinct among RNA polymerases because of the presence of a repetitive heptapeptide sequence within its Carboxyl Terminal Domain (CTD) ([9]; Figure 1). This sequence, Tyr-Ser-Pro-Thr-Ser-Pro-Ser ($Y_1S_2P_3T_4S_5P_6S_7$), is repeated 52 times in mammals, and has been found to be necessary for the transcription of endogenous genes ([10]). The potential for large amounts of post-translational modification (PTM), especially phosphorylation, exists on the pol II CTD, especially phosphorylation. In fact, the phosphorylation of two specific serine residues (Ser2 and Ser5) within the RNA pol II CTD is directly related to transcription initiation and elongation, as well as pre-mRNA capping and polyadenylation ([11]). In terms of initiation, phosphorylation of Ser5 on the promoter-bound RNA pol II CTD is accomplished by cyclin-dependent kinase 7 (cdk7) which is a component of the basal transcription factor TFIIH ([12]). At this point, additional components of the transcription machinery are able to assemble. However, another phosphorylation event, this time on Ser2, is necessary for promoter "clearance" and pol II elongation. The transcription elongation factor P-TEFb (Positive Transcription Elongation Factor b) is the kinase responsible for Ser2 phosphorylation, as it relieves the elongation-inhibitory effects of the factors DSIF (DRB-Sensitive Inducing Factor) and NELF (Basal Embryonic LHRH Factor) ([13]). The presence of 46 Ser2 residues and 51 Ser5 residues allows for a control mechanism of the rate of elongation, a main principle of the kinetic model of transcription-splicing coupling, discussed in-depth later in this chapter.

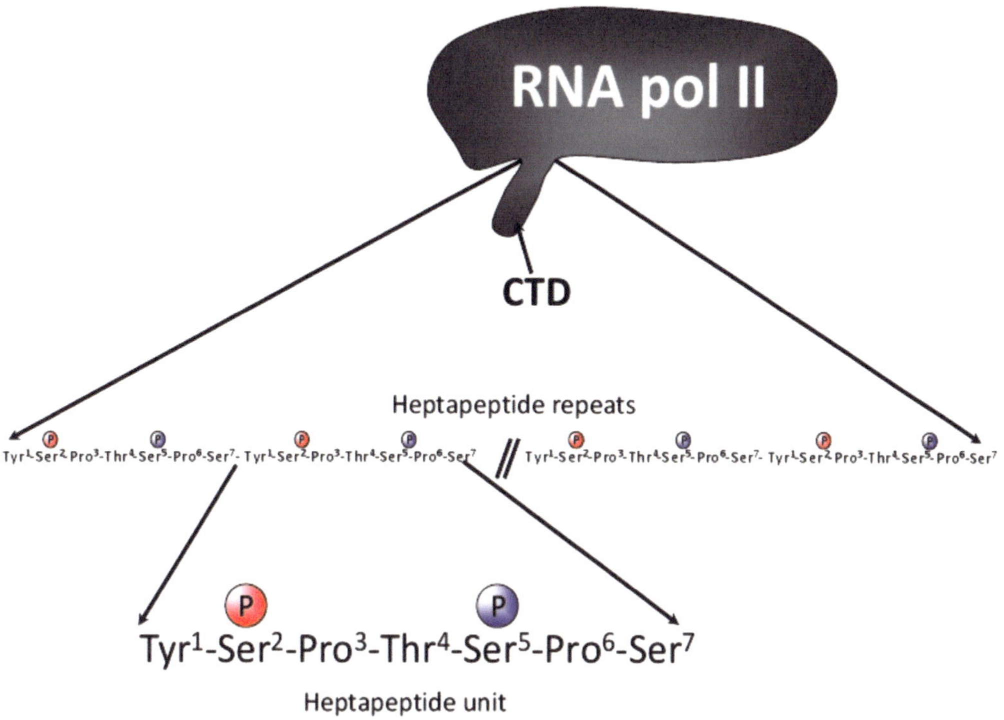

Fig. 1. Structure and composition of the RNA pol II large subunit.
The C-Terminal Domain (CTD) contains up to 52 repeats of the heptapeptide unit YSPTSPS. Note that the consensus sequence of the heptapeptide repeats 26-52 is often degenerated. Post-translational modifications of heptade residues affect the RNA pol II functions. Phosphorylation of Serine 5 (by TFIIH and cyclin-dependent kinase 7) is important for promoter clearance during initiation and elongation. Phosphorylation of Serine 2 (by P-TEFb and cyclin-dependent kinase 9) is associated with elongation and transcriptional termination.

4. Control of RNA splicing.

RNA splicing, catalyzed by the spliceosome, a large RNA-protein complex composed of five small nuclear ribonucleoproteins (snRNPs), provides the cell with an additional level of phenotypic complexity without the need for additional transcript generation ([14]). Control of splicing can occur in "cis" through regulatory sequences in pre-mRNA, as well as "trans" by factors that bind and act upon these sequences. An example of these factors is the SR proteins which act in the control of splice site recognition by affecting spliceosome assembly ([15]). It is the control of splice site recognition which provides the major mechanism by which RNA splicing is regulated. Splice sites within introns have been found to have differing "strengths" which affect their ability to be recognized and acted upon by components of the splicing machinery. This form of splicing regulation is directly related to the control of transcription elongation, both through the kinetic and recruitment models mentioned earlier. Therefore, "co-transcriptional" splicing provides the cell with the advantages of increased efficiency of transcript generation and processing, preventing mRNA degradation and back-hybridization with DNA ([16]).

5. Kinetic model of co-transcriptional splicing.

The kinetic model of co-transcriptional splicing revolves around the concept that the rate of RNA pol II elongation directly affects splice site recognition and spliceosome assembly ([17]; Figure 2). The rate by which RNA pol II transcribes along the length of a gene can be affected by two factors: the phosphorylation level of Ser5 and Ser2 on the RNA pol II CTD, as well as the chromatin structure which encapsulates the gene being transcribed. In a nutshell, fast elongation, which occurs when the RNA pol II CTD is hyperphosphorylated and/or the chromatin of the gene being transcribed has a low nucleosome density, favors the inclusion of downstream exons with "strong" splice sites (Figure 3). In contrast, when the RNA pol II CTD is hypophosphorylated and/or the nucleosome density of the transcribed gene is increased, a slow elongation rate allows enough temporal flexibility for the splicing machinery to assemble on upstream, "weaker" splice sites. Initial experiments supporting this concept showed that using "slow" RNA pol II mutants or inserting pausing

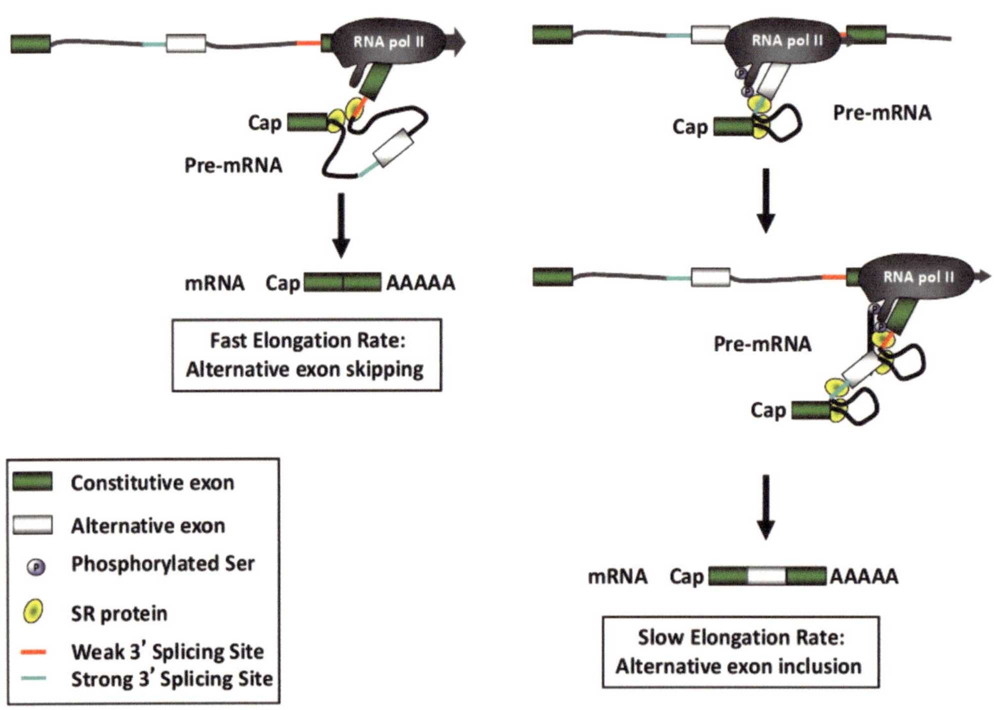

Fig. 2. Kinetic model for co-transcriptional splicing.
The regulation of alternative splicing is modulated by the rate of elongation of RNA pol II. Fast elongation rate (Left panel) results in more frequent exon skipping. The rate of elongation can be influenced by the level of CTD Ser 2 and Ser 5 phosphorylation. The weak 3' splicing site is indicated in blue and the strong 3' splicing site in red. Slower elongation (Right panel) results in inclusion of the alternative exon (Grey rectangle) between the two constitutive exons (Green rectangles). Cap: 7'methyl guanosine; AAAAA: poly A tail

elements in reporter minigenes favors "weak" exon inclusion in the fibronectin and fibroblast growth factor receptor 2 (FGFR2) genes ([18], [19]). The fact that there are 46 Ser2 and 51 Ser5 residues in mammalian CTDs provide a sort of "gas pedal" mechanism for the control of elongation rate, and therefore splicing decisions. In an intriguing example, the chromatin remodeling factor SWI/SNF which interacts with RNA pol II, splicing factors, and spliceosome-associated proteins, can cause inclusion of a block of exons in the middle of the CD44 gene by stalling RNA pol II through a phosphorylation status switch from phospho-Ser2 to phospho-Ser5 ([20]). Further evidence for this intragenic "brake" control mechanism comes from the transient accumulation of phospho-serine 5 on the RNA pol II CTD around the 3' end of yeast introns ([21]). This pausing before an exon is suggestive of a splicing-dependent transcriptional checkpoint which holds any further transcription until spliceosome assembly is accomplished.

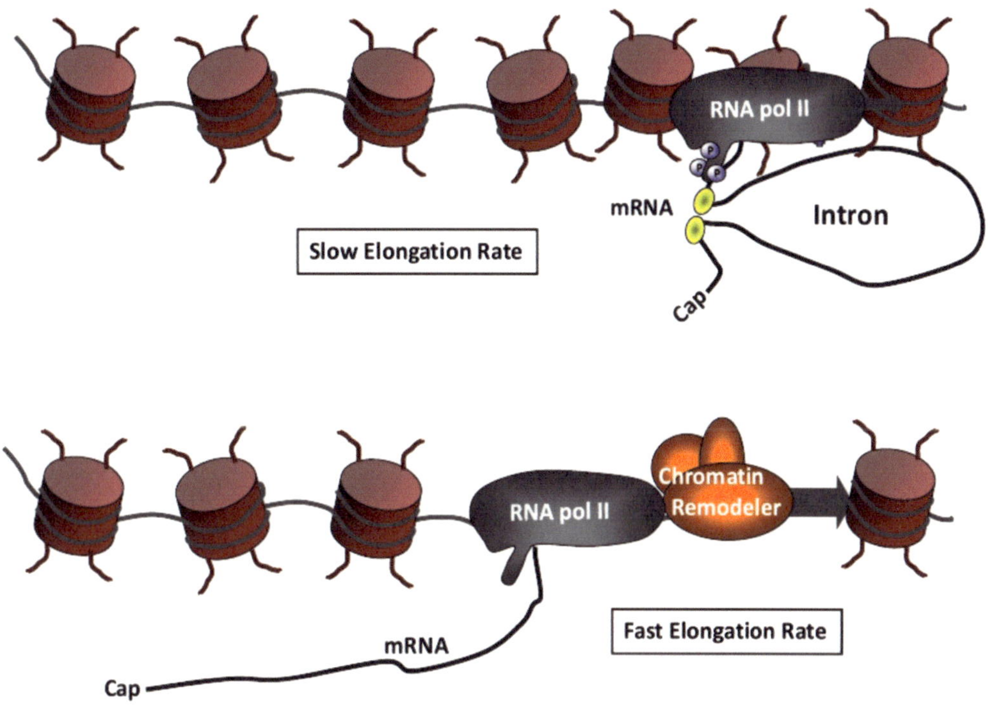

Fig. 3. Modulation of RNA pol II elongation rate is related to nucleosome density. Nucleosomes, through their position and/or density can affect the RNA pol II elongation rate. Low density would privilege a fast elongation rate and lead to exon skipping. This may be facilitated by the presence of chromatin remodeling complexes that can promote nucleosome displacement through sliding or partial loss of histones. The higher nucleosome density would reduce the RNA pol II elongation rate and favor exon inclusion.

In terms of chromatin structure altering elongation rate and splicing, on genes regulated by the chromatin-remodeler SWI/SNF, the ATPase subunit Brahma (Brm) has been shown to contribute to transcription-splicing crosstalk by decreasing the elongation rate (through alterations in nucleosome density patterns) and facilitating recruitment of the splicing machinery to variant exons with suboptimal splice sites ([20]). Conversely, treatment with the histone deacetylase inhibitor, Trichostatin A (TSA) facilitates a more "open" chromatin conformation, stimulating elongation rates and causing inhibition of the fibronectin exon EDI inclusion ([22]). Much more evidence exists that relates chromatin structure and composition to the regulation of both transcription and splicing, independent of elongation rate and the kinetic model of "co-transcriptionality". These concepts, including chromatin as a recruiter of both transcription and splicing factors, nucleosome positioning in delineating critical transcription and splice sites, and the involvement of chromatin modifications and modifiers in both transcription and splicing, will be discussed later in detail in this chapter.

6. Recruitment model of co-transcriptional splicing.

The recruitment model of co-transcriptional splicing is similar to the kinetic model in the sense that it revolves around the RNA pol II CTD (Figure 4). Specifically, the recruitment model involves the allosteric regulation of splicing decisions through interactions with the elongation machinery mediated by the RNA pol II CTD ([23]). The most clear-cut example of the recruitment model involves the RNA pol II CTD, the SR protein SRp20, and the alternative exon EDI of the fibronectin gene ([24]). SRp20 has an inhibitory effect on the

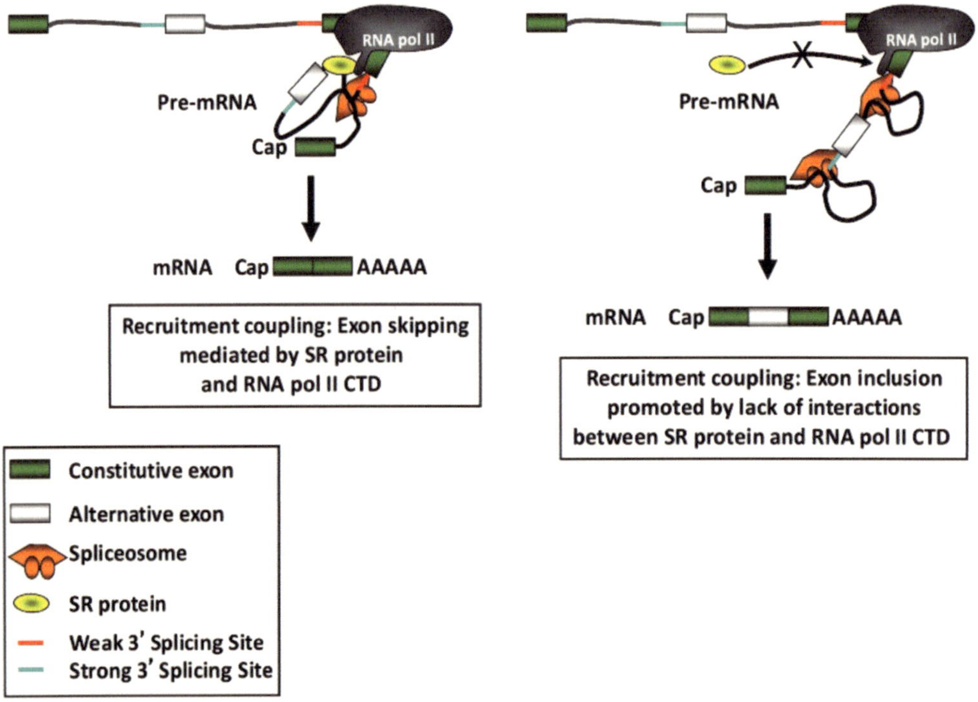

Fig. 4. Recruitment model for co-transcriptional splicing.
In this model, the recruitment of splicing factors SR protein(s) (yellow ovals) is mediated by interactions with the RNA pol II CTD. Binding of SR proteins, such as SRp20, to the CTD favors alternative exon skipping (Left panel). Loss of SR protein interactions with the CTD prevents formation of a proper ternary complex and leads to alternative exon inclusion (right panel). This model is based on work by de la Mata et al. ([24]).

inclusion of the *fibronectin* EDI exon, and this effect is mediated by the RNA pol II CTD. When a RNA pol II mutant lacking the CTD is present, SRp20 is not recruited to the site, and EDI inclusion is greatly enhanced. Long before this evidence was presented, a trend connecting the recruitment of splicing factors with transcript elongation mediated by the RNA pol II CTD was emerging. When genes are placed under the control of RNA polymerase I, III, or bacteriophage T7 RNA polymerase promoters, transcription occurs, but splicing is greatly affected ([25]; [26]; [27]). Logically, the recruitment of splicing factors to proper slice sites is dependent on the RNA pol II CTD ([28]) and deletion of the CTD affects all aspects of RNA processing in the β-globin gene ([29]). The most obvious factor(s) playing a role in the recruitment model of co-transcriptional splicing are the SR proteins. Virtually all members of the SR family are known to interact with RNA pol II, as well as other splicing factors and components of the spliceosome ([30]). Additional factors which interact with both the pol II CTD (phorphorylated or un-phosphorylated), as well as integral components of the spliceosome include the elongation factors CA150 ([31]) and SPT6 ([32]), as well as the transcriptional regulators TRAP150/Med23 ([33]), TFII H ([34]), PSF/p54nrb ([35]), and EWS-Fli and NOR1 ([36]).

Many factors that affect chromatin structure and composition also interact with members of both the elongation and splicing machinery, consequently playing a role in the recruitment model of co-transcriptionality as well. These factors primarily include chromatin remodelers and histone modifiers. Evidence for these chromatin-associated factors acting as "adaptor" molecules, bridging both processes and playing roles in both proposed models for the coupling of transcription and splicing is overwhelming. Therefore, additional sections in this chapter have been included to explore their multi-faceted activity in full detail.

7. Incorporation of both kinetic and recruitment models of co-transcriptionality.

Just as the nuclear processes of transcription and splicing have proven to be non mutually-exclusive, the two models proposed to explain the coupling of both mechanisms have to be integrated to fully understand the concept. For example, the modulation of RNA pol II's elongation rate is directly linked to the recruitment of specific factors involved in altering CTD phosphorylation status and/or nucleosomal density at a particular locus. In the same vein, increasing or decreasing the rate of RNA pol II elongation has an unequivocal impact on the temporal requirement for spliceosome assembly at a particular splice site. An excellent example of this kinetic/recruitment "feedback loop" involves the CD44 gene and the chromatin-remodeling factor SWI/SNF ([20]). SWI/SNF interacts with the U1 and U5 snRNPs (two essential components of the spliceosome), as well as the splicing factor Sam68, at a block of alternative exons inside *CD44*. This binding promotes RNA pol II stalling through a CTD phosphorylation switch from Ser 2 to Ser 5, favoring the inclusion of the block of exons in mature *CD44*. In a similar mechanism, membrane depolarization of neural cells affects splicing of the NCAM gene by altering intragenic histone acetylation patterns, affecting the local chromatin structure, rate of RNA pol II elongation, and the distribution of RNA pol II and splicing machinery surrounding splice sites ([37]).

2. Chromatin as a dynamic active structure

A. Nucleosome density and position

1. Nucleosome position and exon location.

After more than 20 years of research, the role of chromatin as a dynamic structure necessary to regulate the initiation, elongation and termination phases of transcription has now been clearly established ([38]; [39]; [40]). However, despite this vast effort to understand the intricate events leading to these regulatory events, the precise role of chromatin and the location and density of nucleosomes has remained fairly elusive during the process of splicing. Nucleosomes are composed of a stretch of 146 bp of DNA wrapped around an octamer of histone proteins (two H2A, two H2B, two H3, and two H4 histones) generating the basic unit of chromatin, and contribute to chromatin compaction and structure. Clear evidence have been presented to indicate that the two events, transcription and splicing, are coordinated. As early as 1988, electron microscopy of *Drosophila* embryo showed that nascent transcripts were undergoing active splicing ([6]). Direct evidence of co-transcriptional splicing of a specific gene (human *dystrophin*) was later confirmed ([7]). The link with chromatin was later established through the demonstration of preferential association of efficiently excised introns with the chromatin-bound nuclear fraction ([41]). But, in order to get a better understanding of the relationship between nucleosome location and density, we have had to wait until technological advances provided us with an efficient way of mapping nucleosomes, first on an individual gene basis, then over the entire genome. Next-generation sequencing, using various technical platforms (Illumina™, Roche 454 sequencing, pyrosequencing), following microccocal nuclease (MNase) digestion of chromatin from various organisms and cell types, has allowed precise mapping of nucleosome distribution over the entire genome ([42]; [43]; [44]; [45]; [46]). The results demonstrated that there is indeed a higher nucleosome occupancy around exons, an occurrence that was observed across kingdoms from plants to mammals in both gametes and somatic cells ([44]). This strongly advocate for a role for both nucleosome positioning and density in defining exons and introns locations and boundaries.

The presence of single nucleosome units at specific locations overlapping with single exons appears to correlate with the evolutionary conserved average size of ~150 bp observed in mammalian exons ([42]; [43]). This may indicate a role for conserved exon-specific nucleosome positioning sequences aimed at maintaining and defining the identity of exonic regions. The strength of the splice site (likelihood to have efficient splicing) appears to be proportional to the nucleosome density, arguing that nucleosome positioning and density not only affect exon definition and identity, but also contribute to splicing efficiency.

2. Role for DNA sequence in nucleosome positioning.

The possibility of a loosely defined set of "exon-specific DNA sequences" is suggested by computational modeling experiments that were capable of predicting "exon-associated" nucleosome locations matching the ones determined using genome-wide sequencing ([42]; [43]). These exon-specific sequences, with increased nucleosome density over exons, displayed a higher GC content when compared to their counterpart intron sequences ([42]; [43]). As CpG dinucleotides can undergo methylation, a modification that can affect both nucleosome positioning ([47]; [48]) and transcription elongation rate, it appears reasonable to envision a role for CpG methylation in splicing. Supporting this observation, several recent studies have indicated a correlation between DNA methylation and the levels of exon-specific histone post-translational modifications (positive correlation with H3K36me3 and negative correlation with H3K4me2; ([48]; [49]; see next section on "Histone PTMs").

3. Nucleosome density and RNA pol II elongation rate.

The ability to control splicing by modulating RNA pol II elongation rate, referred to as the kinetic model, where slower transcription equates to more efficient splicing of alternative exons, is likely to be influenced by all above-mentioned epigenetic regulatory events. An obvious connection between the "chromatin effect", mediated by nucleosome position and/or density, and the rate of elongation of transcription on alternative splicing (Figure 3) is supported by the comparison of experimental results obtained from *in vitro* splicing assay performed using cell-free extracts and *in vivo*-based experiments ([50]). The rate of transcription was demonstrated to affect the size of RNA loops generated and to also influence the use of alternative splicing sites. The effect of elongation rate on alternative splicing has since been confirmed using RNA Pol II mutants displaying a slow rate of elongation ([24]; [51]) or cells harboring a mutated form of the elongation factor TFIIS ([52]). The presence of nucleosomes has long been known to affect efficiency of transcription. Based on the nucleosome position mapping with regard to transcribed regions, the increased nucleosome density observed at exon locations is expected to significantly decrease the RNA pol II elongation rate, and therefore favor efficient splicing. However, to this day, the ultimate experiment to fully determine the precise nature of the relationship between nucleosome position and splicing involving the simultaneous relocation of nucleosomes and the precise mapping of splicing sites has not been performed.

B. Histone Post-Translational Modifications (PTM).

1. Identification of exon-specific histone PTMs.

The complex nature of chromatin can be significantly modulated by altering the position of nucleosomes through sliding, loss of histone subsets, or re-location of complete histone octamers ([53]) (See "Chromatin Remodelers and Splicing"). In addition to these histone composition changes, the dynamic nature of chromatin and the recruitment of specific factors are strongly dependent on histone post-translational modifications ([1]). These modifications include lysine acetylation, lysine methylation, serine phosphorylation, ADP ribosylation, and ubiquitination. Specific lysine and serine modifications have been associated with genes actively transcribed or repressed. For example, histones H3 and H4 lysine acetylation, histone H3 lysine 4 di- or tri-methylation (H3K4me2; H3K4me3) and histone H3 Serine 10 and Serine 28 phosphorylation (H3S10P, H3S28P) are strongly associated with actively transcribed genes, and histone H3 lysine 9 and lysine 27 di- and tri-methylation (H3K9 me2, H3K9me3, H3K27me2, H3K27me3) are considered to be markers of repressed genes ([54]). A connection between RNA splicing and changes in histone PTMs was demonstrated in the early 2000's. Using Trichostatin A, a histone deacetylase inhibitor, researchers demonstrated that changes in the status of histone lysine acetylation was influencing the regulation of alternative splicing of *fibronectin* exon 33 ([55]; [22]) and of a CD44 reporter gene ([56]). As histone acetylation is considered a marker of actively transcribed genes, this result was by no mean surprising. It can provide support to, both the kinetic model, where histone acetylation can influence the rate of RNA pol II elongation, as well as the model where timing of splicing is described as regulated by the timing of splicing factors recruitment, an event likely to be affected by histone PTMs. But, as was the case for nucleosome positioning, the use of genome-wide analysis of the distribution of histone PTMs has provided a much clearer image of the role of these events in splicing. To date genome-wide maps for 42 different histone PTMs have been generated and matched to exon-intron locations ([57]). After normalization to account for increased nucleosome density over exonic regions, the results show enrichment at exon of tri-methylated histone H3 Lysine 36 (H3K36me3), tri-methylated histone H3 Lysine 4 (H3K4me3), and di-methylated histone H3 Lysine 27 (H3K27me2), and depletion of tri-methylated histone H3 Lysine 9 (K3K9me3) ([58]; [46]) over exonic sequences. The role of H3K36me3 in splicing was further confirmed by studies indicating its association with actively transcribed regions enriched in constitutive exons ([59]; [58]) with a concomitant increased nucleosome occupancy ([58]; [42]). Additional evidence for the role of H3K36me3 and H3K4me3 were provided by experiments monitoring splicing efficiency as a function of methylation levels of H3K36 and H3K4 (over-expression or down-regulation of H3K36- or H3K4-specific methyl-transferases; [60]).

In addition to the well-characterized H3K36me3, H3K4me3, H3K27me2, and H3K9me3, several other histone PTMs (H3K79me1, H4K20me1, H2BK5me1, H3K27 me1, 2, 3) have been occasionally reported to be differentially enriched or depleted in exons ([43]; [61]). However, these PTMs have not been consistently identified as consensus exon markers. These differences in histone PTM patterns observed may reflect different cell types, tissues, or variations in the technical analysis and normalization.

2. Synergy between DNA methylation and histone PTMs.

Based on genome-wide sequencing results, a correlation between the pattern of histone methylation and that of DNA methylation over exonic region suggests that these two epigenetic markers may act synergically to mark exons ([62]; [48]). More specifically, enrichment of H3K36me3 and depletion of H3K4me2 appear to correlate with increased CpG methylation over exonic regions ([48]; [49]).

3. Histone PTMs can mediate interactions between chromatin, splicing factors, and RNA.

Histone PTMs have been demonstrated to act as targets promoting the recruitment of specific regulatory factors for transcription, DNA repair, and other DNA-related events (for review, see [54]). Not surprisingly, a similar role for histone PTMs has been described in the context of RNA splicing, linking chromatin, RNA, and splicing factors (See Figure 5).

The intricacies of the interactions between RNA and chromatin remain poorly defined. Physical interactions between chromatin components and RNA, mediated by the Xist RNA, have been demonstrated to occur in the context of inactive X-chromosome (review by [63]). However, early work by chromatin research pioneers such as Drs. van Holde, Bradbury, and Kornberg, exploring the possibility of RNA-histone interactions in the context of individual or arrays of nucleosomes, failed to clearly identify defined mechanisms leading to specific interactions between core histones and RNA transcripts. Based on the physical properties and inherent charge of mRNA, electrostatic interactions would be predicted, even if they are transient, as suggested by studies showing an impeded mobility of pre-mRNA associated with the presence of nucleosomes affecting pre-mRNA diffusion away from the transcription site ([64]; [65]). The presence of histone tails that can protrude from the nucleosomes and the fact that these tails are highly positively charged provides additional support for conditions conducive to electrostatic interactions between mRNA and chromatin. As early work on investigating the mechanism of splicing had been performed using artificial transcription systems and *in vitro*-assembled chromatin, the importance and the role of histone PTMs in the process was not directly addressed in the interpretation of the results. The presence of multiple types of PTMs, that have now been clearly identified as contributing to various aspects of transcription, is extremely likely to affect RNA-histone interactions. In addition to the potential for direct physical contact between histone and mRNA, researchers suspected and started to investigate the involvement of bridging proteins or complexes, referred to as chromatin-adaptors acting, in regulating the process of RNA splicing. These chromatin-adaptors would provide a scaffold linking DNA, histones, and the RNA splicing machinery. To date, four such chromatin-adaptors have been identified to interact with specific histone PTMs and splicing factors (see Table 1). Two of these chromatin-adaptors are associated with histone PTMs enriched in exons. MORF-related Gene 15 (MRG15), a transcription factor involved in embryonic development and cell proliferation, bridges pre-mRNA through interactions between its chromo-domain, H3K36me3, and the polypyridine tract-binding protein (PTB) splicing factor ([60]). The Chromo-Domain-Helicase-DNA-binding 1 protein (CHD1) mediates pre-mRNA interactions through contacts between H3K4me3 and U2 snRNP ([66]). The other two identified chromatin-adaptors mediate interactions through binding acetylated H3 (Gcn5 contacts U2snRNP, [67]), or H3K9me3 (Heterochromatin Protein 1 -HP1- recognizes hnRNPs, [68]). As genome-wide maps of histone PTMs, chromatin-associated proteins, and location of specific alternative splicing sites continue to be generated, we expect the number of identified chromatin-adaptors involved in splicing to increase.

Chromatin-Adaptor	Matching histone PTM	Splicing Factor
MRG15	H3K36me3	PTB
Gcn5	Acetylated H3	U2snRNP
CHD1	H3K4me3	U2snRNP
HP1α	H3K9me3	hnRNPs

Table 1. Chromatin-Adaptors, target PTMs, and Splicing Factors

C. Chromatin remodelers and splicing.

1. SWI/SNF and splicing.

Two separate chromatin remodeling factors have proven to play an integral role in not only transcription, but also splicing. First, the SWI/SNF chromatin remodeling complex was initially characterized as an ATP-driven motor that disrupts protein-DNA interactions, more specifically histone-DNA contacts within nucleosomes ([69] [70]). Because of this activity, SWI/SNF has proven to be inherently involved in the process of transcription, altering the accessibility of DNA to transcription factors. However, recent evidence has shown SWI/SNF to have an important role in splicing activity, mainly independent of its remodeling capability. Brahma (Brm), the catalytic subunit of SWI/SNF, was found to interact with several components of the spliceosome, as well as Sam68, a splicing enhancer ([20]). It also increased the accumulation of RNA pol II (Ser2 phosphorylated) on regions encoding variant exons of several genes including E-cadherin, BIM, cyclin D1, and CD44. It is postulated that Brm exerts its regulatory activity on splicing by slowing the RNA pol II elongation rate which facilitates recruitment of the splicing machinery to exons with "weaker" splice sites. In a perhaps more surprising role, Brm was shown to affect splicing at the RNA level ([71]). It was found to be incorporated into nascent pre-mRNPs, and human Brm and Brg1 (another SWI/SNF component) associate with RNPs. In addition, depleting SWI/SNF affects the abundance of alternative transcripts from a subset of genes. Overall, SWI/SNF has a role in both transcription and splicing, regulating not only the amount, but also the type of transcript generated.

2. Chd1 and Splicing.

The chromatin-remodeler CHD1, which display significant similarities to the SWI/SNF complex, is a multi-faceted factor with roles in transcription activation, repression, elongation, termination, as well as the deposition of variant histones ([72]). Not surprisingly, novel research has emerged which links CHD1 activity to splicing as well. Yeast two-hybrid assays proved an interaction between CHD1 and the splicing proteins mKIAA0164, Srp20, and SAF-B ([73]). Also, splicing assays showed that Chd1 over-expression can affect alternative splicing. More convincingly, CHD1 was found to interact with the U2snRNP component of the spliceosome ([66]). This interaction was found to be facilitated by CHD1 binding to the tri-methylated histone H3 lysine 4 (H3K4me3) mark generally associated with transcriptional activation. Knockdown of both CHD1 and decreased H3K4me3 reduced the association with U2snRNP and affected splicing efficiency. These results led to the proposal of the existence of "chromatin-adaptor complexes" described earlier in this chapter.

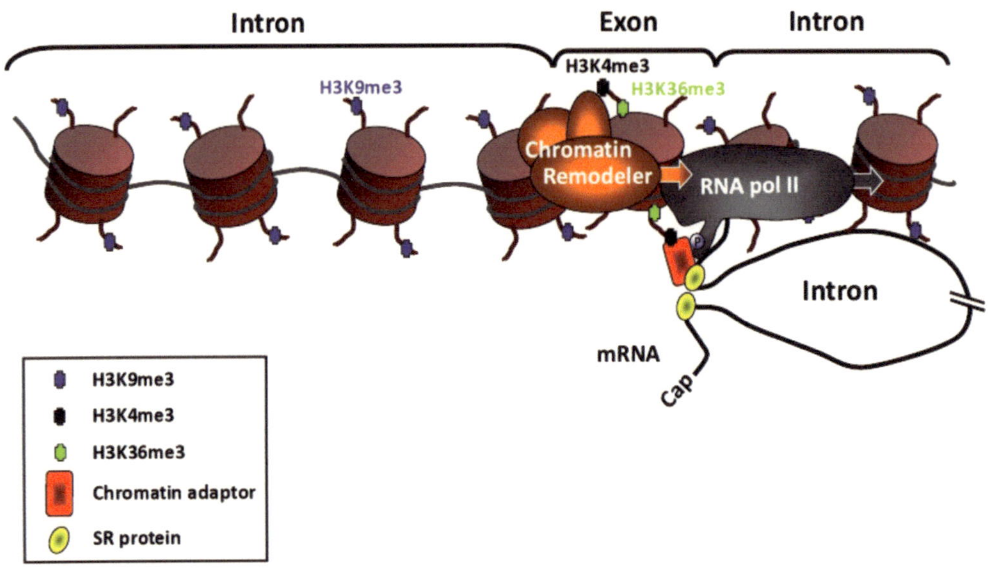

Fig. 5. Chromatin dynamics alter elongation and splicing activity mediated by RNA Pol II CTD.
Nucleosome's position and histone post-translational modifications affect the recruitment of chromatin-associated proteins (chromatin adaptors), which in turn can modulate the recruitment and/or binding of splicing factors to the pre-mRNA. Histone PTMs act as markers of introns (K3K9me3, blue oval) and exons (H3K4me3, black oval and H3K36me3, green oval). The exon-enriched modifications can contribute to the recruitment of splicing factors (yellow oval) and chromatin adaptors (red rectangle), resulting in a significant alteration in splicing efficacy. Chromatin remodelers (orange complex) can regulate the overall or local nucleosome density and position. Such variations can lead to changes in chromatin higher-order structure and modulation of the RNA pol II elongation rate ", affecting splicing decisions (see Figure 3).

3. Conclusion

By now, a distinct niche for chromatin and its interactors in the process of splicing has been established. The cellular process most commonly associated with chromatin, transcription, has been found to act in concert with splicing, increasing the efficiency and accuracy of mature transcript genesis. Two models have been proposed for the coupling of transcription and splicing, kinetic and recruitment, both orchestrated through the modulation and interactions of the RNA pol II C-terminal domain (see Figure 5 for an integrated model). In terms of chromatin structure, nucleosome density and positioning have both been found to have a direct impact on the location, recognition, and selection of splice sites. Post-translational modifications of histone tail residues also have a role in the delineation of splice sites. They are also known to be beacons and docking sites for factors that can simultaneously regulate both transcription and splicing. Chromatin remodelers have shown to interact with the transcriptional and splicing machinery, and are necessary for proper splicing efficiency. In sum, the role of chromatin in splicing is an ever-expanding subject of research and will prove to be for many years to come, as technology allows for a more precise determination of all involved players.

4. References

[1] Jenuwein T, Allis CD (2001) Translating the histone code. Science 293: 1074-1080.
[2] Saha A, Wittmeyer J, Cairns BR (2006) Chromatin remodelling: the industrial revolution of DNA around histones. Nat Rev Mol Cell Biol 7: 437-447.
[3] Crick F (1970) Central dogma of molecular biology. Nature 227: 561-563.
[4] Croft L, Schandorff S, Clark F, Burrage K, Arctander P, et al. (2000) ISIS, the intron information system, reveals the high frequency of alternative splicing in the human genome. Nat Genet 24: 340-341.
[5] Pan Q, Shai O, Lee LJ, Frey BJ, Blencowe BJ (2008) Deep surveying of alternative splicing complexity in the human transcriptome by high-throughput sequencing. Nat Genet 40: 1413-1415.
[6] Beyer AL, Osheim YN (1988) Splice site selection, rate of splicing, and alternative splicing on nascent transcripts. Genes Dev 2: 754-765.
[7] Tennyson CN, Klamut HJ, Worton RG (1995) The human dystrophin gene requires 16 hours to be transcribed and is cotranscriptionally spliced. Nat Genet 9: 184-190.
[8] Munoz MJ, de la Mata M, Kornblihtt AR The carboxy terminal domain of RNA polymerase II and alternative splicing. Trends Biochem Sci 35: 497-504.
[9] Corden JL, Cadena DL, Ahearn JM, Jr., Dahmus ME (1985) A unique structure at the carboxyl terminus of the largest subunit of eukaryotic RNA polymerase II. Proc Natl Acad Sci U S A 82: 7934-7938.
[10] Meininghaus M, Chapman RD, Horndasch M, Eick D (2000) Conditional expression of RNA polymerase II in mammalian cells. Deletion of the carboxyl-terminal domain of the large subunit affects early steps in transcription. J Biol Chem 275: 24375-24382.
[11] Egloff S, Murphy S (2008) Cracking the RNA polymerase II CTD code. Trends Genet 24: 280-288.
[12] Buratowski S (2009) Progression through the RNA polymerase II CTD cycle. Mol Cell 36: 541-546.
[13] Peterlin BM, Price DH (2006) Controlling the elongation phase of transcription with P-TEFb. Mol Cell 23: 297-305.

[14] Matlin AJ, Clark F, Smith CW (2005) Understanding alternative splicing: towards a cellular code. Nat Rev Mol Cell Biol 6: 386-398.
[15] Zahler AM, Lane WS, Stolk JA, Roth MB (1992) SR proteins: a conserved family of pre-mRNA splicing factors. Genes Dev 6: 837-847.
[16] Allemand E, Batsche E, Muchardt C (2008) Splicing, transcription, and chromatin: a menage a trois. Curr Opin Genet Dev 18: 145-151.
[17] Luco RF, Misteli T More than a splicing code: integrating the role of RNA, chromatin and non-coding RNA in alternative splicing regulation. Curr Opin Genet Dev.
[18] de la Mata M, Alonso CR, Kadener S, Fededa JP, Blaustein M, et al. (2003) A slow RNA polymerase II affects alternative splicing in vivo. Mol Cell 12: 525-532.
[19] Robson-Dixon ND, Garcia-Blanco MA (2004) MAZ elements alter transcription elongation and silencing of the fibroblast growth factor receptor 2 exon IIIb. J Biol Chem 279: 29075-29084.
[20] Batsche E, Yaniv M, Muchardt C (2006) The human SWI/SNF subunit Brm is a regulator of alternative splicing. Nat Struct Mol Biol 13: 22-29.
[21] Alexander RD, Innocente SA, Barrass JD, Beggs JD Splicing-dependent RNA polymerase pausing in yeast. Mol Cell 40: 582-593.
[22] Nogues G, Kadener S, Cramer P, Bentley D, Kornblihtt AR (2002) Transcriptional activators differ in their abilities to control alternative splicing. J Biol Chem 277: 43110-43114.
[23] Bentley DL (2005) Rules of engagement: co-transcriptional recruitment of pre-mRNA processing factors. Curr Opin Cell Biol 17: 251-256.
[24] de la Mata M, Kornblihtt AR (2006) RNA polymerase II C-terminal domain mediates regulation of alternative splicing by SRp20. Nat Struct Mol Biol 13: 973-980.
[25] McCracken S, Rosonina E, Fong N, Sikes M, Beyer A, et al. (1998) Role of RNA polymerase II carboxy-terminal domain in coordinating transcription with RNA processing. Cold Spring Harb Symp Quant Biol 63: 301-309.
[26] Sisodia SS, Sollner-Webb B, Cleveland DW (1987) Specificity of RNA maturation pathways: RNAs transcribed by RNA polymerase III are not substrates for splicing or polyadenylation. Mol Cell Biol 7: 3602-3612.
[27] Smale ST, Tjian R (1985) Transcription of herpes simplex virus tk sequences under the control of wild-type and mutant human RNA polymerase I promoters. Mol Cell Biol 5: 352-362.
[28] Misteli T, Spector DL (1999) RNA polymerase II targets pre-mRNA splicing factors to transcription sites in vivo. Mol Cell 3: 697-705.
[29] McCracken S, Fong N, Yankulov K, Ballantyne S, Pan G, et al. (1997) The C-terminal domain of RNA polymerase II couples mRNA processing to transcription. Nature 385: 357-361.
[30] Das R, Yu J, Zhang Z, Gygi MP, Krainer AR, et al. (2007) SR proteins function in coupling RNAP II transcription to pre-mRNA splicing. Mol Cell 26: 867-881.
[31] Goldstrohm AC, Albrecht TR, Sune C, Bedford MT, Garcia-Blanco MA (2001) The transcription elongation factor CA150 interacts with RNA polymerase II and the pre-mRNA splicing factor SF1. Mol Cell Biol 21: 7617-7628.
[32] Yoh SM, Cho H, Pickle L, Evans RM, Jones KA (2007) The Spt6 SH2 domain binds Ser2-P RNAPII to direct Iws1-dependent mRNA splicing and export. Genes Dev 21: 160-174.
[33] Merz C, Urlaub H, Will CL, Luhrmann R (2007) Protein composition of human mRNPs spliced in vitro and differential requirements for mRNP protein recruitment. RNA 13: 116-128.

[34] O'Gorman W, Thomas B, Kwek KY, Furger A, Akoulitchev A (2005) Analysis of U1 small nuclear RNA interaction with cyclin H. J Biol Chem 280: 36920-36925.
[35] Emili A, Shales M, McCracken S, Xie W, Tucker PW, et al. (2002) Splicing and transcription-associated proteins PSF and p54nrb/nonO bind to the RNA polymerase II CTD. RNA 8: 1102-1111.
[36] Knoop LL, Baker SJ (2001) EWS/FLI alters 5'-splice site selection. J Biol Chem 276: 22317-22322.
[37] Schor IE, Rascovan N, Pelisch F, Allo M, Kornblihtt AR (2009) Neuronal cell depolarization induces intragenic chromatin modifications affecting NCAM alternative splicing. Proc Natl Acad Sci U S A 106: 4325-4330.
[38] van Holde KE, Lohr DE, Robert C (1992) What happens to nucleosomes during transcription? J Biol Chem 267: 2837-2840.
[39] Kornberg RD, Lorch Y (1999) Twenty-five years of the nucleosome, fundamental particle of the eukaryote chromosome. Cell 98: 285-294.
[40] Cairns BR (2009) The logic of chromatin architecture and remodelling at promoters. Nature 461: 193-198.
[41] Pandya-Jones A, Black DL (2009) Co-transcriptional splicing of constitutive and alternative exons. RNA 15: 1896-1908.
[42] Tilgner H, Nikolaou C, Althammer S, Sammeth M, Beato M, et al. (2009) Nucleosome positioning as a determinant of exon recognition. Nat Struct Mol Biol 16: 996-1001.
[43] Schwartz S, Meshorer E, Ast G (2009) Chromatin organization marks exon-intron structure. Nat Struct Mol Biol 16: 990-995.
[44] Nahkuri S, Taft RJ, Mattick JS (2009) Nucleosomes are preferentially positioned at exons in somatic and sperm cells. Cell Cycle 8: 3420-3424.
[45] Chen W, Luo L, Zhang L The organization of nucleosomes around splice sites. Nucleic Acids Res 38: 2788-2798.
[46] Dhami P, Saffrey P, Bruce AW, Dillon SC, Chiang K, et al. Complex exon-intron marking by histone modifications is not determined solely by nucleosome distribution. PLoS One 5: e12339.
[47] Lister R, Pelizzola M, Dowen RH, Hawkins RD, Hon G, et al. (2009) Human DNA methylomes at base resolution show widespread epigenomic differences. Nature 462: 315-322.
[48] Hodges E, Smith AD, Kendall J, Xuan Z, Ravi K, et al. (2009) High definition profiling of mammalian DNA methylation by array capture and single molecule bisulfite sequencing. Genome Res 19: 1593-1605.
[49] Chodavarapu RK, Feng S, Bernatavichute YV, Chen PY, Stroud H, et al. Relationship between nucleosome positioning and DNA methylation. Nature 466: 388-392.
[50] Eperon LP, Graham IR, Griffiths AD, Eperon IC (1988) Effects of RNA secondary structure on alternative splicing of pre-mRNA: is folding limited to a region behind the transcribing RNA polymerase? Cell 54: 393-401.
[51] Kornblihtt AR (2006) Chromatin, transcript elongation and alternative splicing. Nat Struct Mol Biol 13: 5-7.
[52] Howe KJ, Kane CM, Ares M, Jr. (2003) Perturbation of transcription elongation influences the fidelity of internal exon inclusion in Saccharomyces cerevisiae. RNA 9: 993-1006.
[53] Smith CL, Peterson CL (2005) ATP-dependent chromatin remodeling. Curr Top Dev Biol 65: 115-148.
[54] Izzo A, Schneider R Chatting histone modifications in mammals. Brief Funct Genomics 9: 429-443.

[55] Kadener S, Cramer P, Nogues G, Cazalla D, de la Mata M, et al. (2001) Antagonistic effects of T-Ag and VP16 reveal a role for RNA pol II elongation on alternative splicing. EMBO J 20: 5759-5768.
[56] Auboeuf D, Honig A, Berget SM, O'Malley BW (2002) Coordinate regulation of transcription and splicing by steroid receptor coregulators. Science 298: 416-419.
[57] Luco RF, Pan Q, Tominaga K, Blencowe BJ, Pereira-Smith OM, et al. Regulation of alternative splicing by histone modifications. Science 327: 996-1000.
[58] Spies N, Nielsen CB, Padgett RA, Burge CB (2009) Biased chromatin signatures around polyadenylation sites and exons. Mol Cell 36: 245-254.
[59] Kolasinska-Zwierz P, Down T, Latorre I, Liu T, Liu XS, et al. (2009) Differential chromatin marking of introns and expressed exons by H3K36me3. Nat Genet 41: 376-381.
[60] Luco RF, Allo M, Schor IE, Kornblihtt AR, Misteli T Epigenetics in alternative pre-mRNA splicing. Cell 144: 16-26.
[61] Andersson R, Enroth S, Rada-Iglesias A, Wadelius C, Komorowski J (2009) Nucleosomes are well positioned in exons and carry characteristic histone modifications. Genome Res 19: 1732-1741.
[62] Meissner A, Mikkelsen TS, Gu H, Wernig M, Hanna J, et al. (2008) Genome-scale DNA methylation maps of pluripotent and differentiated cells. Nature 454: 766-770.
[63] Prasanth KV, Spector DL (2007) Eukaryotic regulatory RNAs: an answer to the 'genome complexity' conundrum. Genes Dev 21: 11-42.
[64] Custodio N, Carmo-Fonseca M, Geraghty F, Pereira HS, Grosveld F, et al. (1999) Inefficient processing impairs release of RNA from the site of transcription. EMBO J 18: 2855-2866.
[65] Carmo-Fonseca M, Custodio N, Calado A (1999) Intranuclear trafficking of messenger RNA. Crit Rev Eukaryot Gene Expr 9: 213-219.
[66] Sims RJ, 3rd, Millhouse S, Chen CF, Lewis BA, Erdjument-Bromage H, et al. (2007) Recognition of trimethylated histone H3 lysine 4 facilitates the recruitment of transcription postinitiation factors and pre-mRNA splicing. Mol Cell 28: 665-676.
[67] Gunderson FQ, Johnson TL (2009) Acetylation by the transcriptional coactivator Gcn5 plays a novel role in co-transcriptional spliceosome assembly. PLoS Genet 5: e1000682.
[68] Piacentini L, Fanti L, Negri R, Del Vescovo V, Fatica A, et al. (2009) Heterochromatin protein 1 (HP1a) positively regulates euchromatic gene expression through RNA transcript association and interaction with hnRNPs in Drosophila. PLoS Genet 5: e1000670.
[69] Winston F, Carlson M (1992) Yeast SNF/SWI transcriptional activators and the SPT/SIN chromatin connection. Trends Genet 8: 387-391.
[70] Sudarsanam P, Winston F (2000) The Swi/Snf family nucleosome-remodeling complexes and transcriptional control. Trends Genet 16: 345-351.
[71] Tyagi A, Ryme J, Brodin D, Ostlund Farrants AK, Visa N (2009) SWI/SNF associates with nascent pre-mRNPs and regulates alternative pre-mRNA processing. PLoS Genet 5: e1000470.
[72] Hall JA, Georgel PT (2007) CHD proteins: a diverse family with strong ties. Biochem Cell Biol 85: 463-476.
[73] Tai HH, Geisterfer M, Bell JC, Moniwa M, Davie JR, et al. (2003) CHD1 associates with NCoR and histone deacetylase as well as with RNA splicing proteins. Biochem Biophys Res Commun 308: 170-176.

Part 2

RNA Processing and Viral Systems

4

The Regulation of HIV-1 mRNA Biogenesis

Massimo Caputi
Charles E. Schmidt College of Medicine, Florida Atlantic University USA

1. Introduction

The machinery regulating the transcription and processing of the human immunodeficiency virus type 1 (HIV-1) genome has been extensively studied for the past two decades, leading to the characterization of a complex set of interactions between viral and cellular factors. Our understanding of the basic molecular mechanisms regulating the expression of cellular genes has been greatly advanced by the lessons learned from this virus. Studies aimed at the understanding of transcription, capping, polyadenylation, splicing and export of the viral transcripts have helped in modeling the mechanisms regulating transcriptional and post-transcriptional events in the cell. Recent developments in the field have also shown that, similarly to cellular genes, transcription and processing of the viral mRNAs are functionally coupled and can potentially be regulated by small non-coding RNAs.

HIV replication is a complex multistep process whereby, following the recognition of specific receptors and co-receptors on the host cell membrane, the virus enters the cell where the viral RNA genome is reverse transcribed and integrated into the cellular DNA. The integrated proviral genome is than transcribed by the host transcription machinery into a 9.2 kb primary transcript, which is alternatively spliced in mRNAs coding for the 9 viral genes. *Tat* and *rev* gene products are shuttled into the nucleus to aid the transcription process, the former, and export of unspliced transcripts, the later. Unspliced transcripts are packaged as viral genome into the nascent virions. *Gag* and *env* gene products code for the structural components of the new virions while the *pol* gene codes for key enzyme required for viral integration into the target host cell, which are than packaged within the virions. The products of the *Vif, Vpr, Vpu* and *Nef* genes are not essential for viral replication but are required for HIV pathogenesis and infectivity *in-vivo*.

HIV-1 has developed a number of strategies to regulate the transcription and processing of its primary transcript. Interactions between viral RNA sequences, the host cell and viral proteins are necessary to express the nine gene products required for its replication. Alteration of the delicate balance between spliced and unspliced RNAs, or disruption of the viral RNA export pathway, can dramatically affect HIV-1 infectivity and pathogenesis (Amendt, et al., 1994, Jablonski & Caputi, 2009, Pollard & Malim, 1998, Purcell & Martin, 1993, Stoltzfus & Madsen, 2006, Wentz, et al., 1997). A better understanding of the mechanisms regulating the transcription and processing of the viral RNA may provide us with novel therapeutic targets.

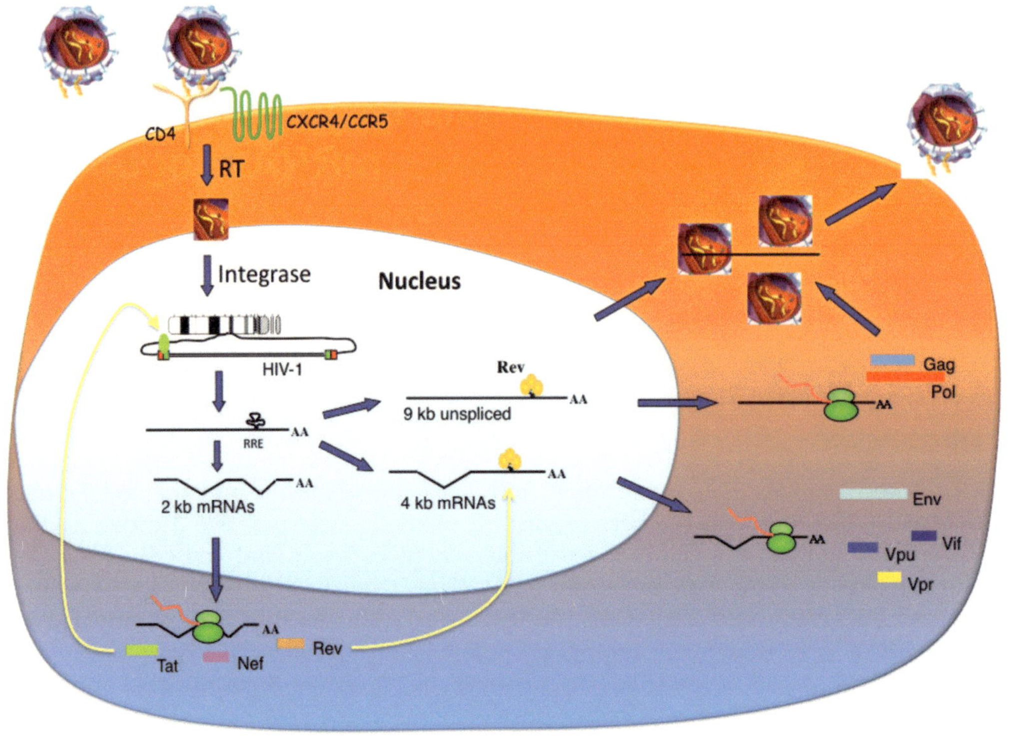

Fig. 1. The HIV-1 replication cycle. The key steps in the viral replication cycle: entry, integration, transcription, splicing export and assembly of the new virions are schematically shown together with the main viral gene products and their functions.

2. HIV-1 transcription regulation

Once the virus is integrated into the host cell chromosome the viral genome is transcribed into a single pre-mRNA from a complex promoter located within the 5′ long terminal repeat (LTR) of the viral genome. The HIV-1 LTR promoter contains two Sp1 binding motifs and two nuclear factor NF-kB binding sites which serves to regulate basal HIV-1 transcription (Pereira, et al., 2000). The LTR also contains binding elements for positive nuclear factor of activated T cells, AP-1, and negative, YY1 and LSF, transcriptional regulators. Tumor necrosis factor-α (TNF-α) and other cytokines can induce NF-kb and activate HIV-1 transcription in infected cells (Van Lint, et al., 2004). Transcription regulation of the HIV-1 genome is mediated by RNA polymerase II (RNAP II) and a combination of basal and promoter specific factors (Fig. 2) (Brady & Kashanchi, 2005, Pereira, et al., 2000).

Shortly after transcription begins RNAP II activity is paused. Before transcription is halted a short (nucleotides +1 to +82) stem loop sequence, the transactivation responsive (TAR) RNA, is synthesized. Binding of the 101 amino acid viral regulatory protein Tat to TAR stimulates transcription elongation and possibly initiation of the viral transcription complex (Fig. 2) (Berkhout, et al., 1989, Gaynor, 1995, Raha, et al., 2005). The Tat-TAR interaction promote the recruitment of the cyclin T1 (CycT1) component of the human positive transcription elongation factor b (P-TEFb) (Garber, et al., 1998, Wei, et al., 1998). CycT1 recruits Cdk9, the catalytic subunit of P-TEFb, which phosphorylates the C-terminal domain (CTD) of RNAP II to facilitate elongation of the viral transcript (Bres, et al., 2008, Peterlin & Price, 2006). The mammalian RNAPII CTD is composed of 52 tandemly repeated heptads with a consensus, Tyr-1-Ser-2-Pro-3-Thr-4-Ser-5-Pro-6-Ser-7. Ser-2 and Ser-5 are targets of phosphorylation and dephosphorylation during transcription (Hirose & Ohkuma, 2007). Phosphorylation of RNAPII CTD is essential for transcription. RNAPII CTD is phosphorylated at Ser-5 by TFIIH (CDK7) during transcription initiation through the promoter clearance stage (Hengartner, et al., 1998) and changes to Ser-2 phosphorylation during elongation when the polymerase is associated with the coding region (Komarnitsky, et al., 2000, Ni, et al., 2004). In addition to promoting Ser-2 phosphorylation, Tat modifies the activity of CDK9 to phosphorylate Ser-5 following release of TFIIH (Zhou, et al., 2000). Furthermore, P-TEFb targets cofactors such as the human homologoue of SPT5 (TAT-CT1), which together with SPT4 constitutes the 5,6-dichloro-1-ß-D-ribofuranosylbenzimidazole sensitivity-inducing factor (DSIF) and the negative elongation factor (NELF) Rd protein (Yamaguchi, et al., 1999). The cooperative interaction of DSIF and NELF induce polymerase pausing near promoter start sites (Wada, et al., 2000, Wada, et al., 1998b). This pausing event can be reversed by a CDK9-dependent phosphorylation of SPT5 (Kim & Sharp, 2001) and the RD protein, which causes a dissociation of NELF from the stem of TAR RNA (Fujinaga, et al., 2004).

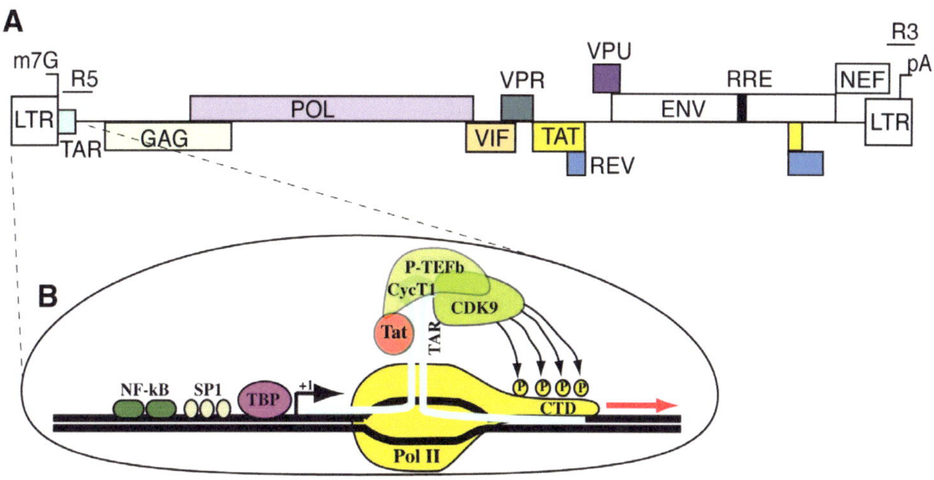

Fig. 2. A) The map shows the genomic organization of the HIV-1 provirus indicating the position of the various viral genes and key features of the viral genome. B) Schematic representation of viral transcription. A number of cellular transcription factors assemble onto the LTR promoter. Binding of Tat onto the TAR sequence promotes assembly of the components of P-TEFb (CycT1 and CDK9). The kinase activity of CDK9 phosphorylates the RNAPII CTD to facilitate elongation.

Tat role in viral transcription is not limited to the recruitment of RNAP II cofactors. Once integrated into the host cell genome, nucleosomes are deposited at specific positions within the viral promoter and exert a strong repression of transcriptional initiation. After Tat activates transcription, the chromatin associated with sequences immediately downstream of the transcription start site becomes accessible to nucleases (Verdin, et al., 1993). The

chromatin remodeling induced by Tat is dependent on the recruitment of enzymes with histone acetyl transferase (HAT) activity, which modify chromatin conformation (Marcello, et al., 2001). These factors include the transcriptional co-activators p300 and the cAMP-responsive binding protein (CREB)-binding protein (CBP) (Marzio, et al., 1998), the p300/CBP-associated factor (P/CAF) (Benkirane, et al., 1998), the general control non-derepressible-5 (GCN5) factor (Col, et al., 2001), the transcription factor TAFII250 (Weissman, et al., 1998) and the TIP60 protein (Kamine, et al., 1996). HATs acetylate the N-terminal tails of histones to stimulate chromatin remodeling and modify specific lysines of transcription factors to modulate DNA-binding affinity (Li, et al., 2007, Yang & Seto, 2008). In addition to histones, Tat itself is a substrate for acetylation by HATs. Lysines at positions 50 and 51 are major substrates for acetylation by p300 and hGCN5 (Col, et al., 2001, Deng, et al., 2001, Kiernan, et al., 1999). Acetylation of lysine 50 of Tat promotes the dissociation of Tat from TAR RNA during early transcription elongation and recruitment of the SWI/SNF chromatin-remodeling complex (Treand, et al., 2006), which synergize with p300 acetyltransferase and acetylated Tat to remodel the nucleosome at the HIV promoter in order to activate transcription (Mahmoudi, et al., 2006). Furthermore, acetylation of lysine 50 triggers the recruitment of P/CAF to the elongating RNA Pol II (Dorr, et al., 2002). P/CAF acetylates Tat on Lys28 (Kiernan, et al., 1999), which enhances the Tat-CycT1 interaction (Bres, et al., 2002). Besides acetylation other post-translational modifications appear to regulate Tat activity. Phosphorylation of Tat Ser16 and Ser46 by the cell cycle regulator Cdk2/cyclin E appears to be required for efficient HIV-1 transcription and replication (Ammosova, et al., 2006). Methylation of Tat on arginine residues by PRMT6 has been shown to inhibit transcriptional activity (Boulanger, et al., 2005), while non-proteolytic ubiquitination of Tat by Hdm2 appears to enhance viral transcription (Bres, et al., 2003).
In addition to its role in viral transactivation, Tat has also been shown to regulate the rate of transcription and expression of host cellular genes (Caldwell, et al., 2000, Gibellini, et al., 2002, Huang, et al., 1998, Ott, et al., 1998, Secchiero, et al., 1999). Furthermore, Tat function appears not to be restricted to infected cells, which actively secrete large amounts of Tat in the bloodstream (Ensoli, et al., 1990). Extracellular Tat can generate a wide array of cell responses ranging from T-cell activation (Wu, et al., 2007) to stimulation of cytokine secretion, cell death in neurons and cell proliferation in endothelial and T-cells (Huigen, et al., 2004, King, et al., 2006, Rubartelli, et al., 1998). The mechanism by which Tat exerts these pleiotropic effects is still unclear.

3. HIV-1 mRNA processing

Before a gene transcript is ready to be transported out of the nucleus it has to be processed by acquiring a cap structure at the 5′ terminus, introns have to be spliced out and a 3′ end is generated by adding a poly(A) tail. Although these reactions are biochemically distinct processes, they are interlinked and influence one another's specificity and efficiency. Most mechanisms regulating the processing of viral transcripts are common to most cellular mRNAs, nevertheless some processes, such as the export of the unspliced and partially spliced mRNAs to the cytoplasm, are unique for the virus.

3.1 Capping

mRNA capping is carried out by a series of enzymatic reactions in which the 5′ triphosphate terminus of the pre-mRNA is cleaved to a diphosphate by a RNA triphosphatase (RTP), then capped with GMP by RNA guanylyltransferase (GT), and methylated by RNA (guanine-N7) methyltransferase (MT). Targeting of Cap formation to transcripts made by RNAP II is achieved through the interaction of the capping enzymes with the phosphorylated RNAPII CTD. The Cap structure is recognized by the Cap binding complex (CBC), which contains the proteins, CBP20 and CBP80 (Proudfoot, et al., 2002, Shatkin & Manley, 2000). HIV-1 capping takes place during the transition from transcription initiation to elongation when the nascent pre-mRNA is only 20–40 nucleotides long. Tat promotes viral mRNA Cap formation by inducing TAR-dependent phosphorylation of RNAPII CTD (Chiu, et al., 2002, Zhou, et al., 2003) Phosphorylation of the CTD Ser-2 and Ser-5 residues has differential effects on recruitment and activation of capping enzymes (Bentley, 2002, Proudfoot, et al., 2002). Although Ser-2 phosphorylation of CTD heptads is sufficient for mammalian GT binding, its activation requires Ser-5 phosphorylated CTD (Ho & Shuman, 1999).

3.2 3' end formation

In higher eukaryotes, with the exception of histone genes, all protein encoding mRNAs contain a uniform 3' end consisting of 200-400 adenosine residues. The poly(A) tail regulates degradation of the mRNA and translation. The formation of the poly (A) tail is directed by sequences present on the pre-mRNA and the mammalian polyadenylation machinery. Prior to the addition of poly(A), the pre-mRNA must be cleaved. The site of cleavage, in most pre-mRNAs, lies between a highly conserved AAUAAA hexamer and a downstream sequence element (DSE), which is a U- or GU-rich motif. The cleavage/ poly(A) complex consists of cleavage factors (CPSF, CstF, CF) and the poly(A) polymerase (PAP). RNA is first cleaved ~10 to 30 nts 3' to AAUAAA, predominantly at a CA dinucleotide, than the PAP synthesizes a polyA tail using ATP as substrate (Proudfoot, et al., 2002, Shatkin & Manley, 2000).

HIV-1 encodes the polyadenylation signal within the repeat (R) region, which is present at the extreme 5' and 3' end of the viral transcript. Thus the 5' polyadenylation signal needs to be repressed while usage of the 3' one needs to be enhanced. Usage of the 3' polyadenylation site is promoted by an upstream enhancer (USE) motif, which stabilizes binding of the cleavage polyadenylation specificity factor (CPSF) to the AAUAAA (Gilmartin, et al., 1995). The 5' HIV-1 polyadenylation site is repressed because it is positioned too close to the transcription initiation site and polyadenylation factors have not yet gained access to the nascent transcript through the RNAP II complex (Cherrington & Ganem, 1992, Weichs an der Glon, et al., 1991). Moreover, binding of U1 snRNP to the major splice donor site, which is located downstream of 5' R, represses polyadenylation at the 5' polyadenylation signal (Ashe, et al., 1995, Ashe, et al., 1997). Cellular proteins can play a role in regulating cleavage and polyadenylation of HIV-1 RNA. hnRNP U has been shown to be involved in the post-transcriptional regulation of viral RNA via interactions with the 3' UTR (Valente & Goff, 2006). The STAR (signal transduction and activation of RNA) protein family member Sam68 enhances HIV-1 gene expression and this effect may be due in part to Sam68's ability to stimulate cleavage of unspliced viral RNA (McLaren, et al., 2004, Reddy, et al., 1999). Experimental evidence also indicates a role for viral proteins in regulating the host polyadenylation machinery to render the cell more supportive of virus replication. The accessory protein Vpr induces polyA polymerase dephosphorylation and its subsequent activation (Mouland, et al., 2002), while Tat increases the expression of the cleavage and polyadenylation specificity factor (CPSF) (Calzado, et al., 2004).

3.3 mRNA Splicing

The removal of intronic sequences in the nascent transcript is carried out by large multicomponent ribonucleoprotein complex, the spliceosome, constituted by five small nuclear ribonucleoprotein complexes (snRNPs, U1, U2, U4, U5, U6), which assembly onto the pre-mRNA requires auxiliary proteins called splicing factors (Moore, et al., 1993). The process of splicing involves recognition of short loosely conserved sequences flanking the introns. The U1 snRNP recognizes the 5′ splice site (5′ss) while the U2 snRNP in combination with the splicing factor U2AF65/35 recognizes sequences at the 3′ splice site (3′ss). 5' and 3' splice sites are required for splicing but alone are not sufficient for the proper recognition of exonic and intronic sequences.

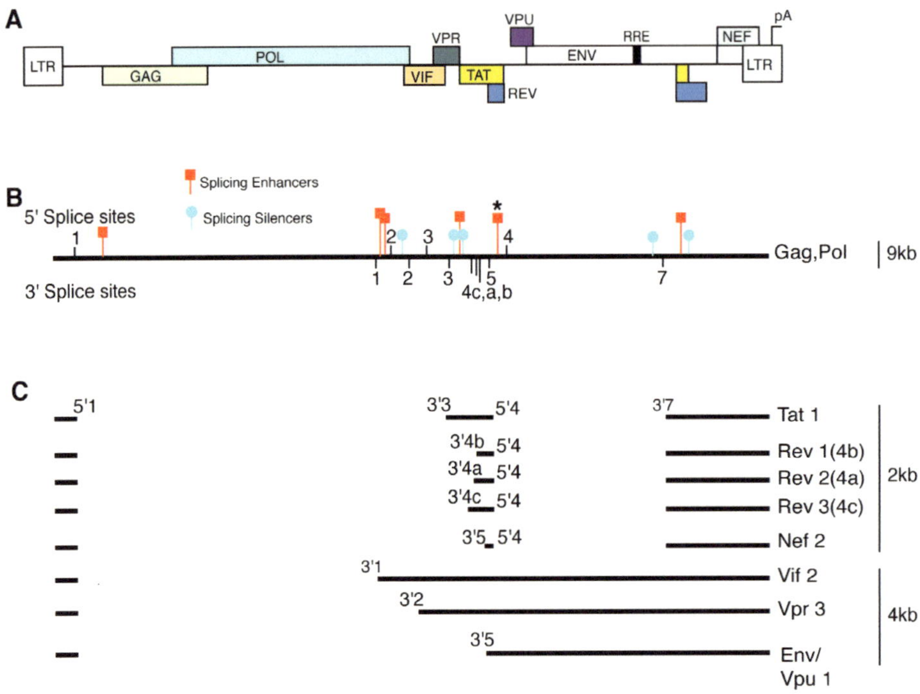

Fig. 3. A) The map shows the HIV-1 open reading frames. B) A single pre-mRNA of 9.2 kb is transcribed by the virus. 5′ and 3′ splice sites are indicated The unspliced viral mRNA codes for the Gag/Pol gene products. 5′ and 3′ splice sites are indicated. Splicing silencers (intronic and exonic) and splicing enhancers (intronic and exonic) are indicated. (*) marks the location of the GAR splicing enhancer (see Fig 5). C) Prevalent spliced viral mRNas. Over 40 alternatively spliced mRNAs are originated by the alternative usage of the multiple 5′ and 3′ splice sites, the most abundant mRNA isoforms are indicated with their approximate size and the splice site utilized to generate them.

Additional regulatory elements are classified as either exonic and intronic splicing enhancers (ESE and ISE) or exonic and intronic splicing silencers (ISS and ESS). These sequences can interact with factors that promote proper recognition of the splice sites and regulate splicing in response to physiological stimuli. Among the best-characterized ESEs are purine-rich sequences that recruit members of the serine/arginine-rich (SR) family of splicing activators (Blencowe, 2000). SR proteins regulate splicing by binding enhancer elements and recruiting and stabilizing components of the core splicing machinery to nearby splice sites (Graveley, 2000). Recent work implicates SR proteins in additional steps of gene expression, including mRNA export, stability, quality control and translation (Huang & Steitz, 2005). The best-known ESSs are dependent on interactions with members of the heterogenous ribonucleoprotein A/B family (hnRNPs A/B) (Krecic & Swanson, 1999). Positive and negative *cis*-acting sequences are often organized in multipartite control elements where SR proteins and hnRNPs often play counteracting roles (Caceres, et al., 1994, Han, et al., 2005, Zahler, et al., 2004).

Alternative splicing is a process common to most cellular mRNAs by which exons from a primary transcript (pre-mRNA) can be spliced in different arrangements to yield mRNAs that will produce functionally different protein variants (Black, 2003). The primary viral transcript undergoes a complex series of splicing events to generate over 40 mRNA isoforms, thus, the same viral protein is encoded by multiple mRNAs that vary for their 5′ and 3′ untranslated regions. Spliced viral mRNAs can be classified in a group of approximately 4kb in length, coding for the Env, Vpu, Vpr and Vif proteins, and a group of approximately 2 kb in length, coding for the Tat, Rev, Vpr and Nef proteins (Fig. 3C) (Purcell & Martin, 1993). Furthermore, approximately 50% of the viral pre-mRNAs leave the nucleus without being spliced. The unspliced 9 kb mRNA codes for the Gag and Gag-Pol polyprotein and is packaged within the nascent virions as viral genome. Alteration of this complex splicing pattern can have profound effects on viral replication and infectivity (Amendt, et al., 1994, Jablonski, et al., 2008, Jacquenet, et al., 2005, Purcell & Martin, 1993). HIV-1 splicing regulation relies on the presence of multiple viral regulatory sequences as well as cellular splicing factors that interact with these elements. To date, 4 exonic splicing silencers (ESS), 1 intronic splicing silencer (ISS), 1 intronic splicing enhancer (ISE) and 6 splicing exonic enhancers (ESE) have been identified (Fig. 3B) (Exline, et al., 2008, McLaren, et al., 2008, Schaub, et al., 2007). Several SR proteins (SC35, SF2, SRp40, 9G8) have been shown to bind the viral splicing enhancers and regulate splicing, while members of the hnRNP A/B (A1, A2 and A3) family have been shown to inhibit the usage of viral splice sites by binding viral spicing silencer elements and counteracting the activity of SR proteins (McLaren, et al., 2008). A third group of proteins interacts with both, enhancer and silencer sequences, is the hnRNP H family (H′, F, 2H9 and GRSF1). These are highly homologous and ubiquitously expressed factors, which regulate splicing, polyadenylation, capping, export and translation of cellular and viral mRNAs (Fogel & McNally, 2000, Han, et al., 2005, Jablonski & Caputi, 2009, Min, et al., 1995, Schaub, et al., 2007).

Cis-acting splicing regulatory elements within the HIV genome are highly heterogenous, redundant and provide for ample regulation of viral genome expression. In addition, the virus appears to directly regulate the relative amount and activity of cellular splicing factors in infected cells. HIV-1 infection has been shown to induce alteration in SR protein subcellular distribution, and activity via modificaton of their phosphorylation state by SR-specific kinases (Fukuhara, et al., 2006). Furthermore, data obtained from infected monocyte-derived macrophages demonstrate that a peak in viral production results in down-regulation of members of the hnRNP A/B, H and SR family, thus confirming the critical role that these proteins may play in viral replication. (Dowling, et al., 2008).

3.4 mRNA export and stability

In the early phase of viral infection the 2 kb class of viral RNAs (translated into Tat, Rev and Nef) is exported to the cytoplasm while 9 and 4 kb viral RNAs are retained in the nucleus.

Nuclear retention of 9 and 4 kb HIV-1 RNAs has been attributed to either partial spliceosome assembly (Chang & Sharp, 1989) or to a series of of poorly characterized sequences called the instability (INS) or *cis*-acting repressor (CRS) sequences (Maldarelli, et al., 1991, Mikaelian, et al., 1996, Nasioulas, et al., 1994, Olsen, et al., 1992) present within the viral mRNA. These sequences restrict the expression of the 9 kb and 4 kb mRNA species. The mechanistic details of inhibition of gene expression by INS/CRS remains obscure, it has been proposed to involve increased splicing efficiency, prevention of nuclear export and degradation of INS/CRS containing RNAs or a combination thereof (Boris-Lawrie, et al., 2001, Reddy, et al., 2000, Wodrich & Krausslich, 2001). The fully spliced 2 kb mRNAs are exported from the nucleus to the cytoplasm with a mechanism similar to the one utilized by the assembly of a protein complex at the junctions between exons (exon junction complex, EJC) during splicing (Rodriguez, et al., 2004). Additionally, factors directly binding to sequences within the RNA may contribute to efficient export (Huang & Steitz, 2005).

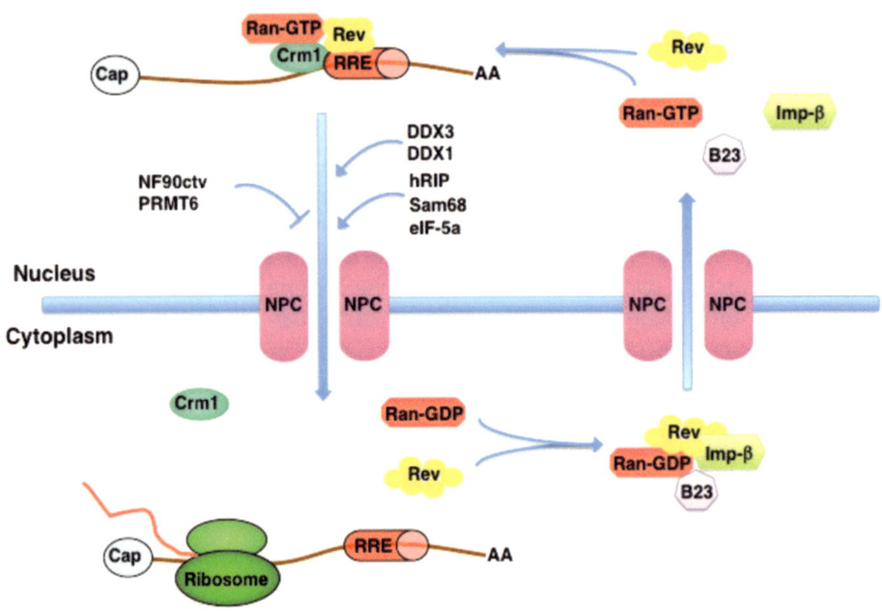

Fig. 4. HIV-1 RNA export to the cytoplasm. 9 and 4 kb viral RNAs are exported to the cytoplasm upon interaction of the Rev/Crm1/RanGTP complex with the RRE sequence within the RNA. The DDX1 and DDX3 helicases facilitate translocation of the Rev-RNA complex to the cytoplasm through the nuclear pore complex (NPC). Other host cell factors have positive (hRIP, SAM68, eIF-5a) or negative (NF90ctv, PRMT6) effects on the Rev-dependent export of the viral RNA but their role is less understood. Importin-b, RanGDP and B24 are required for import of Rev into the nucleus.

Nuclear retention of the unspliced and partially spliced viral mRNAs (9 and 4 kb) is overcome by the viral protein Rev, which is imported into the nucleus and binds to an RNA element within the *env* gene, called the Rev Responsive Element (RRE), and mediates nuclear export and efficient expression of its target RNAs (Fig. 4) (Cullen, 2000, Cullen, 2003). All the 4kb and 9kb viral mRNA species contain the RRE element and in the absence of Rev are poorly expressed in the cytoplasm. Rev import from the cytoplasm into the nucleus is aided by importin-β and the nuclear phosphoprotein B23. Following Rev binding to the RRE, the nuclear export factors CRM1 and Ran-GTP are recruited to the complex to promote export of the viral RNA into the cytoplasm. The Rev-RRE-CRM1-RanGTP RNA complex is finally dissociated in the cytoplasm upon conversion of RanGTP to RanGDP (Suhasini & Reddy, 2009).

Little is known of cellular co-factors required by Rev-RRE other than the general nuclear export factors exportin CRM1 and RAN-GTP. RNA helicases DDX1 and DDX3 are known to associate with the Rev-CRM1-RRE complex and are postulated to aid the egress of the viral RNA through the nuclear pore by remodeling its structure (Fang, et al., 2004, Yedavalli, et al., 2004). Other factors such as the eukaryotic initiation factor eIF-5A (Bevec, et al., 1996, Ruhl, et al., 1993), the human Rev interacting protein (hRIP) (Bogerd, et al., 1995, Fritz, et al., 1995) and Sam68 (Reddy, et al., 1999) have also been shown to enhance Rev activity although their mechanism is still unclear. Cellular factors may also play an inhibitory role in Rev-dependent RNA export. The C-terminal variant of nuclear factor 90 (NF90ctv) has been shown to reduce Rev function by binding and partially relocalizing Rev to the cytoplasm (Urcuqui-Inchima, et al., 2006), while Rev methylation by the arginine methylase PRMT6 reduces Rev binding to the RRE and blocks viral RNA export (Invernizzi, et al., 2006).

4. Transcription and mRNA processing coupling

In recent years our view of gene expression has changed significantly. While a growing number of genetic studies have revealed functional links between the factors that carry out the different steps in the gene expression pathway, conventional biochemical approaches and large-scale mapping of protein-protein interaction networks have uncovered physical interactions between the various machineries (Orphanides & Reinberg, 2002, Proudfoot, et al., 2002). The transcriptional apparatus plays an active role in recruiting the machinery that processes the nascent RNA transcript (Bentley, 2002, Bentley, 2005). The RNAPII CTD operates as a binding platform for components of the RNA processing machineries and its phosphorylation regulates the activity of the capping enzymes, assembly of the spliceosome and the binding of the cleavage/polyadenylation complex (Buratowski, 2003, Fong & Bentley, 2001, Hirose & Ohkuma, 2007, Komarnitsky, et al., 2000, Proudfoot, et al., 2002).

The mechanism coupling 5′ RNA capping with transcription has been well studied. Binding of the DSIF factor (Wada, et al., 1998a, Wada, et al., 1998b) to RNAPII shortly after initiation recruits NELF (Yamaguchi, et al., 1999), which arrests transcription. The cdk7 subunit of the initiation factor TFIIH phosphorylates the RNAPII CTD Ser-5 between initiation and arrest (Woychik & Hampsey, 2002). The paused RNAP II is then joined by the capping enzymes through interactions with the Ser-5 phosphorylated CTD and DSIF (Wada, et al., 1998b, Wen & Shatkin, 1999). Following the addition of the Cap, the kinase activity of P-TEFb phosphorylates DSIF (Ivanov, et al., 2000, Kim & Sharp, 2001), this neutralizes the repressive action of NELF and allows the polymerase to resume elongation. Similary 3' End formation is also linked to transcription. The cleavage/polyadenylation factors CPSF and CstF are transferred by the RNAP II CTD to their specific pre-mRNA-binding sites to produce the mRNA 3' end (Buratowski, 2005). Splicing and 3′ end formation machineries are also connected since repression of the polyadenylation signal within the R5 region is dependent on proximity to the promoter and recognition of the major 5′ splice site by the U1 snRNP (Ashe, et al., 1995, Ashe, et al., 1997).

Several studies have also shown that transcription and splicing are closely connected processes. The rate of elongation, the promoter type, transcriptional activators and the chromatin remodeling factors nearby can all affect splicing of a pre-mRNA (Batsche, et al., 2006, de la Mata, et al., 2003, Kornblihtt, 2005, Kornblihtt, 2007). Again, the RNAPII CTD assumes a central role in the regulation of RNA splicing. Phosphorylation at Ser-2 position of the RNAPII CTD stimulates pre-mRNA splicing (Hirose, et al., 1999, Misteli & Spector, 1999). Studies have identified several splicing factors that interact either directly or indirectly with the transcription machinery (Kameoka, et al., 2004, Kwek, et al., 2002). Many of the works published indicate processes that link the transcription machinery to pre-mRNA splicing. However, a "reverse coupling" mechanism, whereby pre-mRNA splicing exerts an influence on transcription has also been described. Indeed, the SR protein SC35 has been shown to affect transcription elongation (Lin, et al., 2008) and promoter-proximal 5′ splice sites increase transcription initiation via recruitment of the transcription preinitiation complex (PIC) (Damgaard, et al., 2008).
Studies on the association between the viral transcription and splicing machinery are still in their infancy. Research indicates that the cellular factor Tat-SF1, which is required for efficient transcriptional transactivation of the viral genome (Parada & Roeder, 1999, Zhou & Sharp, 1996), is also interacting with spliceosomal components (Fong & Zhou, 2001). The association with both elongation and splicing factors has led to the suggestion that Tat-SF1 can couple these two processes. Tat-SF1 also binds to another transcription-splicing coupling factor, CA150 (TCERG1) (Smith, et al., 2004). Over-expression of CA150 has been shown to reduce the ability of Tat to mediate viral transcription (Sune & Garcia-Blanco, 1999). This function is dependent on the association of CA150 with pre-mRNA splicing factors and RNAPII CTD (Carty, et al., 2000, Goldstrohm, et al., 2001) and may bridge splicing complexes to actively transcribing RNAPII (Sanchez-Alvarez, et al., 2006). The cellular protein c-Ski-interacting protein, SKIP, has been shown to regulate Tat-dependent viral transcription and interact with the splicing associated U5 snRNP and the tri-snRNP 110K protein (Bres, et al., 2005). Studies also indicate the presence of a reverse coupling mechanism in HIV-1. U1 snRNA binding to a specific 5′ splice site within the viral genome appears to overcome a checkpoint for elongation present in the *env* gene intron (Alexander, et al. 2010).
The viral transactivator Tat has also been shown to regulate viral splicing through the ASF/SF2 inhibitor p32 (Berro, et al., 2006). p32 is recruited to the HIV-1 promoter by the acetylated form of Tat, suggesting a mechanism by which acetylation of Tat promotes binding of p32 and thereby inhibits HIV-1 splicing, thus increasing the amounts of unspliced transcripts available for being translated into *gag/pol* gene products and packaging into the nascent virions as viral genome. More recently we have shown that Tat is also a selective mediator of HIV-1 splicing (Jablonski, et al., 2010) via the recruitment of the cellular co-transcriptional splicing activators Tat-SF1 and CA150 (Fig. 5). The Tat-transcription-splicing complex activates a distal splicing enhancer (GAR), which is required for *env* mRNA expression. In the context of the full-length viral genome, this mechanism promotes an autoregulatory feedback that decreases expression of Tat-coding mRNAs and favors expression of Env-specific mRNAs. Tat-mediated splicing does not appear to be dependent on its transcriptional activity. Substitution of the LTR promoter for the heterologous *β-globin*, promoter or down-regulation of Tat transcription co-factors SKIP and Tat-CT1 blocks Tat-mediated transactivation but not splicing. Tat appears to modulate splicing independent of its ability to functionally engage the transcription machinery and alter phosphorylation of the RNAP II CTD, defining a novel mechanism that couples

transcription and RNA processing via the direct recruitment of splicing factors through transcription activators. We have also shown that, like Tat, mammalian transcriptional co-activators of the Torc family can also activate splicing of endogenous genes and that this activity is independent from their role in transcription (Amelio, et al., 2009). These observations provide support for a general mechanism whereby transcriptional activators, viral or cellular, can selectively regulate splicing processes.

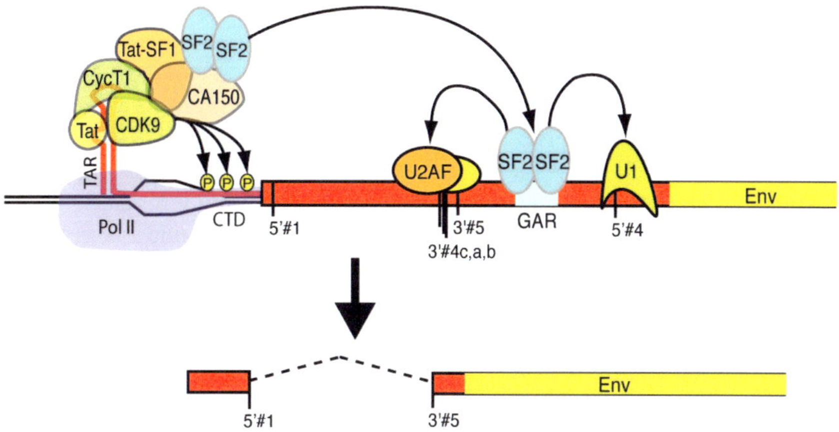

Fig. 5. Model for Tat-mediated splicing. Tat binding to TAR helps the recruitment of Tat-SF1 and CA150, which stimulates the assembly of the splicing factor SF2 onto the GAR enhancer (see Fig. 2). SF2 interaction with GAR promotes the upstream 3'ss and recruitment of U1 snRNP to the downstream 5'ss, which promotes expression of the *env* specific mRNA.

5. HIV-1 derived microRNAs

MicroRNAs (miRNAs) are short non-coding RNA molecules encoded by most eukaryotic life forms ranging from plants to higher order mammals. miRNAs have multiple pre- and post-transcriptional roles in the regulation of gene expression. The first step in the biogenesis of miRNA is the nuclear processing of primary RNA transcripts (pri-miRNAs) approximately 80 nucleotide long into shorter (~60nt) pre-miRNAs, which are exported to the cytoplasm where pre-miRNA are further processed into mature miRNAs and assembled into a ribonucleoprotein complex named RISC (RNA-induced silencing complex) (Chua, et al., 2009, Perron & Provost, 2008, Winter, et al., 2009). The RISC complex and the associated miRNA often contain sequences complementary to the 3' UTR region of the target mRNAs. Perfect complementarity between the target sequence and the miRNA triggers degradation of the target RNA. However, when miRNA and target mRNA sequences are only partially complementary the mRNA is translationaly repressed. Furthermore, miRNA can also operate at chromatine level. miRNAs have been shown to associate with the RNA-induced initiation of transcriptional silencing (RITS) complex and be recruited to complementary sequences in the chromosomal DNA. This promotes the activity of histone modifying enzymes, which alter the chromatin structure and induce transcriptional silencing (Buhler & Moazed, 2007, Verdel, et al., 2004).

Several HIV-1 encoded non-coding RNAs have been identified. In particular, the stem-loop TAR sequence is structurally similar to a pre-miRNA and it has been shown to be processed into two functional miRNAs, the 5′ stem (miR-TAR-5p) and the 3′ stem (miR-TAR-3p) (Klase, et al., 2007, Klase, et al., 2009, Ouellet, et al., 2008). miR-TAR-3p acts as an inhibitor of cellular gene expression targeting genes regulating stress induced cell death (Klase, et al., 2009). The downregulation of the host machinery by viral miRNAs is part of the viral strategies to prolong the life span of an infected cell and allows for efficient viral replication and the emergence of latently infected cells. Additionally, it has been shown that the TAR-derived miRNA can downregulate gene expression by recruiting chromatin remodeling components, thus inducing transcriptional silencing via the RITS mechanism (Purzycka & Adamiak, 2008).

A second miRNA is coded within the viral gene *nef*. Nef is a viral protein required for productive viral infection. It has been shown that miRNAs derived from *nef* transcripts are present in HIV-1 infected cells (Yamamoto, et al., 2002). Nef derived miRNAs appear to down regulate expression of the *nef* gene and they appear to be present in higher amounts in HIV-1 patients that are long time non-progressors and display low viremia.

A third miRNA generated by HIV-1, named miR-H1, is an 81 nucleotide stem loop structure present downstream of the two NF-kB sites in the LTR (Bennasser, et al., 2004). MiR-H1 has been shown to degrade the apoptosis antagonizing transcription factor (AATF) (Kaul, et al., 2009), which leads to lowered cell viability, thus counteracting the anti-apoptotic effect of the TAR-derived miRNAs. Furthermore, miR-H1 down regulates expression of the cellular miRNA miR149, which targets the Vpr gene encoded by HIV-1 (Kaul, et al., 2009). Studies on HIV-1 miRNA variability in different viral isolates have also shown that there is a strong correlation between specific miR-H1 sequences and the development of HIV-1-associated dementia and AIDS related lymphoma (Lamers, et al., 2009).

In addition to generating several viral miRNAs, HIV also regulates the cellular machinery that process small non-coding RNAs. The viral protein Tat appears to act as a generic suppressor of the activity of Dicer (Bennasser, et al., 2005), a key enzyme required for the maturation of small non-coding RNAs. Furthermore, the viral proteins Vpr and Nef have been shown to suppress the cellular miRNA machinery by suppressing production of Dicer (Coley, et al., 2011). Vertebrates have developed RNAi-based antiviral mechanisms. Given the presence in the HIV-1 genome of multiple regions that produce interfering RNAs, the anti-RNA silencing function of several viral proteins appears to be required to sustain viral replication in infected cells.

6. Future prospective

Different aspects of viral replication have been the targets of therapeutics; nevertheless, few efforts have been aimed at the disruption of the mechanism regulating viral RNA biogenesis. Formation of the HIV-1 transcript provides an important model for human RNA processing pathways and can be crucial in the isolation of novel therapeutic targets to block viral replication. Cellular factors regulating HIV RNA are expressed in most cell types and regulate a multitude of cellular splicing events theoretically making them less ideal therapeutic target candidates. Nevertheless, several drugs inhibiting different aspects of Tat transactivation are currently being tested. Different classes of compounds have been shown to specifically inhibit viral transcription by: (i) binding the TAR sequence, (ii) binding Tat, (iii) inhibiting PTEF-b components and (iv) generally inhibiting transactivation by mechanisms not yet well defined (Giacca, 2004). Small molecules that inhibit the splicing activity of SR proteins have also been shown to efficiently repress viral replication in peripheral blood mononuclear cells (PBMC) with little cell toxicity (Bakkour, et al., 2007). Furthermore, the possibility of utilizing delivery systems that specifically target cells infected by the virus (Neff, et al., 2011, Peretti, et al., 2006) suggest that cellular factors regulating the making of the viral RNA can be efficiently targeted to inhibit viral replication.

7. Acknowledgement

I thank Edwin Meagher for advice on the manuscript and Michelle Caputi for help in preparing it. My own work has been supported by the National Institute of Allergy and Infectious Diseases / National Institutes of Health.

8. References

Alexander, M. R.; Wheatley, A. K.; Center, R. J. & Purcell, D. F. (2010). Efficient transcription through an intron requires the binding of an Sm-type U1 snRNP with intact stem loop II to the splice donor. *Nucleic Acids Res,* 38, 3041-53

Amelio, A. L.; Caputi, M. & Conkright, M. D. (2009). Bipartite functions of the CREB co-activators selectively direct alternative splicing or transcriptional activation. *Embo J,* 28, 2733-47

Amendt, B. A.; Hesslein, D.; Chang, L. J. & Stoltzfus, C. M. (1994). Presence of negative and positive cis-acting RNA splicing elements within and flanking the first tat coding exon of human immunodeficiency virus type 1. *Mol. Cell. Biol.,* 14, 3960-3970

Ammosova, T.; Berro, R.; Jerebtsova, M.; Jackson, A.; Charles, S.; Klase, Z.; Southerland, W.; Gordeuk, V. R.; Kashanchi, F. & Nekhai, S. (2006). Phosphorylation of HIV-1 Tat by CDK2 in HIV-1 transcription. *Retrovirology,* 3, 78

Ashe, M. P.; Griffin, P.; James, W. & Proudfoot, N. J. (1995). Poly(A) site selection in the HIV-1 provirus: inhibition of promoter-proximal polyadenylation by the downstream major splice donor site. *Genes Dev,* 9, 3008-25

Ashe, M. P.; Pearson, L. H. & Proudfoot, N. J. (1997). The HIV-1 5' LTR poly(A) site is inactivated by U1 snRNP interaction with the downstream major splice donor site. *Embo J,* 16, 5752-63

Bakkour, N.; Lin, Y. L.; Maire, S.; Ayadi, L.; Mahuteau-Betzer, F.; Nguyen, C. H.; Mettling, C.; Portales, P.; Grierson, D.; Chabot, B.; Jeanteur, P.; Branlant, C.; Corbeau, P. & Tazi, J. (2007). Small-molecule inhibition of HIV pre-mRNA splicing as a novel antiretroviral therapy to overcome drug resistance. *PLoS Pathog,* 3, 1530-9

Batsche, E.; Yaniv, M. & Muchardt, C. (2006). The human SWI/SNF subunit Brm is a regulator of alternative splicing. *Nat Struct Mol Biol,* 13, 22-9

Benkirane, M.; Chun, R. F.; Xiao, H.; Ogryzko, V. V.; Howard, B. H.; Nakatani, Y. & Jeang, K. T. (1998). Activation of integrated provirus requires histone acetyltransferase. p300 and P/CAF are coactivators for HIV-1 Tat. *J Biol Chem,* 273, 24898-905

Bennasser, Y.; Le, S. Y.; Benkirane, M. & Jeang, K. T. (2005). Evidence that HIV-1 encodes an siRNA and a suppressor of RNA silencing. *Immunity,* 22, 607-19

Bennasser, Y.; Le, S. Y.; Yeung, M. L. & Jeang, K. T. (2004). HIV-1 encoded candidate micro-RNAs and their cellular targets. *Retrovirology,* 1, 43

Bentley, D. (2002). The mRNA assembly line: transcription and processing machines in the same factory. *Curr Opin Cell Biol,* 14, 336-42

Bentley, D. L. (2005). Rules of engagement: co-transcriptional recruitment of pre-mRNA processing factors. *Curr Opin Cell Biol,* 17, 251-6

Berkhout, B.; Silverman, R. H. & Jeang, K. T. (1989). Tat trans-activates the human immunodeficiency virus through a nascent RNA target. *Cell,* 59, 273-82

Berro, R.; Kehn, K.; de la Fuente, C.; Pumfery, A.; Adair, R.; Wade, J.; Colberg-Poley, A. M.; Hiscott, J. & Kashanchi, F. (2006). Acetylated Tat regulates human immunodeficiency virus type 1 splicing through its interaction with the splicing regulator p32. *J Virol,* 80, 3189-204

Bevec, D.; Jaksche, H.; Oft, M.; Wohl, T.; Himmelspach, M.; Pacher, A.; Schebesta, M.; Koettnitz, K.; Dobrovnik, M.; Csonga, R.; Lottspeich, F. & Hauber, J. (1996). Inhibition of HIV-1 replication in lymphocytes by mutants of the Rev cofactor eIF-5A. *Science,* 271, 1858-60

Black, D. L. (2003). Mechanisms of alternative pre-messenger RNA splicing. *Annu Rev Biochem,* 72, 291-336

Blencowe, B. J. (2000). Exonic splicing enhancers: mechanism of action, diversity and role in human genetic diseases. *Trends Biochem Sci,* 25, 106-10

Bogerd, H. P.; Fridell, R. A.; Madore, S. & Cullen, B. R. (1995). Identification of a novel cellular cofactor for the Rev/Rex class of retroviral regulatory proteins. *Cell,* 82, 485-94

Boris-Lawrie, K.; Roberts, T. M. & Hull, S. (2001). Retroviral RNA elements integrate components of post-transcriptional gene expression. *Life Sci,* 69, 2697-709

Boulanger, M. C.; Liang, C.; Russell, R. S.; Lin, R.; Bedford, M. T.; Wainberg, M. A. & Richard, S. (2005). Methylation of Tat by PRMT6 regulates human immunodeficiency virus type 1 gene expression. *J Virol,* 79, 124-31

Brady, J. & Kashanchi, F. (2005). Tat gets the "green" light on transcription initiation. *Retrovirology,* 2, 69

Bres, V.; Gomes, N.; Pickle, L. & Jones, K. A. (2005). A human splicing factor, SKIP, associates with P-TEFb and enhances transcription elongation by HIV-1 Tat. *Genes Dev,* 19, 1211-26

Bres, V.; Kiernan, R.; Emiliani, S. & Benkirane, M. (2002). Tat acetyl-acceptor lysines are important for human immunodeficiency virus type-1 replication. *J Biol Chem,* 277, 22215-21

Bres, V.; Kiernan, R. E.; Linares, L. K.; Chable-Bessia, C.; Plechakova, O.; Treand, C.; Emiliani, S.; Peloponese, J. M.; Jeang, K. T.; Coux, O.; Scheffner, M. & Benkirane, M. (2003). A non-proteolytic role for ubiquitin in Tat-mediated transactivation of the HIV-1 promoter. *Nat Cell Biol,* 5, 754-61

Bres, V.; Yoh, S. M. & Jones, K. A. (2008). The multi-tasking P-TEFb complex. *Curr Opin Cell Biol,* 20, 334-40

Buhler, M. & Moazed, D. (2007). Transcription and RNAi in heterochromatic gene silencing. *Nat Struct Mol Biol,* 14, 1041-1048

Buratowski, S. (2003). The CTD code. *Nat Struct Biol,* 10, 679-80

Buratowski, S. (2005). Connections between mRNA 3' end processing and transcription termination. *Curr Opin Cell Biol,* 17, 257-61

Caceres, J. F.; Stamm, S.; Helfman, D. M. & Krainer, A. R. (1994). Regulation of alternative splicing in vivo by overexpression of antagonistic splicing factors. *Science,* 265, 1706-1709

Caldwell, R. L.; Egan, B. S. & Shepherd, V. L. (2000). HIV-1 Tat represses transcription from the mannose receptor promoter. *J Immunol,* 165, 7035-41

Calzado, M. A.; Sancho, R. & Munoz, E. (2004). Human immunodeficiency virus type 1 Tat increases the expression of cleavage and polyadenylation specificity factor 73-kilodalton subunit modulating cellular and viral expression. *J Virol,* 78, 6846-54

Carty, S. M.; Goldstrohm, A. C.; Sune, C.; Garcia-Blanco, M. A. & Greenleaf, A. L. (2000). Protein-interaction modules that organize nuclear function: FF domains of CA150 bind the phosphoCTD of RNA polymerase II. *Proc Natl Acad Sci U S A,* 97, 9015-20

Chang, D. D. & Sharp, P. A. (1989). Regulation by HIV rev depends upon recognition of splice sites. *Cell,* 59, 789-795

Cherrington, J. & Ganem, D. (1992). Regulation of polyadenylation in human immunodeficiency virus (HIV): contributions of promoter proximity and upstream sequences. *Embo J,* 11, 1513-24

Chiu, Y. L.; Ho, C. K.; Saha, N.; Schwer, B.; Shuman, S. & Rana, T. M. (2002). Tat stimulates cotranscriptional capping of HIV mRNA. *Mol Cell,* 10, 585-97

Chua, J. H.; Armugam, A. & Jeyaseelan, K. (2009). MicroRNAs: biogenesis, function and applications. *Curr Opin Mol Ther,* 11, 189-99

Col, E.; Caron, C.; Seigneurin-Berny, D.; Gracia, J.; Favier, A. & Khochbin, S. (2001). The histone acetyltransferase, hGCN5, interacts with and acetylates the HIV transactivator, Tat. *J Biol Chem,* 276, 28179-84

Coley, W.; Van Duyne, R.; Carpio, L.; Guendel, I.; Kehn-Hall, K.; Chevalier, S.; Narayanan, A.; Luu, T.; Lee, N.; Klase, Z. & Kashanchi, F. (2011). Absence of DICER in monocytes and its regulation by HIV-1. *J Biol Chem,* 285, 31930-43

Cullen, B. R. (2000). Nuclear RNA export pathways. *Mol. Cell. Biol.,* 20, 4181-4187

Cullen, B. R. (2003). Nuclear mRNA export: insights from virology. *Trends Biochem Sci,* 28, 419-24

Damgaard, C. K.; Kahns, S.; Lykke-Andersen, S.; Nielsen, A. L.; Jensen, T. H. & Kjems, J. (2008). A 5' splice site enhances the recruitment of basal transcription initiation factors in vivo. *Mol Cell,* 29, 271-8

de la Mata, M.; Alonso, C. R.; Kadener, S.; Fededa, J. P.; Blaustein, M.; Pelisch, F.; Cramer, P.; Bentley, D. & Kornblihtt, A. R. (2003). A slow RNA polymerase II affects alternative splicing in vivo. *Mol Cell,* 12, 525-32

Deng, L.; Wang, D.; de la Fuente, C.; Wang, L.; Li, H.; Lee, C. G.; Donnelly, R.; Wade, J. D.; Lambert, P. & Kashanchi, F. (2001). Enhancement of the p300 HAT activity by HIV-1 Tat on chromatin DNA. *Virology,* 289, 312-26

Dorr, A.; Kiermer, V.; Pedal, A.; Rackwitz, H. R.; Henklein, P.; Schubert, U.; Zhou, M. M.; Verdin, E. & Ott, M. (2002). Transcriptional synergy between Tat and PCAF is dependent on the binding of acetylated Tat to the PCAF bromodomain. *Embo J,* 21, 2715-23

Dowling, D.; Nasr-Esfahani, S.; Tan, C. H.; O'Brien, K.; Howard, J. L.; Jans, D. A.; Purcell, D. F.; Stoltzfus, C. M. & Sonza, S. (2008). HIV-1 infection induces changes in expression of cellular splicing factors that regulate alternative viral splicing and virus production in macrophages. *Retrovirology,* 5, 18

Ensoli, B.; Barillari, G.; Salahuddin, S. Z.; Gallo, R. C. & Wong-Staal, F. (1990). Tat protein of HIV-1 stimulates growth of cells derived from Kaposi's sarcoma lesions of AIDS patients. *Nature,* 345, 84-6

Exline, C. M.; Feng, Z. & Stoltzfus, C. M. (2008). Negative and positive mRNA splicing elements act competitively to regulate human immunodeficiency virus type 1 vif gene expression. *J Virol*, 82, 3921-31

Fang, J.; Kubota, S.; Yang, B.; Zhou, N.; Zhang, H.; Godbout, R. & Pomerantz, R. J. (2004). A DEAD box protein facilitates HIV-1 replication as a cellular co-factor of Rev. *Virology*, 330, 471-80

Fogel, B. L. & McNally, M. T. (2000). A cellular protein, hnRNP H, binds to the negative regulator of splicing element from Rous sarcoma virus. *J Biol Chem*, 275, 32371-32378

Fong, N. & Bentley, D. L. (2001). Capping, splicing, and 3' processing are independently stimulated by RNA polymerase II: different functions for different segments of the CTD. *Genes Dev*, 15, 1783-95

Fong, Y. W. & Zhou, Q. (2001). Stimulatory effect of splicing factors on transcriptional elongation. *Nature*, 414, 929-33.

Fritz, C. C.; Zapp, M. L. & Green, M. R. (1995). A human nucleoporin-like protein that specifically interacts with HIV Rev. *Nature*, 376, 530-3

Fujinaga, K.; Irwin, D.; Huang, Y.; Taube, R.; Kurosu, T. & Peterlin, B. M. (2004). Dynamics of human immunodeficiency virus transcription: P-TEFb phosphorylates RD and dissociates negative effectors from the transactivation response element. *Mol Cell Biol*, 24, 787-95

Fukuhara, T.; Hosoya, T.; Shimizu, S.; Sumi, K.; Oshiro, T.; Yoshinaka, Y.; Suzuki, M.; Yamamoto, N.; Herzenberg, L. A. & Hagiwara, M. (2006). Utilization of host SR protein kinases and RNA-splicing machinery during viral replication. *Proc Natl Acad Sci U S A*, 103, 11329-33

Garber, M. E.; Wei, P.; KewalRamani, V. N.; Mayall, T. P.; Herrmann, C. H.; Rice, A. P.; Littman, D. R. & Jones, K. A. (1998). The interaction between HIV-1 Tat and human cyclin T1 requires zinc and a critical cysteine residue that is not conserved in the murine CycT1 protein. *Genes Dev*, 12, 3512-27

Gaynor, R. B. (1995). Regulation of HIV-1 gene expression by the transactivator protein tat. *Curr. Top. Microbiol. Immunol.*, 193, 51-77

Giacca, M. (2004). The HIV-1 Tat protein: a multifaceted target for novel therapeutic opportunities. *Curr Drug Targets Immune Endocr Metabol Disord*, 4, 277-85

Gibellini, D.; Re, M. C.; La Placa, M. & Zauli, G. (2002). Differentially expressed genes in HIV-1 tat-expressing CD4(+) T-cell line. *Virus Res*, 90, 337-45

Gilmartin, G. M.; Fleming, E. S.; Oetjen, J. & Graveley, B. R. (1995). CPSF recognition of an HIV-1 mRNA 3'-processing enhancer: multiple sequence contacts involved in poly(A) site definition. *Genes Dev*, 9, 72-83

Goldstrohm, A. C.; Albrecht, T. R.; Sune, C.; Bedford, M. T. & Garcia-Blanco, M. A. (2001). The transcription elongation factor CA150 interacts with RNA polymerase II and the pre-mRNA splicing factor SF1. *Mol Cell Biol*, 21, 7617-28

Graveley, B. R. (2000). Sorting out the complexity of SR protein functions. *RNA*, 6, 1197-211

Han, K.; Yeo, G.; An, P.; Burge, C. B. & Grabowski, P. J. (2005). A combinatorial code for splicing silencing: UAGG and GGGG motifs. *PLoS Biol*, 3, e158

Hengartner, C. J.; Myer, V. E.; Liao, S. M.; Wilson, C. J.; Koh, S. S. & Young, R. A. (1998). Temporal regulation of RNA polymerase II by Srb10 and Kin28 cyclin-dependent kinases. *Mol Cell*, 2, 43-53

Hirose, Y. & Ohkuma, Y. (2007). Phosphorylation of the C-terminal domain of RNA polymerase II plays central roles in the integrated events of eucaryotic gene expression. *J Biochem,* 141, 601-8

Hirose, Y.; Tacke, R. & Manley, J. L. (1999). Phosphorylated RNA polymerase II stimulates pre-mRNA splicing. *Genes Dev,* 13, 1234-9

Ho, C. K. & Shuman, S. (1999). Distinct roles for CTD Ser-2 and Ser-5 phosphorylation in the recruitment and allosteric activation of mammalian mRNA capping enzyme. *Mol Cell,* 3, 405-11

Huang, L.; Bosch, I.; Hofmann, W.; Sodroski, J. & Pardee, A. B. (1998). Tat protein induces human immunodeficiency virus type 1 (HIV-1) coreceptors and promotes infection with both macrophage-tropic and T-lymphotropic HIV-1 strains. *J Virol,* 72, 8952-60

Huang, Y. & Steitz, J. A. (2005). SRprises along a messenger's journey. *Mol Cell,* 17, 613-5

Huigen, M. C.; Kamp, W. & Nottet, H. S. (2004). Multiple effects of HIV-1 trans-activator protein on the pathogenesis of HIV-1 infection. *Eur J Clin Invest,* 34, 57-66

Invernizzi, C. F.; Xie, B.; Richard, S. & Wainberg, M. A. (2006). PRMT6 diminishes HIV-1 Rev binding to and export of viral RNA. *Retrovirology,* 3, 93

Ivanov, D.; Kwak, Y. T.; Guo, J. & Gaynor, R. B. (2000). Domains in the SPT5 protein that modulate its transcriptional regulatory properties. *Mol Cell Biol,* 20, 2970-83

Jablonski, J. A.; Amelio, A. L.; Giacca, M. & Caputi, M. (2010). The transcriptional transactivator Tat selectively regulates viral splicing. *Nucleic Acids Res,* 38, 1249-60

Jablonski, J. A.; Buratti, E.; Stuani, C. & Caputi, M. (2008). The secondary structure of the human immunodeficiency virus type 1 transcript modulates viral splicing and infectivity. *J Virol,* 82, 8038-50

Jablonski, J. A. & Caputi, M. (2009). Role of cellular RNA processing factors in human immunodeficiency virus type 1 mRNA metabolism, replication, and infectivity. *J Virol,* 83, 981-92

Jacquenet, S.; Decimo, D.; Muriaux, D. & Darlix, J. L. (2005). Dual effect of the SR proteins ASF/SF2, SC35 and 9G8 on HIV-1 RNA splicing and virion production. *Retrovirology,* 2, 33

Kameoka, S.; Duque, P. & Konarska, M. M. (2004). p54(nrb) associates with the 5' splice site within large transcription/splicing complexes. *Embo J,* 23, 1782-91

Kamine, J.; Elangovan, B.; Subramanian, T.; Coleman, D. & Chinnadurai, G. (1996). Identification of a cellular protein that specifically interacts with the essential cysteine region of the HIV-1 Tat transactivator. *Virology,* 216, 357-66

Kaul, D.; Ahlawat, A. & Gupta, S. D. (2009). HIV-1 genome-encoded hiv1-mir-H1 impairs cellular responses to infection. *Mol Cell Biochem,* 323, 143-8

Kiernan, R. E.; Vanhulle, C.; Schiltz, L.; Adam, E.; Xiao, H.; Maudoux, F.; Calomme, C.; Burny, A.; Nakatani, Y.; Jeang, K. T.; Benkirane, M. & Van Lint, C. (1999). HIV-1 tat transcriptional activity is regulated by acetylation. *Embo J,* 18, 6106-18

Kim, J. B. & Sharp, P. A. (2001). Positive transcription elongation factor B phosphorylates hSPT5 and RNA polymerase II carboxyl-terminal domain independently of cyclin-dependent kinase-activating kinase. *J Biol Chem,* 276, 12317-23

King, J. E.; Eugenin, E. A.; Buckner, C. M. & Berman, J. W. (2006). HIV tat and neurotoxicity. *Microbes Infect,* 8, 1347-57

Klase, Z.; Kale, P.; Winograd, R.; Gupta, M. V.; Heydarian, M.; Berro, R.; McCaffrey, T. & Kashanchi, F. (2007). HIV-1 TAR element is processed by Dicer to yield a viral micro-RNA involved in chromatin remodeling of the viral LTR. *BMC Mol Biol,* 8, 63

Klase, Z.; Winograd, R.; Davis, J.; Carpio, L.; Hildreth, R.; Heydarian, M.; Fu, S.; McCaffrey, T.; Meiri, E.; Ayash-Rashkovsky, M.; Gilad, S.; Bentwich, Z. & Kashanchi, F. (2009). HIV-1 TAR miRNA protects against apoptosis by altering cellular gene expression. *Retrovirology,* 6, 18

Komarnitsky, P.; Cho, E. J. & Buratowski, S. (2000). Different phosphorylated forms of RNA polymerase II and associated mRNA processing factors during transcription. *Genes Dev,* 14, 2452-60

Kornblihtt, A. R. (2005). Promoter usage and alternative splicing. *Curr Opin Cell Biol,* 17, 262-8

Kornblihtt, A. R. (2007). Coupling transcription and alternative splicing. *Adv Exp Med Biol,* 623, 175-89

Krecic, A. M. & Swanson, M. S. (1999). hnRNP complexes: composition, structure, and function. *Curr. Opin. Cell. Biol.,* 11, 363-71

Kwek, K. Y.; Murphy, S.; Furger, A.; Thomas, B.; O'Gorman, W.; Kimura, H.; Proudfoot, N. J. & Akoulitchev, A. (2002). U1 snRNA associates with TFIIH and regulates transcriptional initiation. *Nat Struct Biol,* 9, 800-5

Lamers, S. L.; Salemi, M.; Galligan, D. C.; de Oliveira, T.; Fogel, G. B.; Granier, S. C.; Zhao, L.; Brown, J. N.; Morris, A.; Masliah, E. & McGrath, M. S. (2009). Extensive HIV-1 intra-host recombination is common in tissues with abnormal histopathology. *PLoS One,* 4, e5065

Li, A. G.; Piluso, L. G.; Cai, X.; Gadd, B. J.; Ladurner, A. G. & Liu, X. (2007). An acetylation switch in p53 mediates holo-TFIID recruitment. *Mol Cell,* 28, 408-21

Lin, S.; Coutinho-Mansfield, G.; Wang, D.; Pandit, S. & Fu, X. D. (2008). The splicing factor SC35 has an active role in transcriptional elongation. *Nat Struct Mol Biol,* 15, 819-26

Mahmoudi, T.; Parra, M.; Vries, R. G.; Kauder, S. E.; Verrijzer, C. P.; Ott, M. & Verdin, E. (2006). The SWI/SNF chromatin-remodeling complex is a cofactor for Tat transactivation of the HIV promoter. *J Biol Chem,* 281, 19960-8

Maldarelli, F.; Martin, M. A. & Strebel, K. (1991). Identification of postranscriptionally active inhibitory sequences in human immunodeficiency virus type I RNA: novel level of gene regulation. *J. Virol.,* 65, 5732-5743

Marcello, A.; Zoppe, M. & Giacca, M. (2001). Multiple modes of transcriptional regulation by the HIV-1 Tat transactivator. *IUBMB Life,* 51, 175-81

Marzio, G.; Tyagi, M.; Gutierrez, M. I. & Giacca, M. (1998). HIV-1 tat transactivator recruits p300 and CREB-binding protein histone acetyltransferases to the viral promoter. *Proc Natl Acad Sci U S A,* 95, 13519-24

McLaren, M.; Asai, K. & Cochrane, A. (2004). A novel function for Sam68: enhancement of HIV-1 RNA 3' end processing. *Rna,* 10, 1119-29

McLaren, M.; Marsh, K. & Cochrane, A. (2008). Modulating HIV-1 RNA processing and utilization. *Front Biosci,* 13, 5693-707

Mikaelian, I.; Krieg, M.; Gait, M. J. & Karn, J. (1996). Interaction of INS (CRS) elements and the splicing machinery regulate the production of Rev-responsive mRNAs. *J Mol Biol,* 257, 246-264

Min, H.; Chan, R. C. & Black, D. L. (1995). The generally expressed hnRNP F is involved in a neural-specific pre-mRNA splicing event. *Genes Dev.*, 9, 2659-2671

Misteli, T. & Spector, D. L. (1999). RNA polymerase II targets pre-mRNA splicing factors to transcription sites in vivo. *Mol Cell*, 3, 697-705

Moore, M. J.; Query, C. C. & Sharp, P. A. 1993. Splicing of precursors to mRNA by the spliceosome. In The RNA World, ed. R. F. Gesteland and J. F. Atkins, pp. 303-357. New York: Cold Spring Harbor Press

Mouland, A. J.; Coady, M.; Yao, X. J. & Cohen, E. A. (2002). Hypophosphorylation of poly(A) polymerase and increased polyadenylation activity are associated with human immunodeficiency virus type 1 Vpr expression. *Virology*, 292, 321-30

Nasioulas, G.; Zolotukhin, A. S.; Tabernero, C.; Solomin, L.; Cunningham, C. P.; Pavlakis, G. N. & Felber, B. K. (1994). Elements distinct from human immunodeficiency virus type 1 splice sites are responsible for the Rev dependence of env mRNA. *J Virol*, 68, 2986-93

Neff, C. P.; Zhou, J.; Remling, L.; Kuruvilla, J.; Zhang, J.; Li, H.; Smith, D. D.; Swiderski, P.; Rossi, J. J. & Akkina, R. (2011). An aptamer-siRNA chimera suppresses HIV-1 viral loads and protects from helper CD4(+) T cell decline in humanized mice. *Sci Transl Med*, 3, 66ra6

Ni, Z.; Schwartz, B. E.; Werner, J.; Suarez, J. R. & Lis, J. T. (2004). Coordination of transcription, RNA processing, and surveillance by P-TEFb kinase on heat shock genes. *Mol Cell*, 13, 55-65

Olsen, H. S.; Cochrane, A. W. & Rosen, C. (1992). Interaction of cellular factors with intragenic cis-acting repressive sequences within the HIV genome. *Virology*, 191, 709-15

Orphanides, G. & Reinberg, D. (2002). A unified theory of gene expression. *Cell*, 108, 439-51

Ott, M.; Lovett, J. L.; Mueller, L. & Verdin, E. (1998). Superinduction of IL-8 in T cells by HIV-1 Tat protein is mediated through NF-kappaB factors. *J Immunol*, 160, 2872-80

Ouellet, D. L.; Plante, I.; Landry, P.; Barat, C.; Janelle, M. E.; Flamand, L.; Tremblay, M. J. & Provost, P. (2008). Identification of functional microRNAs released through asymmetrical processing of HIV-1 TAR element. *Nucleic Acids Res*, 36, 2353-65

Parada, C. A. & Roeder, R. G. (1999). A novel RNA polymerase II-containing complex potentiates Tat-enhanced HIV-1 transcription. *Embo J*, 18, 3688-701

Pereira, L. A.; Bentley, K.; Peeters, A.; Churchill, M. J. & Deacon, N. J. (2000). A compilation of cellular transcription factor interactions with the HIV-1 LTR promoter. *Nucleic Acids Res*, 28, 663-8

Peretti, S.; Schiavoni, I.; Pugliese, K. & Federico, M. (2006). Selective elimination of HIV-1-infected cells by Env-directed, HIV-1-based virus-like particles. *Virology*, 345, 115-26

Perron, M. P. & Provost, P. (2008). Protein interactions and complexes in human microRNA biogenesis and function. *Front Biosci*, 13, 2537-47

Peterlin, B. M. & Price, D. H. (2006). Controlling the elongation phase of transcription with P-TEFb. *Mol Cell*, 23, 297-305

Pollard, V. W. & Malim, M. H. (1998). The HIV-1 rev protein. *Annu. Rev. Microbiol.*, 52, 491-532

Proudfoot, N. J.; Furger, A. & Dye, M. J. (2002). Integrating mRNA processing with transcription. *Cell*, 108, 501-12.

Purcell, D. F. J. & Martin, M. A. (1993). Alternative splicing of human immunodeficiency virus type 1 mRNA modulates viral protein expression, replication and infectivity. *J. Virol.*, 67, 6365-6378

Purzycka, K. J. & Adamiak, R. W. (2008). The HIV-2 TAR RNA domain as a potential source of viral-encoded miRNA. A reconnaissance study. *Nucleic Acids Symp Ser (Oxf)*, 511-2

Raha, T.; Cheng, S. W. & Green, M. R. (2005). HIV-1 Tat stimulates transcription complex assembly through recruitment of TBP in the absence of TAFs. *PLoS Biol*, 3, e44

Reddy, T. R.; Tang, H.; Xu, W. & Wong-Staal, F. (2000). Sam68, RNA helicase A and Tap cooperate in the post-transcriptional regulation of human immunodeficiency virus and type D retroviral mRNA. *Oncogene*, 19, 3570-5

Reddy, T. R.; Xu, W.; Mau, J. K.; Goodwin, C. D.; Suhasini, M.; Tang, H.; Frimpong, K.; Rose, D. W. & Wong-Staal, F. (1999). Inhibition of HIV replication by dominant negative mutants of Sam68, a functional homolog of HIV-1 Rev. *Nat Med*, 5, 635-42

Rodriguez, M. S.; Dargemont, C. & Stutz, F. (2004). Nuclear export of RNA. *Biol Cell*, 96, 639-55

Rubartelli, A.; Poggi, A.; Sitia, R. & Zocchi, M. R. (1998). HIV-I Tat: a polypeptide for all seasons. *Immunol Today*, 19, 543-5

Ruhl, M.; Himmelspach, M.; Bahr, G. M.; Hammerschmid, F.; Jaksche, H.; Wolff, B.; Aschauer, H.; Farrington, G. K.; Probst, H.; Bevec, D. & et al. (1993). Eukaryotic initiation factor 5A is a cellular target of the human immunodeficiency virus type 1 Rev activation domain mediating trans-activation. *J Cell Biol*, 123, 1309-20

Sanchez-Alvarez, M.; Goldstrohm, A. C.; Garcia-Blanco, M. A. & Sune, C. (2006). Human transcription elongation factor CA150 localizes to splicing factor-rich nuclear speckles and assembles transcription and splicing components into complexes through its amino and carboxyl regions. *Mol Cell Biol*, 26, 4998-5014

Schaub, M. C.; Lopez, S. R. & Caputi, M. (2007). Members of the heterogeneous nuclear ribonucleoprotein H family activate splicing of an HIV-1 splicing substrate by promoting formation of ATP-dependent spliceosomal complexes. *J Biol Chem*, 282, 13617-26

Secchiero, P.; Zella, D.; Capitani, S.; Gallo, R. C. & Zauli, G. (1999). Extracellular HIV-1 tat protein up-regulates the expression of surface CXC-chemokine receptor 4 in resting CD4+ T cells. *J Immunol*, 162, 2427-31

Shatkin, A. J. & Manley, J. L. (2000). The ends of the affair: capping and polyadenylation. *Nat Struct Biol*, 7, 838-42

Smith, M. J.; Kulkarni, S. & Pawson, T. (2004). FF domains of CA150 bind transcription and splicing factors through multiple weak interactions. *Mol Cell Biol*, 24, 9274-85

Stoltzfus, C. M. & Madsen, J. M. (2006). Role of viral splicing elements and cellular RNA binding proteins in regulation of HIV-1 alternative RNA splicing. *Curr HIV Res*, 4, 43-55

Suhasini, M. & Reddy, T. R. (2009). Cellular proteins and HIV-1 Rev function. *Curr HIV Res*, 7, 91-100

Sune, C. & Garcia-Blanco, M. A. (1999). Transcriptional cofactor CA150 regulates RNA polymerase II elongation in a TATA-box-dependent manner. *Mol Cell Biol*, 19, 4719-28

Treand, C.; du Chene, I.; Bres, V.; Kiernan, R.; Benarous, R.; Benkirane, M. & Emiliani, S. (2006). Requirement for SWI/SNF chromatin-remodeling complex in Tat-mediated activation of the HIV-1 promoter. *Embo J*, 25, 1690-9

Urcuqui-Inchima, S.; Castano, M. E.; Hernandez-Verdun, D.; St-Laurent, G., 3rd & Kumar, A. (2006). Nuclear Factor 90, a cellular dsRNA binding protein inhibits the HIV Rev-export function. *Retrovirology*, 3, 83

Valente, S. T. & Goff, S. P. (2006). Inhibition of HIV-1 gene expression by a fragment of hnRNP U. *Mol Cell*, 23, 597-605

Van Lint, C.; Quivy, V.; Demonte, D.; Chariot, A.; Vanhulle, C.; de Walque, S.; Gaudray, G.; Veithen, E.; Bours, V.; Piette, J. & Burny, A. (2004). Molecular mechanisms involved in HIV-1 transcriptional latency and reactivation: implications for the development of therapeutic strategies. *Bull Mem Acad R Med Belg*, 159, 176-89

Verdel, A.; Jia, S.; Gerber, S.; Sugiyama, T.; Gygi, S.; Grewal, S. I. & Moazed, D. (2004). RNAi-mediated targeting of heterochromatin by the RITS complex. *Science*, 303, 672-6

Verdin, E.; Paras, P., Jr. & Van Lint, C. (1993). Chromatin disruption in the promoter of human immunodeficiency virus type 1 during transcriptional activation. *Embo J*, 12, 3249-59

Wada, T.; Orphanides, G.; Hasegawa, J.; Kim, D. K.; Shima, D.; Yamaguchi, Y.; Fukuda, A.; Hisatake, K.; Oh, S.; Reinberg, D. & Handa, H. (2000). FACT relieves DSIF/NELF-mediated inhibition of transcriptional elongation and reveals functional differences between P-TEFb and TFIIH. *Mol Cell*, 5, 1067-72

Wada, T.; Takagi, T.; Yamaguchi, Y.; Ferdous, A.; Imai, T.; Hirose, S.; Sugimoto, S.; Yano, K.; Hartzog, G. A.; Winston, F.; Buratowski, S. & Handa, H. (1998a). DSIF, a novel transcription elongation factor that regulates RNA polymerase II processivity, is composed of human Spt4 and Spt5 homologs. *Genes Dev*, 12, 343-56

Wada, T.; Takagi, T.; Yamaguchi, Y.; Watanabe, D. & Handa, H. (1998b). Evidence that P-TEFb alleviates the negative effect of DSIF on RNA polymerase II-dependent transcription in vitro. *Embo J*, 17, 7395-403

Wei, P.; Garber, M. E.; Fang, S. M.; Fischer, W. H. & Jones, K. A. (1998). A novel CDK9-associated C-type cyclin interacts directly with HIV-1 Tat and mediates its high-affinity, loop-specific binding to TAR RNA. *Cell*, 92, 451-62

Weichs an der Glon, C.; Monks, J. & Proudfoot, N. J. (1991). Occlusion of the HIV poly(A) site. *Genes Dev*, 5, 244-53

Weissman, J. D.; Brown, J. A.; Howcroft, T. K.; Hwang, J.; Chawla, A.; Roche, P. A.; Schiltz, L.; Nakatani, Y. & Singer, D. S. (1998). HIV-1 tat binds TAFII250 and represses TAFII250-dependent transcription of major histocompatibility class I genes. *Proc Natl Acad Sci U S A*, 95, 11601-6

Wen, Y. & Shatkin, A. J. (1999). Transcription elongation factor hSPT5 stimulates mRNA capping. *Genes Dev*, 13, 1774-9

Wentz, P. M.; Moore, B. E.; Cloyd, M. V.; Berget, S. M. & Donehower, L. A. (1997). A naturally arising mutation of a potential silencer of exon splicing in human immunodeficiency virus type I induces dominant aberrant splicing and arrests virus production. *J. Virol.*, 71, 8542-8551

Winter, J.; Jung, S.; Keller, S.; Gregory, R. I. & Diederichs, S. (2009). Many roads to maturity: microRNA biogenesis pathways and their regulation. *Nat Cell Biol*, 11, 228-34

Wodrich, H. & Krausslich, H. G. (2001). Nucleocytoplasmic RNA transport in retroviral replication. *Results Probl Cell Differ,* 34, 197-217

Woychik, N. A. & Hampsey, M. (2002). The RNA polymerase II machinery: structure illuminates function. *Cell,* 108, 453-63

Wu, R. F.; Ma, Z.; Myers, D. P. & Terada, L. S. (2007). HIV-1 Tat activates dual Nox pathways leading to independent activation of ERK and JNK MAP kinases. *J Biol Chem,* 282, 37412-9

Yamaguchi, Y.; Takagi, T.; Wada, T.; Yano, K.; Furuya, A.; Sugimoto, S.; Hasegawa, J. & Handa, H. (1999). NELF, a multisubunit complex containing RD, cooperates with DSIF to repress RNA polymerase II elongation. *Cell,* 97, 41-51

Yamamoto, T.; Omoto, S.; Mizuguchi, M.; Mizukami, H.; Okuyama, H.; Okada, N.; Saksena, N. K.; Brisibe, E. A.; Otake, K. & Fuji, Y. R. (2002). Double-stranded nef RNA interferes with human immunodeficiency virus type 1 replication. *Microbiol Immunol,* 46, 809-17

Yang, X. J. & Seto, E. (2008). Lysine acetylation: codified crosstalk with other posttranslational modifications. *Mol Cell,* 31, 449-61

Yedavalli, V. S.; Neuveut, C.; Chi, Y. H.; Kleiman, L. & Jeang, K. T. (2004). Requirement of DDX3 DEAD box RNA helicase for HIV-1 Rev-RRE export function. *Cell,* 119, 381-92

Zahler, A. M.; Damgaard, C. K.; Kjems, J. & Caputi, M. (2004). SC35 and heterogeneous nuclear ribonucleoprotein A/B proteins bind to a juxtaposed exonic splicing enhancer/exonic splicing silencer element to regulate HIV-1 tat exon 2 splicing. *J Biol Chem,* 279, 10077-84

Zhou, M.; Deng, L.; Kashanchi, F.; Brady, J. N.; Shatkin, A. J. & Kumar, A. (2003). The Tat/TAR-dependent phosphorylation of RNA polymerase II C-terminal domain stimulates cotranscriptional capping of HIV-1 mRNA. *Proc Natl Acad Sci U S A,* 100, 12666-71

Zhou, M.; Halanski, M. A.; Radonovich, M. F.; Kashanchi, F.; Peng, J.; Price, D. H. & Brady, J. N. (2000). Tat modifies the activity of CDK9 to phosphorylate serine 5 of the RNA polymerase II carboxyl-terminal domain during human immunodeficiency virus type 1 transcription. *Mol Cell Biol,* 20, 5077-86

Zhou, Q. & Sharp, P. A. (1996). Tat-SF1: cofactor for stimulation of transcriptional elongation by HIV-1 Tat. *Science,* 274, 605-10

5

Subversion of RNA Processing Pathways by the Hepatitis *delta* Virus

Yasnee Beeharry and Martin Pelchat
University of Ottawa
Canada

1. Introduction

Viruses are the most opportunistic pathogens, since they extensively use host cell components for their replication. Among the various host factors usurped by viruses, proteins involved in RNA processing pathways are frequently used to regulate their own replication and to affect host protein expression (Lai, 1998). Over the years, the study of viral replication led to discoveries on how cellular RNA processing pathways are complex and how each step is crucial and extremely regulated. In addition to provide a better understanding of viral pathogenesis, investigation of viruses continue to be used as tools to understand the normal cellular RNA processing pathways and to identify new actors or new functions of known components.

The hepatitis *delta* virus (HDV) is a fascinating model. This virus is the smallest known pathogenic RNA capable of infecting human cells, and has to rely more heavily than any other viruses on host proteins for its replication (for general reviews of HDV biology and replication, see (Lai, 2005; Taylor, 2006, 2009; Tseng & Lai, 2009; Pascarella & Negro, 2011)). In this chapter, we present the current knowledge of the use of host proteins involved in RNA processing pathways by HDV, from RNA synthesis to RNA maturation. In addition, we discuss the potential contribution of these proteins to the life cycle of HDV, and possible impacts these interactions might have on natural host processes during an HDV infection.

2. The hepatitis *delta* virus

HDV is a defective RNA virus that requires the hepatitis B virus (HBV) envelope proteins for encapsidation and dissemination (Rizzetto et al., 1977). Co- and super-infection of HBV carriers by HDV causes acute exacerbation of the disease and subsequent chronic hepatitis. People with HDV superinfection have a much greater risk of developing fulminant hepatitis, hepatocellular carcinoma, cirrhosis, and liver failure than people infected with HBV alone (Fattovich et al., 2004; Su et al., 2006; Taylor, 2006; Romeo et al., 2009).

As stated above, HDV is the smallest known human RNA pathogen. It consists of a circular negative single-stranded RNA of about 1,680 nucleotides. This RNA can fold on itself using 74% intra-molecular base-pairing to form an unbranched, rod-like structure that can be divided into two domains (Fig. 1; reviewed by (Chen et al., 1986; Lai, 2005; Taylor, 2006, 2009; Tseng & Lai, 2009)). The left-terminal domain (~360 nt) includes both genomic and antigenomic self-cleaving motifs (i.e. *delta* ribozymes or δRz). The right-terminal domain contains a single open reading frame (ORF) encoding two viral proteins produced alternatively: the small HDAg (HDAg-S) and the large HDAg (HDAg-L; Weiner et al., 1988). The difference between these two proteins is that HDAg-L contains 19 additional amino acids at its C-terminus. During replication, post-transcriptional editing of HDV antigenomic RNA results in transcriptional read-through from the HDAg-S gene (24 kDa; 195 amino acids) and to the production of HDAg-L (27 kDa; 214 amino acids; Casey et al., 1992; Casey & Gerin, 1995; Wong & Lazinski, 2002). Although they are mostly identical, each protein has a distinct function. HDAg-S is essential for HDV replication (Kuo et al., 1989; Yamaguchi et al., 2001), while the HDAg-L is necessary for virion assembly and is reported to be a dominant negative inhibitor of replication (Chao et al., 1990; Chang et al., 1991; Ryu et al., 1992; Sureau et al., 1992; Lee et al., 1995).

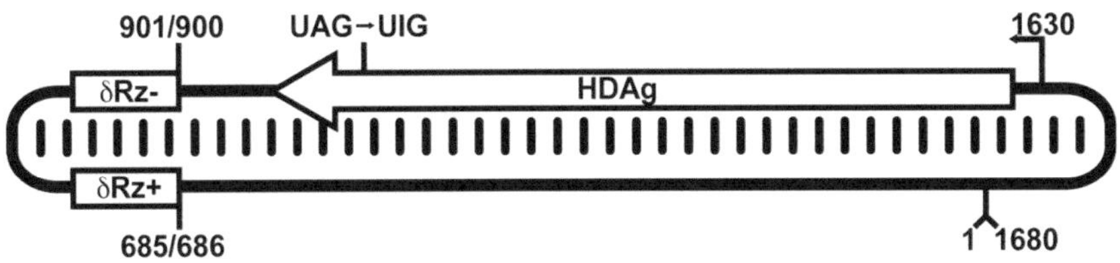

Fig. 1. The Hepatitis *delta* virus RNA genome. The HDV genome is depicted as a superposition of both genomic and antigenomic polarities. The *delta* ribozyme motifs (δRz) and their respective cleavage sites are indicated. The post-transcriptional editing performed by ADAR-1 is also indicated on the top stand. The arrows indicate the proposed HDAg mRNA initiation site. Numbering is in accordance with (Kuo et al., 1988).

HDAgs are RNA binding proteins that associate with HDV genomic RNA to form ribonucleoprotein (RNP) complexes in the HDV-containing HBV virion and in transfected cells (Chang et al., 1988; Niranjanakumari et al., 2002; Chang et al., 2008). This binding is likely facilitated by the rod-like structure adopted by the HDV RNA genome. In addition, HDAg-S can function as an RNA chaperone and modulate the ribozyme activity of HDV RNA (Wang et al., 2003), and is proposed to shuttle HDV RNA to the nucleus for replication, to the cytosol for packaging and export (Ryu et al., 1993; Lai, 2005; Taylor, 2006), and to modulate both HDV transcription and replication (Yamaguchi et al., 2001). Both HDAgs are post-translationally modified (i.e. serine and threonine phosphorylation (Chang et al., 1988; Mu et al., 1999; Mu et al., 2001), arginine methylation (Li et al., 2004), lysine acetylation (Mu et al., 2004), and cysteine farnesylation (Glenn et al., 1992; Otto & Casey, 1996)). These modifications regulate intermolecular interactions affecting subcellular localization of HDAgs and HDV RNA synthesis (Mu et al., 2001; Li et al., 2004; Mu et al., 2004).

Replication of HDV RNA is considered to take place in the nucleus of the infected cells using a symmetrical rolling cycle mechanism (Fig. 2; Taylor, 2009). Replication of the infectious circular RNA monomer (which is assigned genomic polarity by convention and accumulates to a greater intracellular abundance than the antigenomic species) produces linear, multimeric strands which are subsequently cleaved by endogenous ribozymes and ligated, yielding antigenomic circular RNA monomers (~30,000 copies). Using the latter RNAs as templates, the same three steps are repeated to generate the genomic RNA progeny (~300,000 copies). A third RNA also accumulates during replication, which corresponds to the unique HDV mRNA (~600 copies).

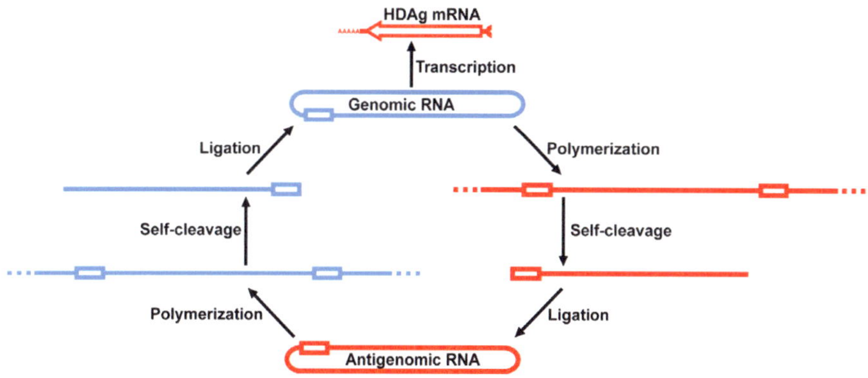

Fig. 2. Symmetrical rolling cycle mechanism used by HDV to replicate its RNA genome. Genomic RNA (blue) serves as a template for the synthesis of antigenomic RNA (red) multimers, which self-cleave and are ligated to form circular antigenomic RNA monomers. The antigenomic RNA monomers are used to synthetize circular genomic RNA monomers using the same steps. Genomic RNA also serve as a template for the transcription of HDAg mRNA.

3. The pathogenesis of hepatitis *delta* virus

Despite its apparent simplicity, HDV causes one of the most serious and rapidly progressive viral hepatitis. It provokes severe acute and chronic liver diseases, and it is associated with the development of hepatocellular carcinoma (Fattovich et al., 2004; Su et al., 2006; Taylor, 2006; Romeo et al., 2009). Interestingly, it was found that HBV replication is repressed in the presence of HDV (Krogsgaard et al., 1987; Farci et al., 1988), suggesting that the induced liver damage is likely caused by HDV replication rather than by HBV.

Since the genome of HDV can replicate in animal cells independently of HBV, many experimental systems using transfection of mammalian cells have examined the impact of the accumulation of HDAg and/or HDV RNA on the phenotype of cells in culture. It has been suggested that expression of HDAg-S or HDAg-L in mammalian cells might cause HDV pathogenesis (Cole et al., 1991; Cole et al., 1993). In contrast, some reports have shown that HDV RNA replication, rather than expression of the HDAgs, might be responsible for the cytopathic effects (Wang et al., 2001). At low concentrations of HDAg-S and without HDAg-L, low levels of HDV genome replication was reported to be able to proceed for at least 2 years without any deleterious effects on the host cell (Chang et al., 2005). When higher level of HDV RNA was induced, cell-cycle arrest in G1/G0 was observed followed by cell death (Chang et al., 2005). Using such systems, experiments have shown that when HDAg and/or HDV RNA are over-expressed, host proteins involved in regulation of cell metabolism and energy pathways, nucleic acid and protein metabolism, transport, signal transduction, apoptosis, and cell growth and maintenance are differentially produced (Mota et al., 2008; Mota et al., 2009). During viral replication, interaction of host factors with both HDAg and the HDV RNA genome might thus affect normal cellular activities.

4. Hijacking of cellular RNA processing machinery by HDV

Because HDV has an extremely limited protein coding capacity, it is completely dependent on its host cell for its replication. HDV has to interact and divert several proteins during its life cycle, including those in the nucleus involved in both viral replication and transcription and those in the cytoplasm that are required for the production of HDAgs. The high accumulation of HDV RNA in infected cells (Chen et al., 1986) suggests that the interaction of HDV RNA with host factors might interfere with several of the normal cellular functions, thereby eliciting the virus' pathogenic effect. Over the last few years, studies have investigated cellular proteins that might interact with either HDAgs or HDV RNA. Several of these proteins are involved in RNA processing, including RNA polymerase subunits, heterogeneous ribonucleoproteins (hnRNPs), RNA helicases, RNA-binding proteins, and both transcription and splicing factors (for a review, see (Greco-Stewart & Pelchat, 2010)). However, the physiological significance of the interaction of most of these proteins remains enigmatic and the identification of additional host factors involved in viral replication is still required to gain a better understanding of both HDV replication and the associated pathogenicity.

4.1 HDV uses host RNA polymerase(s) for both its replication and transcription.

Because HDV does not encode its own replicase, host DNA-dependent RNA polymerases (RNAPs) are considered to be involved in the replication and transcription of HDV RNAs. Several approaches have been used to identify the host RNAP(s) involved in HDV replication/transcription and to study how this redirection from DNA to RNA templates occurs. However, it is largely unknown how the RNA-dependent RNA synthesis of HDV proceeds and there is still controversy on the identity of the RNAP(s) involved in HDV replication.

Many studies using cultured cells and cell extracts have provided evidence of the involvement of RNAP II in HDV replication based on the sensitivity of the accumulation of HDV mRNA and processed unit-length genomic HDV RNAs to low levels of α-amanitin, a mycotoxin that inhibits DNA-dependent RNA synthesis by RNAP II (MacNaughton et al., 1991; Fu & Taylor, 1993; Filipovska & Konarska, 2000; Moraleda & Taylor, 2001; Chang et al., 2008). These results were substantiated by experiments using cells containing an α-amanitin-resistant allele of the largest subunit of RNAP II, which partially relieved transcription inhibition by α-aminitin (Filipovska & Konarska, 2000). RNAP II is furthermore speculated to be involved in the transcription of the HDAg mRNA because, *in vivo*, this mRNA was shown to be post-transcriptionally processed with a 5'-cap and a 3'-poly(A) tail, which are typical features of transcripts generated by RNAP II (Gudima et al., 1999).

Synthesis of complementary strands was possible in transcription assays using nuclear extract (NE) from HeLa cells and RNA derived from the left terminal stem-loop domain of antigenomic HDV RNA (Filipovska & Konarska, 2000). Accumulation of this RNA product was highly sensitive to α-amanitin. This sensitivity was partially abrogated in experiments conducted in NE from cells containing an α-amanitin-resistant allele of the largest subunit of RNAP II, suggesting the involvement of RNAP II in this reaction. Interestingly, the transcription did not proceed by *de novo* initiation, but rather by cleavage of the RNA template followed by extension of the new 3′ end, generating a chimeric template/transcript RNA product. In addition, transcription stopped after the elongation of only 41 nucleotides, and addition of HDAg-S allowed the RNA synthesis to resume (Filipovska & Konarska, 2000). Although not believed to be required for the initiation of RNA synthesis, HDAg-S was suggested to be implicated in the regulation of the elongation reaction through direct binding to RNAP II and displacement of the elongation repressors NELF and DSIF

(Yamaguchi et al., 2001; Yamaguchi et al., 2007). Interestingly, HDAg has been shown to affect transcription from numerous bacterial and eukaryotic promoters (Brazas & Ganem, 1996; Lo et al., 1998; Wei & Ganem, 1998). For example, transcription from the serum response element (SRE) pathway was reported to be stimulated by HDAg-L in a manner independent of the binding of the serum response factor (SRF) protein (Goto et al., 2000; Goto et al., 2003). Because HDAg directly binds RNAP II and stimulates transcription elongation (Yamaguchi et al., 2001), it is possible that this protein affects the rate of host mRNA transcription, and consequently some RNA processing events.

Recently, RNAP II was reported to interact with HDV-derived RNAs at sites located within the terminal stem-loop domains of both polarities of HDV RNA (Greco-Stewart et al., 2007; Abrahem & Pelchat, 2008; Chang et al., 2008). Mutagenesis near these tips of the rod affects both HDV accumulation in cells and RNAP II binding *in vitro* (Beard et al., 1996; Greco-Stewart et al., 2007; Abrahem & Pelchat, 2008). To obtain insights into the recognition of HDV RNA promoter by RNAP II, an RNA fragment derived from the right terminal stem-loop region of genomic HDV RNA was used. This RNA fragment includes the reported initiation site for HDAg mRNA transcription (i.e. position 1630; Gudima et al., 2000) and it has been used in several investigations as templates for *in vitro* transcription using NE (Beard et al., 1996; Abrahem & Pelchat, 2008). Inhibition of HDV transcription by an antibody raised against the C-terminal domain of RNAP II, and direct binding of the RNA polymerase II confirmed that this HDV-derived RNA acts as a promoter for RNAP II (Abrahem & Pelchat, 2008). Using RNA affinity chromatography, it was established that an active RNAP II pre-initiation complex forms on this RNA promoter, and that this complex contains the same RNAP II subunits as those found on a typical DNA promoter during promoter recognition (i.e. RNAP II, TFIIA, TFIIB, TFIID, TFIIE, TFIIF, TFIIH, and TFIIS; Abrahem & Pelchat, 2008). In addition, analogous to what is observed to occur on DNA promoters during transcription (Yudkovsky et al., 2000), it was found that a re-initiation complex (i.e. TFIIA, TFIID, and TFIIE) might remain on the RNA promoter following transcription initiation (Abrahem & Pelchat, 2008). Furthermore, the direct binding of the TATA-binding protein was demonstrated, and it was suggested that this protein might be required to nucleate the RNAP II pre-initiation complex on the RNA promoter (Abrahem & Pelchat, 2008). Finally, the tertiary structure of purified RNAP II engaged in transcription on an HDV-RNA promoter has been reported (Lehmann et al., 2007). Superposing the DNA and RNA template-product crystal structures on the RNAP II transcription active site showed that they both occupied the same site. This finding suggests that RNAP II is recognizing RNA and DNA templates in similar way.

In contrast to the genomic RNA and HDAg mRNA, the synthesis of the antigenomic species has been shown to be resistant to higher doses of α-amanitin and to take place in the nucleolus, suggesting the involvement of another yet unknown RNAP in the life cycle of HDV (Modahl et al., 2000; Macnaughton et al., 2002; Li et al., 2006). It has been hypothesized that RNAP I or an RNAP I-like polymerase might be involved in HDV replication, because *in vitro* antigenomic HDV RNA synthesis is significantly decreased upon immunodepletion of the NE with an α-SL1 antibody (Li et al., 2006), and both polarities of HDV RNA were shown to associate with RNAP I in cells replicating HDV RNA (Greco-Stewart et al., 2009). Similarly, a role for RNAP III was also suggested based on its association with the HDV RNA genome in cells replicating HDV (Greco-Stewart et al., 2009). However, whether or not these associations are relevant for HDV replication is uncertain.

4.2 Interaction of host proteins with HDAgs.

Several RNA helicases were found to interact with HDAgs, including nucleolin, nucleophosmin, DDX1 and DHX15 (Lee et al., 1998; Huang et al., 2001; Cao et al., 2009). Nucleolin is a multifunctional nuclear phosphoprotein with both DNA/RNA helicase and ATPase activities, and is involved in several processes, including synthesis and maturation of the ribosome, cell proliferation and growth, nuclear trafficking, cytokinesis, nucleogenesis, transcriptional repression, replication, signal transduction, and chromosome remodelling (Tuteja & Tuteja, 1998). The nucleolin-binding domain of HDAgs is conserved among HDV variants, and it was shown that this domain is required for nucleolar targeting and accumulation of HDV RNA. Like Nucleolin, nucleophosmin is another multifunctional nuclear phosphoprotein that has been shown to interact with both HDAg-S and HDAg-L (Huang et al., 2001). This protein is involved in cell growth and proliferation, nuclear shuttling, and ribosome biogenesis. Nucleophosmin was reported to be upregulated in cells replicating HDV and to co-localize with HDAg in the nucleolus (Okuwaki, 2008). Both DDX1 and DHX15 are ATP-dependent RNA helicases involved in cellular processes such as alteration of RNA secondary structure during translation initiation, splicing, and both ribosome and spliceosome assembly (de la Cruz et al., 1999; Wen et al., 2008). Although the function of all these RNA helicases in HDV replication is unknown, their levels correlates with the amount of HDV RNA present in cells (Huang et al., 2001; Cao et al., 2009), suggesting that they might enhance HDV replication by affecting the localization of HDV RNPs. Alternatively, they might assist to the refolding of the HDV RNA genome during viral replication (Ghisolfi et al., 1992; Tuteja & Tuteja, 1998). However, it is possible that their interaction with HDAgs might be indirect since all the interactions were also observed in the absence of HDV replication (Hiscox, 2002; Cao et al., 2009; Han et al., 2009).

HDAg-S was also found to interact with many proteins capable of associating with the Argonaute (Ago) proteins, and suspected to be involved in miRNA-mediated silencing (Haussecker et al., 2008; Cao et al., 2009). Using a combined proteomic-RNAi screen, several RNA-binding proteins (IMP2, IMP3, RALY, RBM14, ILF2, and ILF3), the polyadenylate-binding protein 4 (BABPC4), and the putative RNA helicase MOV10 were found to be required for efficient HDV replication (Haussecker et al., 2008; Cao et al., 2009). Interestingly, HDV accumulation was found to be diminished only when Ago4 expression wass prevented, but not in the absence of Ago1-3 (Haussecker et al., 2008). Although the precise function of all these proteins for HDV is unclear, it was suggested that some uncharacterized downstream effectors in the microRNA (miRNA) interference pathway might remodel HDV RNA and facilitate HDV replication/transcription (Haussecker et al., 2008). It is also possible that during HDV replication, specific miRNA pathways might be deregulated.

4.3 Interaction of host proteins with the HDV RNA genome.

An essential host protein for the progression of HDV infection is the adenosine deaminase that acts on RNA (ADAR). This enzyme is involved in site-selective RNA editing, by changing specific adenosine residues to inosine (Fig. 1; Casey et al., 1992; Casey & Gerin, 1995). The small isoform of adenosine deaminase acting on RNA (ADAR-1) performs the post-transcriptional RNA editing of the HDV antigenome leading to the production of HDAg-L (Wong & Lazinski, 2002). Specifically, during HDV replication, the UAG amber termination codon of HDAg-S is converted to UIG on the antigenomic RNA genome. When genomic RNA is generated from the modified antigenome, inosine is read as guanine yielding a codon for tryptophan instead of a stop codon. This modification is retained in subsequent rounds of replication and results in translational readthrough which produces HDAg-L. HDAg-S was shown to inhibit this editing event (Polson et al., 1998), thus delaying HDAg-L production and regulating HDV life cycle. As stated above, HDV RNA accumulating at high levels was shown to be pathogenic to the cell (Chang et al., 2005). Thus, it is possible that during a typical HDV infection, HDV RNA-editing by ADAR-1, with the appearance of HDAg-L and the resulting down-regulation of viral RNA replication might have been selected to insure cell survival.

Recently, several approaches were used to identify additional host proteins that might be involved in HDV replication using HDV-derived RNA fragments as baits (Sikora et al., 2009). These studies led to the identification of SC35, ASF/SF2, the heterogeneous ribonucleoproteins L (hnRNP-L), the polypyrimidine tract-binding (PTB) protein-associated splicing factor (PSF), p54nrb, the glyceraldehyde 3-phosphate dehydrogenase (GAPDH), and the eukaryotic translation elongation factor 1 alpha 1 (eEF1A1). Due to their specific interactions with both polarities of HDV RNA (Sikora et al., 2009), it is possible that these RNA processing proteins could play a role in HDV RNA biology.

SC35, ASF/SF2 and hnRNP-L are abundant nuclear proteins playing important roles in pre-mRNA splicing and various RNA metabolism pathways (Hastings & Krainer, 2001). Both ASF/SF2 and hnRNP-L have also been shown to enhance cytoplasmic accumulation of an intronless mRNA (Liu & Mertz, 1995; Huang & Steitz, 2001). For example, hnRNP-L was reported to enhance cytoplasmic export of the herpes simplex virus thymidine kinase intronless mRNA by binding to the pre-mRNA processing enhancer (PPE; Liu & Mertz, 1995). Although SC35, ASF/SF2 and hnRNP-L have the ability to bind to the HDV RNA genome (Sikora et al., 2009), the functions of these proteins in the HDV life cycle is unknown. One possibility is that they might have a role in HDV RNA cellular localization, since HDV RNA is intronless. Furthermore, because hnRNP-L can also interact with HDAg-S (Cao et al., 2009), a complex of these two proteins might modulate HDV RNA shuttling in the cell. HDV RNA was shown to transiently co-localize with SC35 in nuclear speckles, and SC35 was reported to be binding HDV RNA during active transcription by RNAP II (Bichko & Taylor, 1996; Abrahem & Pelchat, 2008). It is thus possible that SC35 might have a role in HDV RNA transcription. The interaction of HDV RNA with these proteins might also give clues to HDV pathogenesis. Dysregulation of the splicing pathways have been associated with cell transformation and tumorogenesis (Castiglioni et al., 2006; Lee et al., 2006; Pospisil et al., 2006). ASF/SF2 is also involved in the maintenance of genome integrity. It was reported that stable RNA-DNA hybrids (R-loops), that form between nascent RNA transcripts and template DNA, accumulate in ASF/SF2-depleted cells (Li & Manley, 2005; Li et al., 2005). Although not tested, it is possible that under high HDV RNA accumulation, ASF/SF2 might be diverted from protecting chromosomal DNA, which in turn could lead to accumulation of R-loops, ultimately leading to genomic instability, a characteristic of almost all human cancers.

Two additional host proteins known to be involved in splicing were also found to bind HDV RNA: PSF and p54nrb (Greco-Stewart et al., 2006; Sikora et al., 2009). PSF is a multifunctional protein involved in many processes such as splicing, polyadenylation, transcriptional regulation, retention of defective RNAs, nucleic acid unwinding and annealing, nuclear shuttling, and pH homeostasis (Shav-Tal & Zipori, 2002). P54nrb is related to PSF, and both proteins share homology within their C-terminal portions (Dong et al., 1993). PSF forms a heterotetramer with p54nrb, and together they were shown to interact with the C-terminal domain (CTD) of RNAP II during both transcription initiation and elongation (Emili et al., 2002). It is also suggested that PSF might be able to interact with RNA and the CTD of RNAP II simultaneously (Emili et al., 2002). Using co-immunoprecipitations and electrophoretic mobility shift assays of a series of HDV-derived RNAs with purified, recombinant hexahistidine-tagged PSF, it was determined that PSF binds directly to terminal stem-loop domains of both polarities of HDV RNA at locations corresponding to the regions bound by RNAP II (Greco-Stewart et al., 2006), including a section of the HDV RNA genome reported to have RNA promoter activity (Beard et al., 1996; Abrahem & Pelchat, 2008). Recent results indicate that RNAP II interaction with HDV RNA might require both the PSF-HDV RNA interaction and the RNAP II-PSF interaction (Greco-Stewart and Pelchat, unpublished data). This suggests that PSF might provide a direct physical link between HDV RNA and RNAP II to promote initial binding of RNAP II and subsequent transcription on an HDV RNA template. The interaction of PSF with HDV RNA might also provide a mechanism for HDV pathogenesis. PSF mutations have been identified in both cervical cancer and papillary renal carcinoma cell lineages, and PSF dysregulation is associated with induction of several oncogenes (Clark et al., 1997; Benn et al., 2000; Song et al., 2004; Song et al., 2005; Li et al., 2009; Wang et al., 2009). More importantly, it was shown that noncoding RNAs can bind PSF and reverse PSF-mediated repression of several proto-oncogenes, thus promoting cell proliferation and oncogenesis (Song et al., 2004; Song et al., 2005). Thus, it is possible that the interaction of PSF with HDV RNA can reverse PSF repression and promote liver tumor development.

GAPDH was found to bind to the extremities of both polarities of the HDV RNA genome (Lin et al., 2000; Sikora et al., 2009). GAPDH is an enzyme historically known to be involved in glycolysis. In addition to this metabolic role, GAPDH is a multifunctional protein involved in apoptotic cell death, DNA proofreading, nuclear fusion, telomere maintenance, nuclear translocation, cell entry into S-phase, and hyperglycemic stress (Sirover, 2005). GAPDH might also be involved in transcriptional regulation, as it associates with Schizosaccharomyces pombe RNAP II (Mitsuzawa et al., 2005), stimulates RNAP II transcription in Xenopus laevis oocyte (Morgenegg et al., 1986), and was reported to transcriptionally activate histone H2B (Zheng et al., 2003). Although the precise function of GAPDH in HDV biology is still unknown, this protein was reported to facilitate the shuttling of HDV RNA to the nucleus, and to act as a molecular chaperone enhancing *delta* ribozyme activity almost two-fold (Lin et al., 2000). Interestingly, GAPDH can also bind both the 5′-UTR (+) of the hepatitis A virus and the 3′-UTR (+/-) of the human parainfluenza virus-3 (De et al., 1996; Schultz et al., 1996). These interactions were suggested to have a role in RNA-dependent viral RNA synthesis of these two viruses. Because GAPDH plays essential roles in several cellular processes, it is possible that the high level of HDV RNA occurring during infection might affect one or more GAPDH activities and contribute to liver disease.

Recently, the eukaryotic translation elongation factor 1 alpha 1 (eEF1A1) was reported to interact with both polarities of the HDV RNA genome (Sikora et al., 2009). eEF1A1 is mostly known for its role in translation where it binds and delivers aminoacyl-tRNA to the ribosome (Brands et al., 1986). Interestingly, eEF1A1 is one of the protein repetitively reported to be involved in viral RNA synthesis. eEF1A1 associates and enhances the RNA-dependent RNA polymerase activities of poliovirus, vesicular stomatitis virus, turnip yellow mosaic virus, and West Nile virus (Joshi et al., 1986; Harris et al., 1994; Blackwell & Brinton, 1997; Das et al.,

1998). eEF1A1 has also been reported to be involved in the recruitment of HIV RNA to RNAP II using the HIV TAR element (Wu-Baer et al., 1996). More importantly, eEF1A1 was recently shown to interact with the peach latent mosaic viroid (Dube et al., 2009). Viroids are RNA pathogens very similar to HDV, because they have no replicase and have to rely heavily on their hosts. They are a small, single-stranded, circular RNA pathogens able to infect plants and do not encode any proteins (Flores et al., 2011). Although the function for eEF1A1 interaction with HDV RNA is still unknown, based on its involvement in viral RNA synthesis, it is tempting to speculate that this protein might enhance the RNAP II-mediated replication of HDV RNA. Interaction of HDV RNA with eEF1A1 might also give clues to HDV pathology. In addition to its main role in cellular translation through the binding of tRNAs (Brands et al., 1986), eEF1A1 also binds other highly-structured single-stranded RNA, such as the non-coding RNA HSR1. The eEF1A1-HSR1 complex activates the heat shock transcription factor 1 (HSF1), which binds to DNA elements and induces the expression of heat shock proteins. Although not studied, it is possible that HDV RNA might compete with HSR1 for eEF1A1 binding and block a heat shock response. In agreement with this hypothesis, hsp105, which belongs to the heat shock protein 70 family which is regulated by HSF1, was found to be downregulated in Huh7 cells expressing HDV mRNA (Mota et al., 2008).

5. Conclusion

The mechanisms by which HDV infection contributes to clinical hepatitis are poorly understood. HDV is unique among human viral pathogens in that it has a very limited coding capacity and must rely heavily on host proteins for its life cycle. Over the last few years, several host proteins have been shown to interact with either HDAgs or HDV RNA. Similar to what is observed for other RNA viruses, normal cellular components associated with RNA-processing pathways appear to be exploited by HDV. However, it is likely that several of these proteins interact indirectly with the HDV components, either through host RNA or protein interaction.

Although the normal functions of these proteins are frequently linked to viral replication and/or transcription, their precise roles in both HDV biology and HDV-mediated pathogenesis still need to be clarified. However, their interaction with the HDV RNA genome is consistent with their known biological properties. Several of these proteins are very abundant and are often referred as housekeeping proteins. Nonetheless, it is possible that the high level of HDV RNA occurring during infection could divert some of these proteins from their normal cellular functions, and produce ill effects. Further investigation on these interactions is needed in order to improve our understanding of the mechanisms of both HDV replication and pathogenesis.

6. Acknowledgment

This work was funded by a Canadian Institutes of Health Research grant to M.P.

7. References

Abrahem, A., & Pelchat, M. (2008) *Formation of an RNA polymerase II preinitiation complex on an RNA promoter derived from the hepatitis delta virus RNA genome*, Nucleic Acids Res. 36, 5201-5211

Beard, M. R., MacNaughton, T. B., & Gowans, E. J. (1996) *Identification and characterization of a hepatitis delta virus RNA transcriptional promoter*, J. Virol. 70, 4986-4995

Benn, D. E., Dwight, T., Richardson, A. L., Delbridge, L., Bambach, C. P., Stowasser, M., Gordon, R. D., Marsh, D. J., & Robinson, B. G. (2000) *Sporadic and familial pheochromocytomas are associated with loss of at least two discrete intervals on chromosome 1p*, Cancer Res. 60, 7048-7051

Bichko, V. V., & Taylor, J. M. (1996) *Redistribution of the delta antigens in cells replicating the genome of hepatitis delta virus*, J. Virol. 70, 8064-8070

Blackwell, J. L., & Brinton, M. A. (1997) *Translation elongation factor-1 alpha interacts with the 3' stem-loop region of West Nile virus genomic RNA*, J. Virol. 71, 6433-6444

Brands, J. H., Maassen, J. A., van Hemert, F. J., Amons, R., & Moller, W. (1986) *The primary structure of the alpha subunit of human elongation factor 1. Structural aspects of guanine-nucleotide-binding sites*, Eur. J. Biochem. 155, 167-171

Brazas, R., & Ganem, D. (1996) *A cellular homolog of hepatitis delta antigen: implications for viral replication and evolution*, Science 274, 90-94

Cao, D., Haussecker, D., Huang, Y., & Kay, M. A. (2009) *Combined proteomic-RNAi screen for host factors involved in human hepatitis delta virus replication*, RNA 15, 1971-1979

Casey, J. L., Bergmann, K. F., Brown, T. L., & Gerin, J. L. (1992) *Structural requirements for RNA editing in hepatitis delta virus: evidence for a uridine-to-cytidine editing mechanism*, Proc. Natl. Acad. Sci. USA 89, 7149-7153

Casey, J. L., & Gerin, J. L. (1995) *Hepatitis D virus RNA editing: specific modification of adenosine in the antigenomic RNA*, J. Virol. 69, 7593-7600

Castiglioni, F., Tagliabue, E., Campiglio, M., Pupa, S. M., Balsari, A., & Menard, S. (2006) *Role of exon-16-deleted HER2 in breast carcinomas*, Endocr Relat Cancer 13, 221-232

Chang, F. L., Chen, P. J., Tu, S. J., Wang, C. J., & Chen, D. S. (1991) *The large form of hepatitis delta antigen is crucial for assembly of hepatitis delta virus*, Proc. Natl. Acad. Sci. USA 88, 8490-8494

Chang, J., Gudima, S. O., Tarn, C., Nie, X., & Taylor, J. M. (2005) *Development of a novel system to study hepatitis delta virus genome replication*, J Virol 79, 8182-8188

Chang, J., Gudima, S. O., & Taylor, J. M. (2005) *Evolution of hepatitis delta virus RNA genome following long-term replication in cell culture*, J Virol 79, 13310-13316

Chang, J., Nie, X., Chang, H. E., Han, Z., & Taylor, J. (2008) *Transcription of hepatitis delta virus RNA by RNA polymerase II*, J. Virol. 82, 1118-1127

Chang, M. F., Baker, S. C., Soe, L. H., Kamahora, T., Keck, J. G., Makino, S., Govindarajan, S., & Lai, M. M. (1988) *Human hepatitis delta antigen is a nuclear phosphoprotein with RNA-binding activity*, J. Virol. 62, 2403-2410

Chao, M., Hsieh, S. Y., & Taylor, J. (1990) *Role of two forms of hepatitis delta virus antigen: evidence for a mechanism of self-limiting genome replication*, J. Virol. 64, 5066-5069

Chen, P. J., Kalpana, G., Goldberg, J., Mason, W., Werner, B., Gerin, J., & Taylor, J. (1986) *Structure and replication of the genome of the hepatitis delta virus*, Proc. Natl. Acad. Sci. USA 83, 8774-8778

Clark, J., Lu, Y. J., Sidhar, S. K., Parker, C., Gill, S., Smedley, D., Hamoudi, R., Linehan, W. M., Shipley, J., & Cooper, C. S. (1997) *Fusion of splicing factor genes PSF and NonO (p54nrb) to the TFE3 gene in papillary renal cell carcinoma*, Oncogene 15, 2233-2239

Cole, S. M., Gowans, E. J., Macnaughton, T. B., Hall, P. D., & Burrell, C. J. (1991) *Direct evidence for cytotoxicity associated with expression of hepatitis delta virus antigen*, Hepatology 13, 845-851

Cole, S. M., Macnaughton, T. B., & Gowans, E. J. (1993) *Differential roles for HDAg-p24 and -p27 in HDV pathogenesis*, Prog Clin Biol Res 382, 131-138

Das, T., Mathur, M., Gupta, A. K., Janssen, G. M., & Banerjee, A. K. (1998) *RNA polymerase of vesicular stomatitis virus specifically associates with translation elongation factor-1 alphabetagamma for its activity*, Proc. Natl. Acad. Sci. USA 95, 1449-1454

De, B. P., Gupta, S., Zhao, H., Drazba, J. A., & Banerjee, A. K. (1996) *Specific interaction in vitro and in vivo of glyceraldehyde-3-phosphate dehydrogenase and LA protein with cis-acting RNAs of human parainfluenza virus type 3*, J Biol Chem 271, 24728-24735

de la Cruz, J., Kressler, D., & Linder, P. (1999) *Unwinding RNA in Saccharomyces cerevisiae: DEAD-box proteins and related families*, Trends Biochem Sci 24, 192-198

Dong, B., Horowitz, D. S., Kobayashi, R., & Krainer, A. R. (1993) *Purification and cDNA cloning of HeLa cell p54nrb, a nuclear protein with two RNA recognition motifs and extensive homology to human splicing factor PSF and Drosophila NONA/BJ6*, Nucleic Acids Res. 21, 4085-4092

Dube, A., Bisaillon, M., & Perreault, J. P. (2009) *Identification of Proteins from Prunus persica That Interact with Peach Latent Mosaic Viroid*, Journal of Virology 83, 12057-12067

Emili, A., Shales, M., McCracken, S., Xie, W., Tucker, P. W., Kobayashi, R., Blencowe, B. J., & Ingles, C. J. (2002) *Splicing and transcription-associated proteins PSF and p54nrb/nonO bind to the RNA polymerase II CTD*, RNA 8, 1102-1111

Farci, P., Karayiannis, P., Lai, M. E., Marongiu, F., Orgiana, G., Balestrieri, A., & Thomas, H. C. (1988) *Acute and chronic hepatitis delta virus infection: direct or indirect effect on hepatitis B virus replication?*, J Med Virol 26, 279-288

Fattovich, G., Stroffolini, T., Zagni, I., & Donato, F. (2004) *Hepatocellular carcinoma in cirrhosis: incidence and risk factors*, Gastroenterology 127, S35-50

Filipovska, J., & Konarska, M. M. (2000) *Specific HDV RNA-templated transcription by pol II in vitro*, RNA 6, 41-54

Flores, R., Grubb, D., Elleuch, A., Nohales, M. A., Delgado, S., & Gago, S. (2011) *Rolling-circle replication of viroids, viroid-like satellite RNAs and hepatitis delta virus: Variations on a theme*, RNA Biol 8,

Fu, T. B., & Taylor, J. (1993) *The RNAs of hepatitis delta virus are copied by RNA polymerase II in nuclear homogenates*, J. Virol. 67, 6965-6972

Ghisolfi, L., Joseph, G., Amalric, F., & Erard, M. (1992) *The glycine-rich domain of nucleolin has an unusual supersecondary structure responsible for its RNA-helix-destabilizing properties*, J. Biol. Chem. 267, 2955-2959

Glenn, J. S., Watson, J. A., Havel, C. M., & White, J. M. (1992) *Identification of a prenylation site in delta virus large antigen*, Science 256, 1331-1333

Goto, T., Kato, N., Ono-Nita, S. K., Yoshida, H., Otsuka, M., Shiratori, Y., & Omata, M. (2000) *Large isoform of hepatitis delta antigen activates serum response factor-associated transcription*, J. Biol. Chem. 275, 37311-37316

Goto, T., Kato, N., Yoshida, H., Otsuka, M., Moriyama, M., Shiratori, Y., Koike, K., Matsumura, M., & Omata, M. (2003) *Synergistic activation of the serum response element-dependent pathway by hepatitis B virus x protein and large-isoform hepatitis delta antigen*, J. Infect. Dis. 187, 820-828

Greco-Stewart, V. S., Miron, P., Abrahem, A., & Pelchat, M. (2007) *The human RNA polymerase II interacts with the terminal stem-loop regions of the hepatitis delta virus RNA genome*, Virology 357, 68-78

Greco-Stewart, V. S., & Pelchat, M. (2010) *Interaction of Host Cellular Proteins with Components of the Hepatitis Delta Virus*, Viruses 2, 189-212

Greco-Stewart, V. S., Schissel, E., & Pelchat, M. (2009) *The hepatitis delta virus RNA genome interacts with the human RNA polymerases I and III*, Virology 386, 12-15

Greco-Stewart, V. S., Thibault, C. S., & Pelchat, M. (2006) *Binding of the polypyrimidine tract-binding protein-associated splicing factor (PSF) to the hepatitis delta virus RNA*, Virology 356, 35-44

Gudima, S., Dingle, K., Wu, T. T., Moraleda, G., & Taylor, J. (1999) *Characterization of the 5' ends for polyadenylated RNAs synthesized during the replication of hepatitis delta virus*, J Virol 73, 6533-6539

Gudima, S., Wu, S. Y., Chiang, C. M., Moraleda, G., & Taylor, J. (2000) *Origin of hepatitis delta virus mRNA*, J. Virol. 74, 7204-7210

Han, Z., Alves, C., Gudima, S., & Taylor, J. (2009) *Intracellular localization of hepatitis delta virus proteins in the presence and absence of viral RNA accumulation*, J. Virol. 83, 6457-6463

Harris, K. S., Xiang, W., Alexander, L., Lane, W. S., Paul, A. V., & Wimmer, E. (1994) *Interaction of poliovirus polypeptide 3CDpro with the 5' and 3' termini of the poliovirus genome. Identification of viral and cellular cofactors needed for efficient binding*, J. Biol. Chem. 269, 27004-27014

Hastings, M. L., & Krainer, A. R. (2001) *Pre-mRNA splicing in the new millennium*, Curr Opin Cell Biol 13, 302-309

Haussecker, D., Cao, D., Huang, Y., Parameswaran, P., Fire, A. Z., & Kay, M. A. (2008) *Capped small RNAs and MOV10 in human hepatitis delta virus replication*, Nat. Struct. Mol. Biol. 15, 714-721

Hiscox, J. A. (2002) *The nucleolus--a gateway to viral infection?*, Arch. Virol. 147, 1077-1089

Huang, W. H., Yung, B. Y., Syu, W. J., & Lee, Y. H. (2001) *The nucleolar phosphoprotein B23 interacts with hepatitis delta antigens and modulates the hepatitis delta virus RNA replication*, J. Biol. Chem. 276, 25166-25175

Huang, Y., & Steitz, J. A. (2001) *Splicing factors SRp20 and 9G8 promote the nucleocytoplasmic export of mRNA*, Mol Cell 7, 899-905

Joshi, R. L., Ravel, J. M., & Haenni, A. L. (1986) *Interaction of turnip yellow mosaic virus Val-RNA with eukaryotic elongation factor EF-1 [alpha]. Search for a function*, EMBO J. 5, 1143-1148

Krogsgaard, K., Kryger, P., Aldershvile, J., Andersson, P., Sorensen, T. I., & Nielsen, J. O. (1987) *Delta-infection and suppression of hepatitis B virus replication in chronic HBsAg carriers*, Hepatology 7, 42-45

Kuo, M. Y., Chao, M., & Taylor, J. (1989) *Initiation of replication of the human hepatitis delta virus genome from cloned DNA: role of delta antigen*, J. Virol. 63, 1945-1950

Kuo, M. Y., Goldberg, J., Coates, L., Mason, W., Gerin, J., & Taylor, J. (1988) *Molecular cloning of hepatitis delta virus RNA from an infected woodchuck liver: sequence, structure, and applications*, J. Virol. 62, 1855-1861

Lai, M. M. (1998) *Cellular factors in the transcription and replication of viral RNA genomes: a parallel to DNA-dependent RNA transcription*, Virology 244, 1-12

Lai, M. M. (2005) *RNA replication without RNA-dependent RNA polymerase: surprises from hepatitis delta virus*, J. Virol. 79, 7951-7958

Lee, C. H., Chang, S. C., Chen, C. J., & Chang, M. F. (1998) *The nucleolin binding activity of hepatitis delta antigen is associated with nucleolus targeting*, J. Biol. Chem. 273, 7650-7656

Lee, C. Z., Chen, P. J., & Chen, D. S. (1995) *Large hepatitis delta antigen in packaging and replication inhibition: role of the carboxyl-terminal 19 amino acids and amino-terminal sequences*, J. Virol. 69, 5332-5336

Lee, E. J., Jo, M., Park, J., Zhang, W., & Lee, J. H. (2006) *Alternative splicing variants of IRF-1 lacking exons 7, 8, and 9 in cervical cancer*, Biochem Biophys Res Commun 347, 882-888

Lehmann, E., Brueckner, F., & Cramer, P. (2007) *Molecular basis of RNA-dependent RNA polymerase II activity*, Nature 450, 445-449

Li, L., Feng, T., Lian, Y., Zhang, G., Garen, A., & Song, X. (2009) *Role of human noncoding RNAs in the control of tumorigenesis*, Proc. Natl. Acad. Sci. USA 106, 12956-12961

Li, X., & Manley, J. L. (2005) *Inactivation of the SR protein splicing factor ASF/SF2 results in genomic instability*, Cell 122, 365-378

Li, X., Wang, J., & Manley, J. L. (2005) *Loss of splicing factor ASF/SF2 induces G2 cell cycle arrest and apoptosis, but inhibits internucleosomal DNA fragmentation*, Genes Dev 19, 2705-2714

Li, Y. J., Macnaughton, T., Gao, L., & Lai, M. M. (2006) *RNA-templated replication of hepatitis delta virus: genomic and antigenomic RNAs associate with different nuclear bodies*, J. Virol. 80, 6478-6486

Li, Y. J., Stallcup, M. R., & Lai, M. M. (2004) *Hepatitis delta virus antigen is methylated at arginine residues, and methylation regulates subcellular localization and RNA replication*, J. Virol. 78, 13325-13334

Lin, S. S., Chang, S. C., Wang, Y. H., Sun, C. Y., & Chang, M. F. (2000) *Specific interaction between the hepatitis delta virus RNA and glyceraldehyde 3-phosphate dehydrogenase: an enhancement on ribozyme catalysis*, Virology 271, 46-57

Liu, X., & Mertz, J. E. (1995) *HnRNP L binds a cis-acting RNA sequence element that enables intron-dependent gene expression*, Genes Dev 9, 1766-1780

Lo, K., Sheu, G. T., & Lai, M. M. (1998) *Inhibition of Cellular RNA polymerase II transcription by delta antigen of hepatitis delta virus*, Virology 247, 178-188

MacNaughton, T. B., Gowans, E. J., McNamara, S. P., & Burrell, C. J. (1991) *Hepatitis delta antigen is necessary for access of hepatitis delta virus RNA to the cell transcriptional machinery but is not part of the transcriptional complex*, Virology 184, 387-390

Macnaughton, T. B., Shi, S. T., Modahl, L. E., & Lai, M. M. (2002) *Rolling circle replication of hepatitis delta virus RNA is carried out by two different cellular RNA polymerases*, J. Virol. 76, 3920-3927

Mitsuzawa, H., Kimura, M., Kanda, E., & Ishihama, A. (2005) *Glyceraldehyde-3-phosphate dehydrogenase and actin associate with RNA polymerase II and interact with its Rpb7 subunit*, FEBS Lett 579, 48-52

Modahl, L. E., Macnaughton, T. B., Zhu, N., Johnson, D. L., & Lai, M. M. (2000) *RNA-Dependent replication and transcription of hepatitis delta virus RNA involve distinct cellular RNA polymerases*, Mol. Cell. Biol. 20, 6030-6039

Moraleda, G., & Taylor, J. (2001) *Host RNA polymerase requirements for transcription of the human hepatitis delta virus genome*, J Virol 75, 10161-10169

Morgenegg, G., Winkler, G. C., Hubscher, U., Heizmann, C. W., Mous, J., & Kuenzle, C. C. (1986) *Glyceraldehyde-3-phosphate dehydrogenase is a nonhistone protein and a possible activator of transcription in neurons*, J Neurochem 47, 54-62

Mota, S., Mendes, M., Freitas, N., Penque, D., Coelho, A. V., & Cunha, C. (2009) *Proteome analysis of a human liver carcinoma cell line stably expressing hepatitis delta virus ribonucleoproteins*, J Proteomics 72, 616-627

Mota, S., Mendes, M., Penque, D., Coelho, A. V., & Cunha, C. (2008) *Changes in the proteome of Huh7 cells induced by transient expression of hepatitis D virus RNA and antigens*, J. Proteomics 71, 71-79

Mu, J. J., Chen, D. S., & Chen, P. J. (2001) *The conserved serine 177 in the delta antigen of hepatitis delta virus is one putative phosphorylation site and is required for efficient viral RNA replication*, J. Virol. 75, 9087-9095

Mu, J. J., Tsay, Y. G., Juan, L. J., Fu, T. F., Huang, W. H., Chen, D. S., & Chen, P. J. (2004) *The small delta antigen of hepatitis delta virus is an acetylated protein and acetylation of lysine 72 may influence its cellular localization and viral RNA synthesis*, Virology 319, 60-70

Mu, J. J., Wu, H. L., Chiang, B. L., Chang, R. P., Chen, D. S., & Chen, P. J. (1999) *Characterization of the phosphorylated forms and the phosphorylated residues of hepatitis delta virus delta antigens*, J. Virol. 73, 10540-10545

Niranjanakumari, S., Lasda, E., Brazas, R., & Garcia-Blanco, M. A. (2002) *Reversible cross-linking combined with immunoprecipitation to study RNA-protein interactions in vivo*, Methods 26, 182-190

Okuwaki, M. (2008) *The structure and functions of NPM1/Nucleophsmin/B23, a multifunctional nucleolar acidic protein*, J. Biochem. 143, 441-448

Otto, J. C., & Casey, P. J. (1996) *The hepatitis delta virus large antigen is farnesylated both in vitro and in animal cells*, J. Biol. Chem. 271, 4569-4572

Pascarella, S., & Negro, F. (2011) *Hepatitis D virus: an update*, Liver Int 31, 7-21

Polson, A. G., Ley, H. L., 3rd, Bass, B. L., & Casey, J. L. (1998) *Hepatitis delta virus RNA editing is highly specific for the amber/W site and is suppressed by hepatitis delta antigen*, Mol. Cell. Biol. 18, 1919-1926

Pospisil, H., Herrmann, A., Butherus, K., Pirson, S., Reich, J. G., & Kemmner, W. (2006) *Verification of predicted alternatively spliced Wnt genes reveals two new splice variants (CTNNB1 and LRP5) and altered Axin-1 expression during tumour progression*, BMC Genomics 7, 148

Rizzetto, M., Canese, M. G., Arico, S., Crivelli, O., Trepo, C., Bonino, F., & Verme, G. (1977) *Immunofluorescence detection of new antigen-antibody system (delta/anti-delta) associated to hepatitis B virus in liver and in serum of HBsAg carriers*, Gut 18, 997-1003

Romeo, R., Del Ninno, E., Rumi, M., Russo, A., Sangiovanni, A., de Franchis, R., Ronchi, G., & Colombo, M. (2009) *A 28-year Study of the Course of Hepatitis Delta Infection, a Risk Factor for Cirrhosis and Hepatocellular Carcinoma*, Gastroenterology

Ryu, W. S., Bayer, M., & Taylor, J. (1992) *Assembly of hepatitis delta virus particles*, J. Virol. 66, 2310-2315

Ryu, W. S., Netter, H. J., Bayer, M., & Taylor, J. (1993) *Ribonucleoprotein complexes of hepatitis delta virus*, J. Virol. 67, 3281-3287

Schultz, D. E., Hardin, C. C., & Lemon, S. M. (1996) *Specific interaction of glyceraldehyde 3-phosphate dehydrogenase with the 5'-nontranslated RNA of hepatitis A virus*, J Biol Chem 271, 14134-14142

Shav-Tal, Y., & Zipori, D. (2002) *PSF and p54(nrb)/NonO--multi-functional nuclear proteins*, FEBS Lett. 531, 109-114

Sikora, D., Greco-Stewart, V. S., Miron, P., & Pelchat, M. (2009) *The hepatitis delta virus RNA genome interacts with eEF1A1, p54(nrb), hnRNP-L, GAPDH and ASF/SF2*, Virology 390, 71-78

Sirover, M. A. (2005) *New nuclear functions of the glycolytic protein, glyceraldehyde-3-phosphate dehydrogenase, in mammalian cells*, J. Cell. Biochem. 95, 45-52

Song, X., Sui, A., & Garen, A. (2004) *Binding of mouse VL30 retrotransposon RNA to PSF protein induces genes repressed by PSF: effects on steroidogenesis and oncogenesis*, Proc Natl Acad Sci U S A 101, 621-626

Song, X., Sun, Y., & Garen, A. (2005) *Roles of PSF protein and VL30 RNA in reversible gene regulation*, Proc Natl Acad Sci U S A 102, 12189-12193

Su, C. W., Huang, Y. H., Huo, T. I., Shih, H. H., Sheen, I. J., Chen, S. W., Lee, P. C., Lee, S. D., & Wu, J. C. (2006) *Genotypes and viremia of hepatitis B and D viruses are associated with outcomes of chronic hepatitis D patients*, Gastroenterology 130, 1625-1635

Sureau, C., Moriarty, A. M., Thornton, G. B., & Lanford, R. E. (1992) *Production of infectious hepatitis delta virus in vitro and neutralization with antibodies directed against hepatitis B virus pre-S antigens*, J. Virol. 66, 1241-1245

Taylor, J. M. (2006) *Hepatitis delta virus*, Virology 344, 71-76

Taylor, J. M. (2009) *Chapter 3. Replication of the hepatitis delta virus RNA genome*, Adv. Virus Res. 74, 103-121

Tseng, C. H., & Lai, M. C. (2009) *Hepatitis Delta Virus RNA Replication*, Viruses 1, 818-831

Tuteja, R., & Tuteja, N. (1998) *Nucleolin: a multifunctional major nucleolar phosphoprotein*, Crit. Rev. Biochem. Mol. Biol. 33, 407-436

Wang, C. C., Chang, T. C., Lin, C. W., Tsui, H. L., Chu, P. B., Chen, B. S., Huang, Z. S., & Wu, H. N. (2003) *Nucleic acid binding properties of the nucleic acid chaperone domain of hepatitis delta antigen*, Nucleic Acids Res. 31, 6481-6492

Wang, D., Pearlberg, J., Liu, Y. T., & Ganem, D. (2001) *Deleterious effects of hepatitis delta virus replication on host cell proliferation*, J Virol 75, 3600-3604

Wang, G., Cui, Y., Zhang, G., Garen, A., & Song, X. (2009) *Regulation of proto-oncogene transcription, cell proliferation, and tumorigenesis in mice by PSF protein and a VL30 noncoding RNA*, Proc. Natl. Acad. Sci. USA 106, 16794-16798

Wei, Y., & Ganem, D. (1998) *Activation of heterologous gene expression by the large isoform of hepatitis delta antigen*, J. Virol. 72, 2089-2096

Weiner, A. J., Choo, Q. L., Wang, K. S., Govindarajan, S., Redeker, A. G., Gerin, J. L., & Houghton, M. (1988) *A single antigenomic open reading frame of the hepatitis delta virus encodes the epitope(s) of both hepatitis delta antigen polypeptides p24 delta and p27 delta*, J. Virol. 62, 594-599

Wen, X., Tannukit, S., & Paine, M. L. (2008) *TFIP11 interacts with mDEAH9, an RNA helicase involved in spliceosome disassembly*, Int J Mol Sci 9, 2105-2113

Wong, S. K., & Lazinski, D. W. (2002) *Replicating hepatitis delta virus RNA is edited in the nucleus by the small form of ADAR1*, Proc. Natl. Acad. Sci. USA 99, 15118-15123

Wu-Baer, F., Lane, W. S., & Gaynor, R. B. (1996) *Identification of a group of cellular cofactors that stimulate the binding of RNA polymerase II and TRP-185 to human immunodeficiency virus 1 TAR RNA*, J. Biol. Chem. 271, 4201-4208

Yamaguchi, Y., Filipovska, J., Yano, K., Furuya, A., Inukai, N., Narita, T., Wada, T., Sugimoto, S., Konarska, M. M., & Handa, H. (2001) *Stimulation of RNA polymerase II elongation by hepatitis delta antigen*, Science 293, 124-127

Yamaguchi, Y., Mura, T., Chanarat, S., Okamoto, S., & Handa, H. (2007) *Hepatitis delta antigen binds to the clamp of RNA polymerase II and affects transcriptional fidelity*, Genes Cells 12, 863-875

Yudkovsky, N., Ranish, J. A., & Hahn, S. (2000) *A transcription reinitiation intermediate that is stabilized by activator,* Nature 408, 225-229

Zheng, L., Roeder, R. G., & Luo, Y. (2003) *S phase activation of the histone H2B promoter by OCA-S, a coactivator complex that contains GAPDH as a key component*, Cell 114, 255-266

Part 3

RNA Processing in Diverse Model Systems

6

Alternative Polyadenylation in Yeast: 3´-UTR Elements and Processing Factors Acting at a Distance

Mónica Lamas-Maceiras, Silvia Seoane and María A. Freire-Picos
Facultad de Ciencias, Dpto. Biología Celular & Molecular, Universidade da Coruña, Spain

1. Introduction

One of the key steps necessary to obtain a messenger RNA (mRNA) is 3´-end RNA processing. The two specific 3´-end processing reactions for genes transcribed by RNAP-II (RNA polymerase II) are pre-mRNA cleavage followed by the addition to the cleaved 3´-end of a polyadenine "tail" (polyadenylation) catalyzed by the poly-A polymerase. For some genes this 3´-end processing gets more complex due to the fact that a single gene can be transcribed in two or more mRNAs differing in their 3´-UTR length due to the presence of two or more cleavage and polyadenylation points. This multiple (or alternative) 3´-end processing is also referred to as alternative polyadenylation (APA). In this chapter we will analyze some aspects of alternative RNA processing in eukaryotes using yeast as model. Hence, we will focus on the involvement of RNA processing machinery factors and elements in the UTRs (3´-UnTranslated Regions) necessary for this processing.

1.1 Elements for 3´-end RNA processing

In the yeast *Saccharomyces cerevisiae*, this RNA processing is catalyzed by multi-subunit complexes (Fig. 1): CFIA (Cleavage Factor IA) consists of Rna14, Rna15, Clp1 and Pcf11; CFIB (Cleavage Factor IB) consists of Hrp1/Nab4 factor; Holo-CPF (holo-Cleavage and Polyadenylation Factor) consists of an APT (Associated with Pta1) subcomplex which includes Pti1, Swd2, Syc1, Ref2, two protein phosphatases, Glc7 and Ssu72, and the Pta1 factor, which appears to be a scaffold that bridges holo-CPF sub-complexes (Nedea et al., 2003) but is also involved in different interactions that modulate processing (Ghazy et al., 2009). Regarding the CPF subcomplex it consists of Cft1/Yhh1, Brr5/Ysh1 and Cft2/Ydh1, the last one is able to interact with factors involved in cleavage and also polyadenylation as Pfs2 (Kyburtz et al., 2003).

The RNA 3´-end processing machineries are relatively conserved in eukaryotes, with moderate homologies between yeasts and human processing factors (reviewed by Keller & Minvielle-Sebastia, 1997; Zhao et al., 1999; Kyburz et al., 2003).

The UTR sequences necessary for 3´-end processing (*cis* elements) are less conserved. In the mammalian system 3´-end processing is driven mainly by three elements at the 3´-UTR: the sequence AAUAAA separated 10-30 positions to the cleavage site itself and followed by a

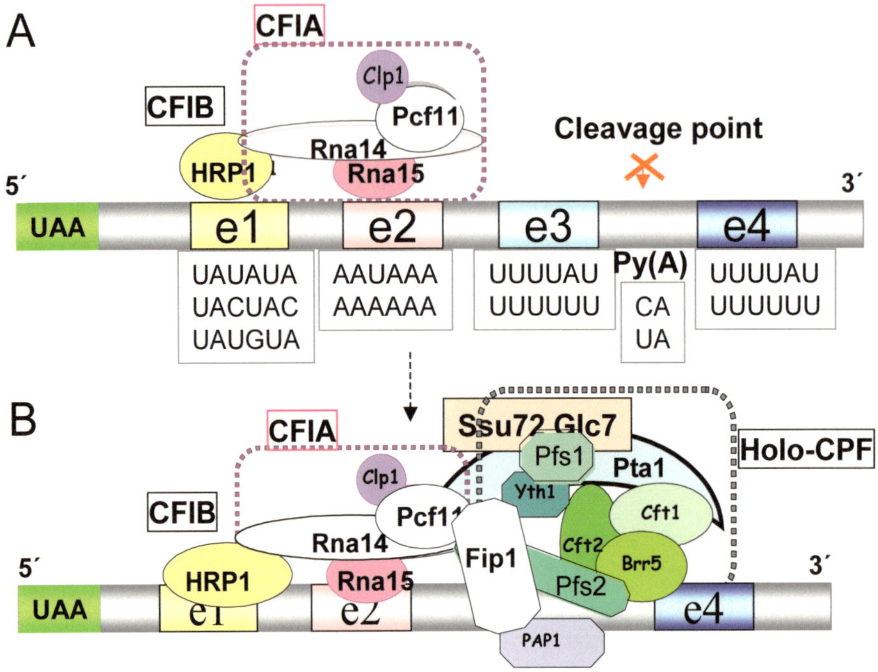

Fig. 1. Model of yeast RNA processing machinery including components of the different sub-complexes. A The UTR elements (e1 to e4) necessary for processing and their interaction with Hrp1 and Rna15 are also indicated. B A further step positioning the 3´-end machinery components at the UTR, indicating the complexes.

Downstream Sequence Element (DSE) located 30 nucleotides downstream of the cleavage site (Bilger et al., 1994).

A recent review (Danckwardt et al., 2008) summarizes variations in this pattern as the Upstream Sequence Elements (USEs). In yeast there is a more complex combination, global analyses of yeast UTRs showed (Van Helden et al., 2000; Graber et al., 1999) five elements as necessary to position the 3´-end machinery, **e1** (positioning, A-rich element), **e2** (efficiency; UA-rich element), **e3** (5´U-rich), the cleavage (Py(A)) site and **e4** (downstream, U-rich element) (reviewed by Graber et al., 2003) (Fig. 1A).

1.2 Genes with alternative polyadenylation

The yeast genes with regulated alternative polyadenylation have in common the presence of a canonical RNA processing element and a second (and in some instances more positions) non-canonical that does not include all the elements. The common feature for the less conserved is the presence of multiple AT-rich regions (Sparks & Dieckerman, 1998).

The biological sense of using regulatory alternatives of RNA processing with complex 3´-UTR is to have an alternative way to modulate gene expression and is described in many eukaryotes. In the yeast *Saccharomyces cerevisiae* APA is associated with differential regulation of gene expression. As examples, the *CBP1* gene is processed in two mRNAs (2.2 and 1.2kb) by alternative 3´-end processing, the predominance being regulated by the carbon source (Sparks et al., 1997). The *SUA7* transcript predominance changes with the growth phase (Hoppes et al., 2000), after a heat shock or when copper concentrations cause stress to cells (Kim Guisbert et al., 2007).

Alternative polyadenylation is a widespread mechanism in eukaryotes. Expressed Sequence Tag analyses estimated that 40-50% of human genes undergo alternative polyadenylation (Tian et al., 2005; Beaudoning et al., 2000), an important regulatory mechanism with implications in different types of illnesses (Edwalds- Gilbert et al, 1997; Hall-Pogar et al., 2005; Dumont et al., 2004; Caballero et al., 2004). More recently (Shepard et al., 2011) developed a method, PAS-Seq (Poly(A) Site Sequencing), to analyze polyadenylation at the transcriptome level showing a dynamic regulation of APA during stem cells differentiation in mammals. In plants APA is also a widespread mechanism; in *Arabidopsis thaliana* the flowering time control pathway depends on the alternative polyadenylation of the FCA pre-mRNA (Simpson et al., 2003). FCA is an RNA-binding protein and required for the alternative polyadenylation of its own pre-mRNA. The FY and FCA factors control these processing positions. Additionally PCFS4 (homolog to yeast Pcf11) also regulates FCA alternative processing (Xing et al., 2008).

The yeast genes with alternative polyadenylation may be classified following several criteria:

i. Regarding the UTR length and the possibility of APA regulation, there are genes processed with regulatory alternatives. In these the alternative processing positions allow to differentiate transcripts (ie, *HIS3* with 13 sites (Mahandevan et al., 1997), *SUA7* with two transcripts (1.2 and 1.4) (Hoopes et al., 2000) or the two *KlCYC1* (1.14 kb and 1.5 kb) (Freire-Picos et al., 2001). The genes with apparently non-regulatory alternatives are where the alternative sites are separated by as few as 10-11 nucleotides in the *ACT1* transcripts (Gallwith et al., 1981) or the seven variants of *YPT1* 3′-end transcripts (Heidmann et al., 1992).

ii. Regarding if the transcript alternatives include truncated coding regions as the *RNA14* or non-truncated ones as *SUA7* (Sparks & Dieckerman 1998).

While analyzing alternative polyadenylation in rice; Shen and coworkers (Shen et al., 2008) defined "microheterogeneity" in processing as the phenomenon of finding alternative poly(A) sites located within 30 nucleotides of another in the same gene due to the probably slack nature of the polyadenylation machinery. We consider that the APA for yeast genes where the alternative sites are separated by as few as 10-11 nucleotides, as the *ACT1,* are examples of microheterogeneity.

1.3 RNA processing factors involved in APA

Some components of the yeast RNA processing machinery have been involved in alternative processing selection. Different groups have described that mutations in the RNA processing factors affect poly(A) choice (Table 1). The involvement of Pcf11 (Licatalosi et al., 2002), Yhh1 (Dichtl et al., 2002), Ydh1 (Kyburz et al 2003) and Rat1 (Wong et al 2003) was studied in the gene *ACT1,* belonging to the non-regulated group and included in Table 1 as examples of microheterogeneity (M). The effects on *RNA14* processing, with truncated alternatives (T), were shown in Ssu72 (He et al., 2003) and Npl3 (Wong et al., 2007) mutants. However, until more recently with Hrp1 (Kim Guisbert et al., 2007) or with Pta1 and Pcf11 (Seoane et al., 2009a), little was known about the factors specifically involved in alternative 3′-end selection in yeast genes with regulated (and non-truncated) 3′-end alternatives, or their possible interaction with specific elements at the 3′-UTR.

Factor /mutation	Processed gene / Type	Reference
ssu72-3	*RNA14* /T	He et al., 2003
Npl3	*RNA14* /T	Wong et al., 2007
Ydh1/Cft2p	*ACT1* /M	Kyburtz et al., 2003
Rat1	*ACT1* /M	Luo et al., 2006
pcf11-2 & *mpe1-1*	*ACT1* /M	Vo et al., 2001
Pcf11	*ACT1* /M	Licatalosi et al., 2002
Yhh1	*ACT1* /M	Ditchll et al., 2002b
Hrp1	*SUA7* /**C**	Kim Guisbert et al., 2007
Pta1& Pcf11	*KlCYC1* /**C** *CBP1* /T	Seoane et al., 2009
fip1-1 & *rna14-2*	*KlCYC1*/ ***C***	Lamas-Maceiras et al., this chapter

Table 1. Yeast factors involved in alternative RNA processing. Type of APA: truncated (T) or non-truncated (C= complete) and microheterogeneity (M).

The proximal *KlCYC1* 3´-UTR contains the AU-rich element important for both proximal and distal processing (at the two wild type positions) showing long distance APA regulation, in which Pta1 and Pcf11 are also involved. Clearly, there must be more factors connecting the ***cis***-elements with the RNA processing machinery. Kim Guisbert and coworkers (Kim Guisbert et al., 2007) previously showed that Hrp1 (an RNA-binding factor and the only component of yeast CFIB) is involved in *SUA7* alternative polyadenylation. Pta1 establishes a physical interaction with Pcf11 (GST pull-down assays) (Ghazy et al., 2009). In the same work the Pta1 does not interact directly with Hrp1. Gross and Moore (2001a) previously had proposed that the Hrp1 binds directly to the e1 element and by means of its interaction with Rna14 directs Rna15 towards the e2 element (Fig. 1). Rna14 also binds Pcf11. All these interactions point out the interest to check if Rna14 is also involved in APA. We also analyzed the effect of Fip1 since this factor has an inhibitory effect on the Pap1 (polyA polymerase) activity (Zhelkovvsky et al., 1998). The *fip1-1* protein extract is defective in the poly(A) addition of *CYC1* substrate; ***in vitro***, *pta1-1* mutants have a 3´-end processing defect very similar to *fip1-1* defects (Zhao et al., 1999).

1.4 APA studies on *KlCYC1*: *cis* elements and factors involved

The long 3´-UTR (1.2 kb) of the *KlCYC1* gene from *Kluyveromyces lactis* is processed at two alternative positions (698 or 1092). The two *KlCYC1* transcripts change their predominance along the growth phase, but not with the carbon source (Freire-Picos et al., 2001). We have shown that when the UTR is split after the first processing point, thereby separating the proximal or distal sequences, they may act as independent processing elements in both *S. cerevisiae* and *K. lactis* yeast species (Seoane et al., 2005). The *KlCYC1* APA is also conserved when expressed in *S. cerevisiae*; the separation of the alternative processing positions (395 nucleotides) is a reason to use it as model to study APA in *S. cerevisiae*.

The role of several alleles of Pta1 and Pcf11 in alternative processing was studied using Pta1 and Pcf11 mutants where the predominance of *KlCYC1* and *CBP1* transcript isoforms was changed (Seoane et al., 2009). In the same work we showed that the *KlCYC1* APA is dependent on the AU-rich element located at the proximal 3´-UTR at positions 670 to 699. Mutations of this element change the transcript predominance and this effect is compensated when the mutated UTR is expressed in *pta1-1*, *pcf11-2* mutant strains. Therefore, the preference for the two alternative processing positions (proximal and distal) is directed through this AU-rich element located at the proximal UTR, and therefore acting at a distance in combination with Pta1 and Pcf11 (Seoane et al., 2009). More information is needed to better understand the mechanism. In *S. cerevisiae* Hrp1 binds to the e1, UTR element, and does not interact with Pta1, therefore, more factors need to be identified to complete the relation of factors involved in APA.

The APA determinants are the intrinsic strength of sequence elements, the concentration or activity of polyadenylation factors and/or tissue or stage-specific regulatory factors (Barabino & Keller, 1999). The involvement of RNA structure in rRNA processing has been well characterized (Rauhé and Planta, 1995). Histone mRNAs 3´-end processing is also dependent on a secondary structure, a stem-loop, positioned upstream of the cleavage site (Marzluff, 2005; Gilmartin 2005). The possible combination of RNA secondary structures with *cis* elements and/or polyadenylation factors constitutes a possible determinant for processing that is not clear in yeast genes with APA.

Taking into account the relevance of the proximal AU-rich element in the *KlCYC1* APA in the present work we analyzed two aspects of alternative RNA processing in yeast: at first an analysis of the changes caused by mutations at the *KlCYC1* proximal AU-rich element (that change transcript predominance) related to changes in the predicted RNA secondary structure and stability. Secondly, we show the involvement and effect of not previously characterized yeast RNA processing factors (Rna14 and Fip1) in *KlCYC1* APA.

2. Methodology

2.1 Strains and growth conditions

Strains FY23 (*MATa ura3-52 trp163 leu2-1*) were described previously (Madison & Winston 1997). Strains XH6 (*MATa ura3-52 leu2Δ1 trp1Δ63 his3Δ200 pta1::TRP1* [*YCpLEU2-PTA1*]) and XH15 (*MATa ura3-52 leu2Δ1 trp1Δ63 his3Δ200 pta1::TRP1* [*YCpLEU2-pta1-3*]) are an isogenic pair that have been disrupted at the chromosomal *pta1* locus (*pta1::TRP1*) (He et al., 2003) and differ from each other only by the plasmid-borne *pta1* allele. *pcf11-2*, *pcf11-9* (Amrani et al., 1997). BMA64 (*MATa ura3 leu2 ade2 his3*) ***rna14-1*** (*MATα ura3-1 trp1-1 ade2-1 leu2-3-112 his3-11,15 rna14-1*); *rna14-2* (*MATa ura3 leu2 trp1 ade2 his3 rna14-2*) (Minvielle-Sebastia et al., 1991) *fip1-1* (*MATa leu2-3 112 ura3-52 trp1 his4 fip1::LEU2/pIA23 (CEN4 TRP1 fip1-1*) (Preker et al., 1997).

Yeasts cultures, manipulations and transformations were done as previously (Seoane et al., 2009).

2.2 Northern analysis

Total RNA extractions and Northern experiments were carried out according to (Zitomer & Hall, 1976). Hybridization signals were quantitated using the Image-Quant program (Molecular Dynamics) and normalized with respect to U3 RNA. The U3 probe, corresponding to *S. cerevisiae* small nuclear RNA (snRNA) R17A, was obtained by PCR amplification with primers U3F: 5´-CGACGTACTTCAGTATGTAA-3´ and U3R: 5´-ATTTGTACCCACCCATAGAG-3'. *ACT1* and *CYC1* probes were prepared by digestion of cloned versions with specific restriction enzymes.

Normalization of mRNA signals: a double normalization was performed for better comparison among the different mutants. First, all transcripts were normalized with respect to U3. Secondly, all signals were normalized with respect to the wild type band (for single transcripts) or with respect to the upper band in the wild type strain (for multiple processing factors).

2.3 mRNA-stability experiments

Cultures of the *rpb1-1* thermosensitive RNA polymerase II mutant strain (Nonet et al., 1987) transformed with different versions of *KlCYC1* 3´-UTR were grown in CM-Ura at 30°C until they reached an OD_{600} of 0.6. Cultures were shifted to 37°C to induce a rapid shutdown of mRNA synthesis, and 10 mL samples were taken, at the times described in Figure 4.

2.4 Site-directed mutagenesis

Specific mutations (M3a) on *KlCYC1* 3´-UTR were introduced using the Stratagene QuickChange™ site-directed mutagenesis kit, using specific oligos:
ossMUT1C-1: 5´- CTATGTACTACTATTCCAAGAATACCAAATTTTATGATTATTTCT TTCTTTTTAACAACTCTACTACTTCTATTATCAAC-3´.
ossMUT1C-2: 5´-GTTGATAATAGAAGTAGTAGAGTTGTTAAAAAGAAAGAAATAA TCATAAAATTTGGTATTCTTGGAATAGTAGTACATAG-3´.
Plasmid pCT2 (Freire-Picos et al., 2001) was used as *KlCYC1* template for the site-directed mutagenesis experiments, and as a source of wild type 3´-UTR in expression experiments.

2.5 Computer programs

For secondary structure analysis the program used was RNA-Draw (Matzura et al., 1996) (http://iubio.bio.indiana.edu/soft/molbio/ibmpc/rnadraw-readme.html)
The *S. cerevisiae* mRNA 3′-processing site predictor was used to search for the yeast RNA processing determinants at 3´-UTRs http://harlequin.jax.org/polyA/ (Graber et al., 2002).

3. Results and discussion

3.1 Analysis of 3´-end processing elements in a secondary structure context

The previous analyses showed that the *KlCYC1* 3´-UTR contains multiple putative processing elements but most of them do not match canonical consensus (Freire-Picos et al., 2001). In Figure 2A the RNA processing prediction output for *KlCYC1* 3´-UTR (*S. cerevisiae* mRNA 3′-processing site predictor) is shown. The graph is combined with the experimental data of real polyadenylation positions (P1 and P2) (Freire-Picos et al., 2001). The *KlCYC1* sequences at the first processing position (P1) are identified by the program showing the highest probability peak, matching the five elements (detailed in Fig. 2B). The location of the determinant elements for processing in the proximal region contrast with the lower probability peaks shown with the sequence near the second polyadenylation position (P2) (Fig. 2A).
The *KlCYC1* complete 3´-UTR secondary structure prediction was calculated (using RNA Draw program) for the wild type sequence (Fig. 2C). As shown in the complete view, the whole UTR forms a complex squiggle structure. There is a central region (CR) where there is a confluence for: the end of the coding region, the end of the distal 3′-UTR (both encircled) and the first polyadenylation point determined experimentally. Part of this region is magnified to show the end-triplet and polyadenylation position. Interestingly, the CR includes the five elements for the proximal processing position. The distal processing point

(P2) is located almost 400 bases downstream in a region structurally different from the proximal one (Fig. 2C). The AU-rich element, previously shown as APA determinant element, partially overlaps with the e2 element and therefore is also located at the CR.

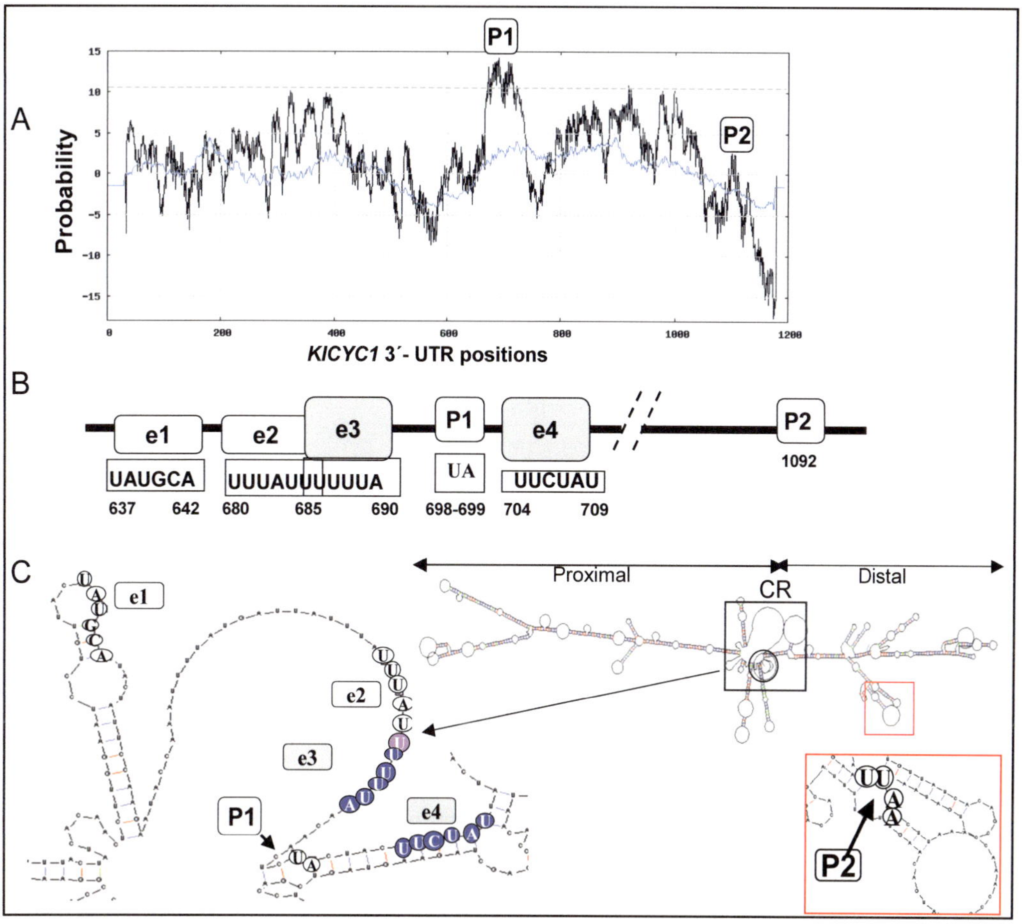

Fig. 2. The *KlCYC1* 3´-UTR. A Processing prediction output using the *S. cerevisiae* site predictor. B Detail of sequences matching the elements for the first (and canonical) processing point (P1). C Processing elements located in the context of the 3´-UTR secondary structure.

In summary, the sequences surrounding the proximal processing point (P1) correspond to canonical RNA processing sequences that are located in a central region of confluence of secondary structures and *cis* elements including the proximal AU-rich element. The sequences surrounding the distal processing point (P2) do not match the canonical consensus and do not share similarity with the secondary structure prediction surrounding P1.

The differences found in both, the *cis*-elements and the putative secondary structures, at the alternative processing points can be an important feature for a differential regulation of *KlCYC1* APA.

3.2 The APA changes caused by AU-rich mutations are more related to Pta1 than to the secondary structure

The involvement of the proximal AU-rich element (wild type and M1 or M2 mutated forms) and the *pta1-1* mutation in switching short or long distance RNA processing has been recently shown (Seoane et al., 2009). To analyze the possible implications of changes in the secondary structure derived of mutations at the AU-rich element, we analyzed the secondary structure prediction for each UTR variant (Fig. 3). In this analysis we also included a new mutant M3b where the substitution was A for C at the same positions as in M1 (Fig. 3A). To complete this analysis, the effects on *KlCYC1* transcript predominance were studied by expressing the gene in either a wild type or a *pta1-1* mutant strain.

As shown in Figure 3C, the punctual mutations in M1 clearly abolish several secondary structures at the CR encompassing the first polyadenylation site. The M2 mutant (3D), despite it having a 5 bp deletion, shows no relevant change in the structure, just a shorter duplex region indicated by an asterisk (Fig. 3D). The new mutant M3a does not change the structure prediction with respect to the wild type (Fig. 3E).

A *KlCYC1* proximal AU-rich sequence

Wt	673	5'-TTTATTTATTTATTTTTTAACAACTCTAC-3´700
M1		5'-TTATTT**T**TTT**T**TTTTTTAACAACTCTAC-3´
M2		5'-TTATTTATTTATTTTTTAACAA....AC-3´
M3a		5'-TTATTT**C**TTT**C**TTTTTTAACAACTCTAC-3´

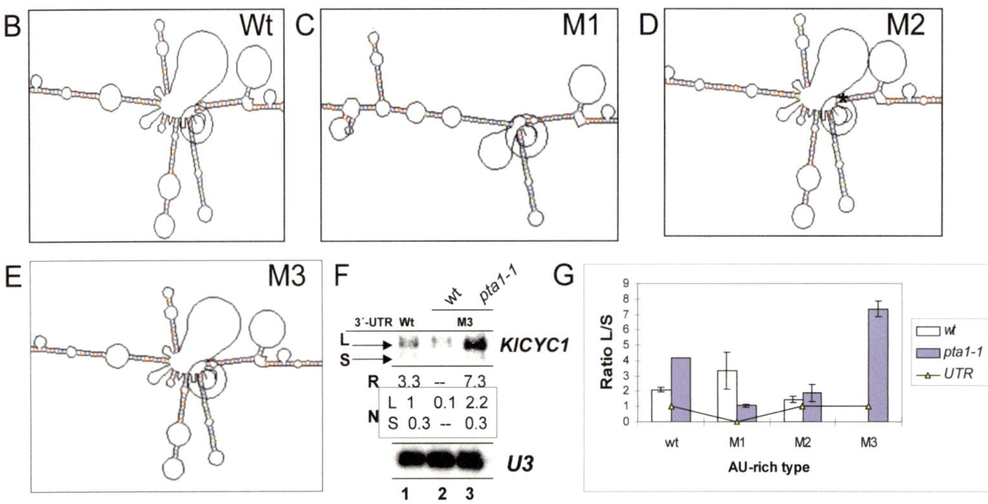

Fig. 3. Study of the predicted secondary structure changes (caused by mutations at the proximal AU-rich element) in relation to *KlCYC1* transcripts ratio. A Sequence of M1 and M2 and M3a mutations. B to E Secondary structures calculated with RNA Draw. F Expression of M3a mutation in either wild type (lane1) or *pta1-1 S. cerevisiae* strains (lanes 2 and 3) compares with the expression of a wild type 3´-UTR in a wildtype strain for Pta1 (XH6). G *KlCYC1* L/S ratios in the different UTR mutations expresed in either a wild type or a *pta1-1* mutant strain. The information of the UTR secondary structure in each mutant was included in the same graph giving to the secondary structure a value of 1 (equal or very similar to wild type) or 0 (different structure).

The M3a mutation causes a strong reduction in the two *KlCYC1* transcripts when expressed in the wild type strain (compare lanes 1 and 2) while there is a strong increase in the long transcript signal in the *pta1-1* mutant strain (lanes 2 and 3). The increase is also two fold respect to the normal expression with a wild type UTR (compare lanes 1 and 3). Therefore we found a clear enhancement in the usage of the distal processing point in the *pta1-1* mutant strain expressing the M3a mutation. This last result can be considered as a gain in the processing efficiency at the distal position only when Pta1 is mutated.

The changes in *KlCYC1* transcripts ratio (L/S) analyzed in strains and 3´-UTR mutants are shown in Figure 3G. To be able to include the secondary structure in the graph we used a binary code where the presence of the wild type UTR was considered as 1 and its absence as 0. By comparing the secondary structure variations and the changes in ratio shown in Figure 3G, we conclude that the changes in the L/S ratios are more dependent on the sequence mutations and the *pta1-1* mutant alelle than on the possible secondary structure alterations.

The *pta1-1* mutation was characterized as a non-sense mutation (*pta1-1 ocre* fragment) in the *PTA1* coding region, however, despite this mutation, a small amount of Pta1 protein is able to maintain cell viability (Zhao et al., 1999). The changes in *KlCYC1* transcript predominance are due to the low Pta1 levels present in the *pta1-1* mutant, a result that was confirmed by using the conditional degradation in Pta1-*td* degron strain (Seoane et al., 2009).

Therefore, the results with the new mutant M3a show that the *KlCYC1* APA is dependent on the AU-rich element and the Pta1 levels. The parallel secondary structure analysis with the AU-rich mutants does not seem to have an effect on *KlCYC1* APA.

3.3 Effect of the *KlCYC1* AU-rich element mutants on transcript stability

Recent stability analysis of *KlCYC1* transcripts revealed the presence of different mRNA turnover mechanisms able to operate on *KlCYC1* mRNAs under different physiological conditions (Seoane-Rosende et al., 2009). The AU-rich elements that match with the consensus UUAUUUAUU are also known as ARE (AU-Rich Elements) acting as signals to determine mRNA stability, not only in higher eukaryotes but also in yeasts (Vasudevan & Peltz., 2001). It is reasonable to consider that the AU-rich element mutated in M1 can be governing *KlCYC1* transcript stability. To determine if the AU-rich sequence present at positions 673 to 686 was also involved in *KlCYC1* transcript stability, the wild type *KlCYC1* plasmid pCT2 (Freire-Picos et al., 2001) or the site-directed mutagenesis derivatives M1 and M2 were expressed in the *rpb1-1* thermosensitive mutant strain, Figure 4 shows the effect of the mutations in *KlCYC1* transcript predominance.

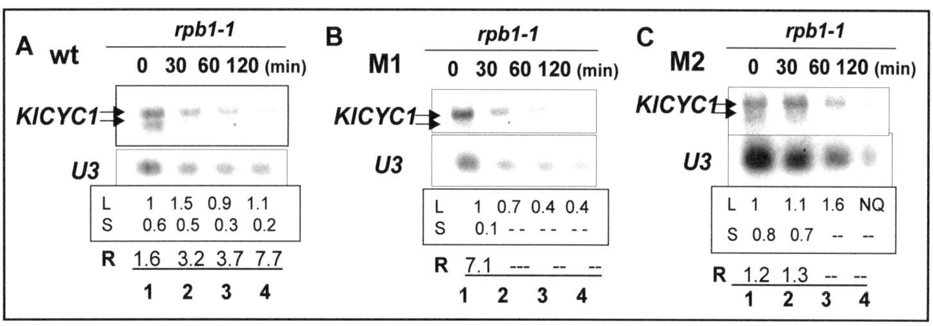

Fig. 4. Involvement of the proximal AU-rich element in transcript stability: expression in an *rpb1-1* thermosensitive mutant. A: Expression of wild type *KlCYC1* 3´-UTR (pCT2), B: Expression of M1 C: Expression of M2. Normalized values were taken with respect to U3. R: L/S Ratio. NQ: not quantitated.

At permissive temperature (30ºC) the wild type *KlCYC1* 3´-UTR expressed in *rpb1-1* has a ratio upper/lower of 1.2 (Figure 4A, lane 1). This ratio increases two-fold when the temperature is changed to 37ºC for 30 min and keeps increasing up to 7.7 after 1 hour (Figure 4A, lanes 1 to 4). This increase is due to a progressive decrease of the shorter transcript, while the longer transcript is almost invariant. Thus, both *KlCYC1* transcripts have different stabilities once transcription is abolished. The distal part of the 3´-UTR region, present only in the long transcript, is important for this stability.

Analyzing expression in the M1 mutant, the signal of the shorter transcript is very low at permissive temperature, due to effects in processing, and after 30 minutes at 37ºC is not possible to detect a signal (Figure 4B). It is important to note that in this mutant, the longer transcript reduces to the half after one hour. Therefore the AU-rich element mutated in M1 is important for the stability of the long transcript since the A to C changes cause a faster degradation of mRNAs. Hence, this AU-rich sequence is not equivalent to an ARE motif since its deletion should have caused the opposite effect.

When the same experiment is performed in M2 (where the AU-rich sequence is not mutated), the longer transcript remains stable at least up to one hour (Figure 4C), which reinforces the idea that the AU-rich element at position 674 to 686 is acting at a distance, affecting the stability of the long 3´-UTR.

3.4 The involvement of other yeast RNA processing factors in APA

Although the interplay between Pta1, Pcf11 and the AU-rich region is clear, the connection between the *cis* and *trans* factors driving APA is unknown. In the *SUA7* system the Hrp1 factor binds to an e1-like element, however, Hrp1 does not interact with Pta1 (Ghazy et al., 2009), and therefore, it is necessary to search for new factors. To identify new RNA processing factors involved in APA, and following the same procedures done previously, we expressed *KlCYC1* in yeast mutants for the RNA processing factors Rna14 and Fip1 belonging to the CFIA and PF1 complexes.

The analysis of *KlCYC1* transcript predominance is shown in Fig. 5 . The *S. cerevisiae CYC1* is included as a gene with a well characterized single processing (Guo & Sherman 1996). The *pcf11-2* and *pcf11-9* alleles, previously characterized as involved in *KlCYC1* and *CBP1* APA (Seoane et al., 2009), were included as a positive controls.

In the *rna14-2* mutant the *KlCYC1* transcripts show a 0.8 L/S ratio (Fig. 5, compare lanes 6 and 7). This ratio change is similar to that obtained by expressing the gene in *pcf11* mutants (compare lane 6 with lanes 3 and 4). Although in this mutant there is a clear reduction in mRNA levels, the results on *CYC1* and *ACT1* also show a lower expression therefore that´s a general processing effect. The *KlCYC1* transcripts are undetectable in the *rna14-1* mutant (lane 5), and from this result we cannot make conclusions on APA, nevertheless, this drastic effect does not affect the other genes tested, suggesting a more relevant role of Rna14 in *KlCYC1* 3´-end processing. Rouillard and Coworkers (2000) characterized two types of *rna14* mutants the poly(A) negatives as *rna14-1* causing defects in 3´-end maturation and those with no apparent effect in polyadenylation. The drastic result with *KlCYC1*, but not with the other analyzed genes, points towards gene specific effects in this mutant.

With respect to the *fip1-1* mutant, this mutation causes a preference of usage of the proximal processing position with respect to the wild type (Fig. 5, compare lanes 2 and 1, respectively). Regarding Fip1 the normalized transcript values with respect to U3 indicate that there is a change in processing preference rather than in upper transcript degradation, especially when comparing the result of the wild type 3′-UTR in a wild type strain.

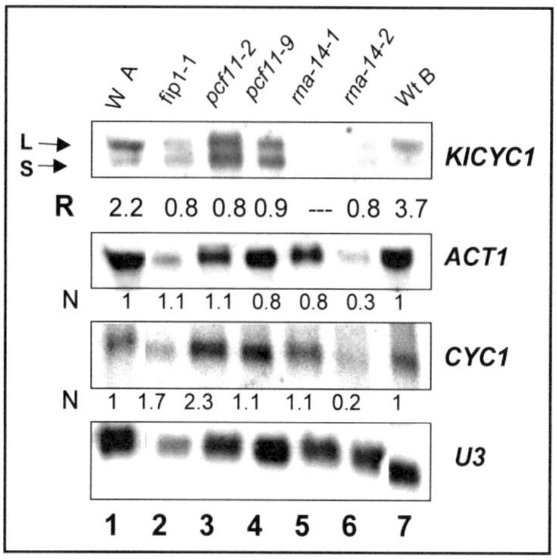

Fig. 5. Effect of RNA processing factors on *KlCYC1* APA. R Long/Short (L/S) ratio, to compare transcript predominance. N Represents the double normalized signals. Two wild type strains were included in the blot: WtA WtB corresponding to XH6 and BMA64 strains, respectively.

Transcription is coupled to RNA-processing (Proufoot, 2004) and is dependent on the carboxy-terminal repeat domain (CTD) of the Rpb1 subunit of RNAP II as reviewed in (Bentley, 2005). The coupling is mediated, in part, by Ssu72, which is a CTD phosphatase with specificity for the serine-5-P of the CTD (Hausmann et al., 2005; Krisnamurthy et al., 2004) and Pcf11, which bridges the CTD to the nascent transcript (Zhang et al., 2005). Pcf11 contains an N-terminus CID (CTD Interaction Domain) able to interact with serine-2-phosphorylated heptapeptide repeats; the *pcf11-9* mutation affects CTD binding, however, mutations in *pcf11-2* (located downstream of the CID) do not (Sadowski et al., 2003). Our results on *KlCYC1* expressed in the two mutants show similar L/S ratios (Fig. 1A), suggesting that the alternative processing effect of *pcf11-2* and *pcf11-9* does not depend on Pcf11-CTD interactions.

Future studies combining APA processing studies and *S. cerevisiae* mutants for specific CTD serine 2 kinases and phosphatases will help to clarify the regulatory role.

The data presented, combined with the information of protein-protein interactions led us to propose a model for APA in the *KlCYC1* system (Fig. 6). The factors involved in APA are shown in white. This model explains the possibility that the relationship of both pta1 and pcf11 with the *KlCYC1* AU-rich element is mediated by Rna14. This possibility is consistent with the result in Figure 4 showing the *rna14-2* effect on *KlCYC1* APA. The role of Rna14 driving Rna15 towards the e2 element (Gross & Moore 2001) makes Rna15 an excellent candidate in binding this proximal AU-rich element (which partially overlaps with the e2 canonical sequence). The specific APA changes in the *pta1-1* mutant can be explained for a more regulatory role of these factors and its specific interactions with phosphatases (as Ssu72 or Glc7) that regulate its activity (Ghazy et al., 2009). This modulation must be in response to changes in cellular conditions as the growth phase, or stress conditions. The involvement of Fip1, as a factor conecting the RNA processing machinery with the polyA polymerase (Pap1), in APA is a new data that, following the model in Figure 6, connects the RNA binding factors as Hrp1 and Rna14, and the HoloCPF, where Pta1 is the regulator, with the actual cleavage and polyadenylation site.

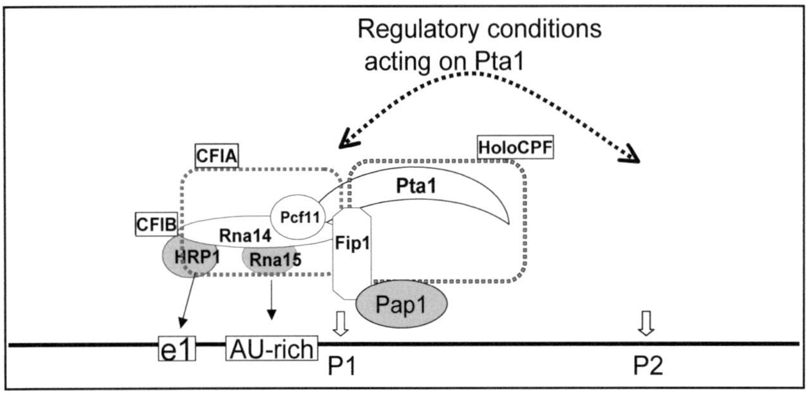

Fig. 6. Model for the interplay between factors of the RNA processing machinery involved in APA and the *KlCYC1* proximal AU-rich element. Those with effect on *KlCYC1* APA are in white. The model includes Hrp1 as factor involved in *SUA7* APA (in grey), and Rna15 as the factor connecting e2 element with the factors characterized for *KlCYC1*. The curved arrow indicates the role of Pta1 in the preferential processing point usage. Small white arrows indicate the two processing points.

4. Conclusions

The complexity of the *KlCYC1* is shown by the multiple elements present in its long 3´-UTR. The secondary structure prediction for the long *KlCYC1* 3´-UTR indicates a complex squiggle structure with a central region where there is a confluence of the 3´- UTR ends and also contains the first processing point, which corresponds with the canonical yeast RNA processing elements. The alternative processing position (P2) is in a suboptimal region and in a separate region of the secondary structure. The parallel analysis of *KlCYC1* processing in different AU-rich mutations and their corresponding secondary structure predictions do not indicate that the structures may play a relevant role in *KlCYC1* APA.

The mutation M3a combined with *pta1-1* mutation causes a strong increase in distal RNA processing, as an example of gain of function in usage of distal processing point. This is clearer when comparing with the transcripts ratio in a wild type context (for both UTR and strain). This result indicates both the importance of Pta1 in selecting proximal position and the fact that low Pta1 levels (RNA processing machineries with subestequiometric changes due to low Pta1 levels) cause an increase in processing efficiency at the distal point only when the proximal AU-rich element is mutated. In the future our goal is to analyze if conditions that regulate Pta1 *in vivo* causing changes in protein levels, phosphorylation status or interactions under different conditions are associated with APA.

KlCYC1 transcripts stability analyses indicate that the changes caused in the AU-rich element affects, the long transcript stability since its mutation causes a faster degradation of the long mRNA. Hence, this AU-rich sequence is not equivalent to an ARE motif since its deletion should have caused the opposite effect.

The analysis of *fip1-1* and *rna14-2* mutations shows an effect in alternative processing with a predominance pattern similar to that in Pcf11 mutants. This information together with the Rna14 ability to connect RNA binding factors (such as Rna15) with other components of the processing machinery is important to understand the effects of 3´-UTR mutations combined with processing factors.

The results obtained allowed us to propose the connection between the factors involved in alternative processing and the proximal AU rich element driving long and short distance 3´-end processing as shown in Figure 6.

5. Acknowledgements

We thank A. Eiroa for proofreading the English in the manuscript. This work was funded by XUGA PGIDIT 06PXIB103086PR.

6. References

Amrani, N.; Minet, N.; Wyers, F.; Dufour, M.; Aggerbeck, L. & Lacroute, F. (1997). *PCF11* encodes a third protein component of the yeast cleavage and polyadenylation factor I. *Mol. Cell. Biol.* Vol.17, No 3, pp. 1102-1109, ISBN 0270-7306

Barabino, S. M. & Keller, W. (1999). Last but not least: regulated poly(A) tail formation. *Cell* Vol. 99, No 1, pp. 9-11, ISBN 0092-8674

Beaudoing, E.; Freier, S.; Wyatt, J.R.; Claverie, J.M. & Gautheret, D. (2000). Patterns of variant polyadenylation signal usage in human genes. *Genome Res.* Vol. 10, No 7, pp. 1001-1010, ISBN 1088-9051.

Bilger, A.; Fox, C.A.; Wahle, E. & Wickens M. (1994). Nuclear polyadenylation factors recognize cytoplasmic polyadenylation elements. *Genes Dev.* Vol. 8, No 9, pp. 1106-16, ISBN 0890-9369

Bentley, D. L. (2005). Rules of engagement: co-transcriptional recruitment of pre-mRNA processing factors. *Curr. Opin. Cell. Biol.* Vol. 17, No. 3, pp. 251-256, ISBN 0955-0674.

Côté, C.A.; Greer, C.L. & Peculis, B. A. (2002). Dynamic conformational model for the role of ITS2 in pre-rRNA processing in yeast. *RNA* Vol.8, No.6, pp 786-97, ISBN 1355-8382.

Danckwardt, S.; Hentze, M. W. & Kulozik, A.E. (2008). 3´-end mRNA processing : Molecular mechanisms and implications for health and disease. *EMBO J.* Vol. 27, No 3, pp. 482-498, ISBN 0261-4189

Dichtl, B.; Blank, D.; Ohnacker, M.; Friedlein, A.; Roeder, D.; Langen, H. & Keller, W. (2002a). A role for Ssu72 in balancing RNA polymerase II transcription elongation and termination. *Mol. Cell* Vol. 10, No. 5, pp. 1139-1150, ISBN 1097-2765.

Dichtl, B., Blank, D.; Sadowski, M.; Hübner, W.; Weiser, S. & Keller, W. (2002b). Yhh1p/Cft1p directly links poly(A) site recognition and RNA polymerase II transcription termination. *EMBO J* Vol 21No15: 4125-4135 ISBN 0261-4189

Caballero, J. J.; Girón, M.D.; Vargas, A.M.; Sevillano, N.; Suárez, M.D. & Salto, R. (2004). *Biochem Biophys Res Commun.*Vol. 319, No 1, pp. 247-55, ISBN 0006-291X.

Dumont, M.; Frank, D.; Moisan, A.M.; Tranchant, M.; Soucy, P.; Breton, R.; Labrie, F.; Tavtigian, S.V. & Simard, J. (2004). Structure of primate and rodent orthologs of the prostate cancer susceptibility gene ELAC2. *Biochim. Biophys. Acta,* Vol. 1679, No. 3, pp. 230-247, ISBN 006-3002.

Edwalds-Gilbert, G.; Veraldi, K.L. & Milcarek, C. (1997). Alternative poly(A) site selection in complex transcription units: means to an end. *Nucleic Acids Res.* Vol.25, No. 13, pp. 2547-2561, ISBN 1362-4962.

Freire-Picos, M.A.; Lombardía-Ferreira, L.J.; Ramil, E.; Gonzalez-Domínguez, M. & Cerdán, M.E. (2001). The *KlCYC1* gene, a downstream region for two differentially regulated transcripts. *Yeast* Vol. 18, No. 14, 1347-1355, ISBN 0749-503X..

Ghazy, M.A.; He, X.; Singh, B.N.; Hampsey, M. & Moore C. (2009). The essential N terminus of the Pta1 scaffold protein is required for snoRNA transcription termination and Ssu72 function but is dispensable for pre-mRNA 3´-end processing. *Mol. Cell Biol* Vol. 29, No. 8, pp. 2296-2307, ISBN 0270-7306.

Gallwitz, D.; Perrin, F. & Seidel, M. (1981). The actin gene in yeast *Saccharomyces cerevisiae*: 5´ and 3´ end mapping, flanking and putative regulatory sequences. *Nucleic Acids Res.* Vol. 9, No. 23, pp. 6339-6350, ISBN 1362-4962.

Gilmartin G.M. (2005) Eukaryotic mRNA 3´pprocessing: a common means to different ends. *Genes Dev.* Vol. 19, No. 21, pp 2517-2521, ISBN 0890-9369

Graber, J.; Cantor, C. R.; Mohr, S. C. and Smith, T. F. (1999). Genomic detection of new yeast pre-mRNA 3'-end-processing signals. *Nucleic Acids Res.* Vol. 27, No. 3, pp. 888-894, ISBN 1362-4962.

Graber, J. H.; McAllister, G. D. & Smith, T.F. (2002). Probabilistic prediction of *Saccharomyces cerevisiae* mRNA 3´-processing sites. *Nucleic Acids Res.* Vol. 30, No. 8, pp. 1851-1858, ISBN 1362-4962.

Graber, J.H. (2003). Variations in yeast 3´-processing *cis*-elements correlate with transcript stability. *Trends Genet. Vol.* 19, No. 3, pp. 473-475, ISBN 0168-9479.

Gross, S. & Moore, CL (2001). Rna15 interaction with the A-rich yeast polyadenylation signal is an essential step in mRNA 3'-end formation. *Mol Cell Biol.* Vol. 21, No. 23, pp. 8045-55, ISBN 0270-7306.

Guo, Z. & Sherman, F. (1996). 3'-end-forming signals of yeast mRNA. *Trends Biochem Sci.* Vol. 21, No. 12, pp. 477-481, ISBN 0968-0004.

Hausmann, S.; Koiwa, H.; Krishnamurthy, S.; Hampsey, M. & Shuman, S. (2005). Different strategies for carboxyl-terminal domain (CTD) recognition by serine 5-specific CTD phosphatases. *JBC. Vol.* 280, No. 45, pp. 37681-37688, ISBN 1083-351X.

He, X.; Khan, A. U.; Cheng, H.; Pappas, D. L. Jr.; Hampsey, M. & Moore, C.L. (2003). Functional interactions between the transcription and mRNA 3' end processing machineries mediated by Ssu72 and Sub1. *Genes Dev.* Vol. 17, No. 8, pp. 1030-1042, ISBN 0890-9369.

Heidmann, S. B.; Obermaier, B.; Vogel, K. & Domdey, H. (1992). Identification of polyadenylation sites in *Saccharomyces cerevisiae. Mol. Cell. Biol.* Vol. 12, No. 9, pp. 4215-4229, ISBN 4215-4229.

Hoopes, B. C.; Bowers, G. D. & DiVisconte, M. J. (2000) .The two *Saccharomyces cerevisiae SUA7* (*TFIIB*) transcripts differ at the 3´-end and respond differently to stress. *Nucleic Acids Res.* Vol. 28, No. 22, pp. 4435-4443, ISBN 1362-4962.

Hall-Pogar, T.; Zhang, H.; Tian, B. & Lutz, C. S. (2005). Alternative polyadenylation of cyclooxyase-2. *Nucleic Acids Res.* Vol. 33, No. 8, pp. 2565-2579, ISBN 1362-4962.

Keller, W. & Minvielle-Sebastia, L. (1997). A comparison of mammalian and yeast 3´-end processing. *Curr Opin Cell. Biol.* Vol.9, No. 3, pp.329-336, ISBN 0955-0674.

Kim Guisbert, K. S.; Li, H. & Guthrie, C. (2007). Alternative 3´pre-mRNA processing in *Saccharomyces cerevisiae* is modulated by Nab4/Hrp1 in vivo. *Plos Biology* Vol. 5, No. 1, pp. 15-22, ISBN 1544-9173.

Krishnamurthy, S.; He, X.; Reyes-Reyes, M.; Moore, C.L. & Hampsey, M. (2004). Ssu72 is an RNA polymerase II CTD phosphatase. *Mol Cell.* Vol. 14, No. 3, pp. 387-394, ISBN 1097-2765.

Kyburz, A.; Sadowski, M.; Dichtl, B. & Keller, W. (2003). The role of the yeast cleavage and polyadenylation factor subunit Ydh1p/Cft2p in pre-mRNA 3'-end formation. *Nucleic Acids Res.* Vol. 31, No. 14, pp. 3936-3945 ISBN 1362-4962.

Licatalosi, D. D.; Geiger, G.; Minet, M.; Schroeder, S.; Cilli, K.; McNeil, J. B. & Bently, D. L. (2002). Functional interaction of yeast pre-mRNA 3' end processing factors with RNA polymerase II. *Mol. Cell* Vol. 9, No. 5, pp. 1101-1111 ISBN 1097-2765.

Luo W.; Johnson, A.W. & Bentley D.L. (2006). The role of Rat1 in coupling mRNA 3'-end processing to transcription termination: implications for a unified allosteric-torpedo model. *Genes Dev.* Vol. 20, No. 8, pp. 954-965, ISBN 0890-9369.

Lutz C. S. & Moreira A. (2011). Altenative mRNA polyadenylation in eukaryotes: an effective regulator of gene expression. *WIREs RNA* Vol. 2, No. 1, pp. 23-31, ISBN 1757-7012.

Madison, J. M. & Winston, F. (1997). Evidence that Spt3 functionally interacts with Mot1, TFIIA and TATA-binding protein to confer promoter-specific transcriptional control in *Saccharomyces cerevisiae. Mol. Cell. Biol.* Vol. 17, No. 1, pp. 287-295, ISBN 4215-4229.

Mahandevan, S.; Raghumand, T. R.; Panicker, S. & Struhl, K. (1997). Characterization of 3´-end formation of the yeast *HIS3* mRNA. *Gene* Vol. 190, No. 1, pp. 69-76, ISBN 0378-1119.

Marzluff, WF. (2005). Metazoan replication-dependent histone mRNAs: a distinct set of RNA polymerase II transcripts. *Curr. Opin Cell Biol.* Vol. 17, No. 3, pp. 274-280, ISBN 0955-0674.

Matzura, O. & Wennborg, A. (1996). RNAdraw: an integrated program for RNA secondary structure calculation and analysis under 32-bit Microsoft Windows. *Comp. Aplic. Biosci.* Vol. 12, No. 3, pp. 247-249, ISBN 0266-7001.

Minvielle-Sebastia, L.; Winsor, B.; Bonneaud, N. & Lacroute F. (1991). Mutations in the yeast RNA14 and RNA15 genes result in an abnormal mRNA decay rate; sequence analysis reveals an RNA-binding domain in the RNA15 protein. *Mol Cell Biol.* Vol. 11, No. 6, pp. 3075-87, ISBN 4215-4229.

Nedea, E.; He, X.; Kim, M.; Pootoolal, J.; Zhong, G.; Canadien, V.; Hughes, T.; Buratowski, S.; Moore, C. L. & Greenblatt, J. (2003). Organization and function of APT, a subcomplex of the yeast cleavage and polyadenylation factor involved in the formation of mRNA and small nucleolar RNA 3'-ends. *J. Biol. Chem.* Vol. 278, No. 35, pp. 33000-33010, ISBN 1083-351X.

Nonet, M.; Scafe, C.; Sexton, J. & Young, R. (1987). Eukaryotic RNA polymerase conditional mutant that rapidly ceases mRNA synthesis. Mol Cell Biol Vol 7, No 5, pp1602-1611, ISBN 4215-4229.

Preker, P. J.; Ohnacker, M.; Minvielle-Sebastia, L. & Keller, W. (1997). A multisubunit 3´ end processing factor from yeast containing poly(A) polymerase and homologues of the subunits of mammalian cleavage and polyadenylation specificity factor the subunits of mammalian cleavage andpolyadenylation specificity factor *EMBO J.* Vol. 164, No. 15, pp. 727-4737, ISBN 0261-4189.

Proudfoot, N. (2004). New perspectives on connecting messenger RNA 3' end formation to transcription. *Curr. Opin. Cell Biol.* Vol. 16, No. 3, pp. 272-278, ISBN 0955-0674.

Raué, H. A. & Panta, R. J. (1995) The pathway to maturity: processing of ribosomal RNA in *Saccharomyces cerevisiae. Gene Expr.* Vol. 5, No. 1, pp. 71-77, ISBN 1052-2166.

Rouillard, J.M.; Brendolise, C. and Lacroute, F. (2000). Rna14p, a component of the yeast nuclear cleavage/polyadenylation factor I, is also localised in mitochondria *Mol. Gen Genet* Vol. 262, No. 6, pp.1103-12, ISBN 0026-8925

Rosonina, E. & Manley, J. L. (2010). Alternative polyadenylation Blooms. *Dev Cell* Vol. 18, No. 2, pp. 172-174, ISBN 1534-5807

Seoane, S.; Guiard, B.; Rodriguez-Torres, A. M. & Freire-Picos, M. A. (2005). Effects of splitting alternative *KlCYC1* 3'-UTR regions on processing: Metabolic consequences and biotechnological applications. *J. Biotechnol.* Vol. 118, No. 2, pp. 49-156, ISBN 0168-1658.

Seoane, S.; Lamas-Maceiras, M.; Rodríguez Torres, A. M & Freire Picos, M. A. (2009). Involvement of Pta1, Pcf11 and a *KlCYC1* AU-rich element in alternative RNA 3'-end processing selection in yeast. *FEBS Letters* Vol. 583, No. 17, pp. 2843-2848, ISBN 0014-5793.

Seoane-Rosende S.; Salgado, T.; Poncelas, M.; Rodríguez Torres, A. M. & Freire-Picos, M. A. (2009) Análisis of stability by elements at the proximal 3´-UTR of two *KlCYC1* mRNAs. *Current research topics in Applied Microbiology and Microbial Biotechnology. Proceedings of the II International Conference on Environmental, Industrial and applied Microbiology (Biomicroworld2007)* pp.565-568, ISBN-13 978981-283-754-7, Seville, Spain, November-December 2007.

Shen, Y.; Ji, G.; Haas, B. J.; Wu, X.; Zheng, J.; Reese, G. J. & Li, Q. Q. (2008). Genome level analysis of rice mRNA 3'-end processing signals and alternative polyadenylation. *Nucleic Acids Res.* Vol. 36, No. 9, pp. 3150-3161, ISBN 1362-4962.

Shepard, P. J.; Choi, E. A.; Lu, J.; Flanagan, L. A; Hertel, Kl. & Shi, Y. (2011). Complex and dynamic landscape of RNA polyadenylation revealed by PAS-seq. *RNA* Vol. 17, No. 4, pp. 761-72, ISBN 1355-8382.

Simpson, G. G.; Dijwel, P. P.; Quesada, V.; Henderson, I. & Dean, C. (2003). FY is an RNA 3´end-processing factor that interacts with FCA to control the *Arabidopsis* floral transition. *Cell* Vol. 13, No. 6, pp. 777-797, ISBN 0092-8674.

Sparks, K. A.; Mayer, S. A. & Dieckerman, C. L. (1997) Premature 3´-end formation of *CBP1* mRNA results in the downregulation of cytochrome *b* mRNA during the induction of respiration in *Saccharomyces cerevisiae*. *Mol Cell. Biol.* Vol. 17, No. 8, pp. 4199-4207, ISBN0270-7306.

Sparks, K. A. & Dieckerman, C. L. (1998). Regulation of poly(A) site choice of several yeast mRNAs. Nucleic Acids Res. Vol. 26, No. 20, pp. 4676-4687, ISBN 1362-4962.

Tian, B.; Hu, J.; Zhang, H. & Lutz, C. S. (2005). A large-scale analysis of mRNA polyadenylation of human and mouse genes. *Nucleic Acids Res.* Vol. 33, No. 1, pp. 201-212, ISBN 1362-4962.

Van Helden, J.; Del Olmo, M. & Pérez-Ortín, J. E. (2000). Statistical analysis of yeast genomic downstream sequences reveals putative polyadenylation signals. *Nucleic Acids Res.* Vol. 28, No. 4, pp. 1000-1010, ISBN 1362-4962.

Vasudevan, S. & Peltz, S.W. (2001). Regulated ARE-mediated mRNA decay in *Saccharomyces cerevisiae*. *Mol Cell* Vol 7, No 6, pp 1191-1200, ISBN 1097-2765.

Vo, L.T.; Minet, M.; Schmitter, J.M.; Lacroute, F. & Wyers, F. (2001). Mpe1, a zinc knuckle protein, is an essential component of yeast cleavage and polyadenylation factor required for the cleavage and polyadenylation of mRNA. *Mol Cell Biol* Vol. 21 No 24 pp.8346-56, ISBN 0270-7306.

Wong, C. M.; Qiu, H.; Hu, C.; Dong, J. & Hinnebusch, A. G. (2007). Yeast cap binding complex impedes recruitment of cleavage factor IA to weak termination sites. *Mol Cell Biol.* Vol. 27, No. 18, pp. 6520-6531, ISBN 0270-7306.

Xing, D.; Zhao, H.; Xu, R. & Li, Q. Q. (2008). Arabidopsis PCFS4, a homologue of yeast polyadenylation factor Pcf11p, regulates *FCA* alternative processing and promotes flowering time. *Plant J.* Vol. 54, No. 5, pp. 899-910, ISBN 0960-7412.

Zhang, Z.; Fu, J. & Gilmour, D. S. (2005). CTD-Dependent dismantling of the RNA polymerase II elongation complex by the pre-mRNA 3´-end processing factor Pcf11. *Genes Dev.* Vol. 19, No. 13, pp. 1572-80, ISBN 0890-9369.

Zhao, J.; Hyman, L. & Moore, C. L. (1999). Formation of mRNA 3' ends in eukaryotes: mechanism, regulation, and interrelation-ships with other steps in mRNA synthesis. *Microbiol. Mol. Biol. Rev.* Vol. 63, No. 2, pp. 405-445, ISBN 1092-2172.

Zhao, J.; Kessler, M.; Helmling, S.; O'Connor, J. P. & Moore C. (1999). Pta1, a component of yeast CF II, is required for both cleavage and poly(A) addition of mRNA precursor. *Mol Cell Biol* Vol. 19, No. 11, pp. 7733-7740, ISBN 0270-7306.

Zhelkovsky, A.; Helmling, S. & Moore, C. (1998). Processivity of the *Saccharomyces cerevisiae* poly(A) polymerase requires interactions at the carboxyl-terminal RNA binding domain. *Mol Cell Bio.l* Vol.18, No.10, pp.5942-51, ISBN 0270-7306.

Zitomer, R. S. & Hall, B. D. (1976). Yeast cytochrome *c* messenger RNA. *In vitro* translation and specific immunoprecipitation of the *CYC1* gene product. *J. Biol. Chem.* Vol. 251, No. 20, pp. 6320-6326, ISBN 0021-9258.

7

RNA Processing Activities of the *Arabidopsis* Argonaute Protein Family

Ki Wook Kim, Andrew L Eamens and Peter M Waterhouse
University of Sydney, School of Molecular Biosciences
Australia

1. Introduction

Stringent regulation of gene expression is essential for all organisms, and eukaryotes rely on diverse RNA silencing mechanisms for this regulation at both the transcriptional and post-transcriptional level. For example, transcriptional gene silencing (TGS) maintains genome integrity by controlling the replication of transposons and other repetitive DNA elements, as well as preserving chromatin states and epigenetic imprinting. Post-transcriptional gene silencing (PTGS) mechanisms on the other hand control the expression of messenger RNA (mRNA) transcripts of protein-coding genes in order to regulate developmental transitions and responses to environmental stresses. In plants, both transcriptional and post-transcriptional RNA silencing mechanisms are also involved in the defence against invading pathogens, especially viruses.

RNA silencing pathways are directed by a specific class of small RNA (sRNA) which are predominantly 20 to 25 nucleotides (nt) in length. These sRNAs are processed from longer precursor molecules of either perfectly or imperfectly double-stranded RNA (dsRNA) by a member of the DICER RNase III-like endonuclease family (Bernstein et al., 2001; Gregory et al., 2005). Once processed from its dsRNA substrate, the sRNA is subsequently modified and loaded into an RNaseH-like Argonaute (AGO) protein to form the catalytic core of an RNA-induced silencing complex (RISC). RISC uses the loaded sRNA as a sequence-specificity guide to direct RNA silencing of the targeted sequence at either the transcriptional or post-transcriptional level depending on; i) the class of sRNA loaded by AGO, and; ii) the AGO protein family member loaded with the sRNA.

Although the effector function mediated by the sRNA-loaded AGO protein is highly conserved amongst eukaryotes, the number of AGO proteins encoded by different species varies widely (Tolia & Joshua-Tor, 2007; Hutvagner & Simard, 2008; Vaucheret, 2008). For example, *Caenorhabditis elegans* (*C. elegans*) has twenty seven AGOs, *Drosophila melanogaster* (*Drosophila*) five, humans four and the yeast *Schizosaccharomyces pombe* one. In *Arabidopsis thaliana* (Arabidopsis), the model dicotyledonous plant species, the AGO protein family consists of ten members, that mediate the parallel RNA silencing pathways of Arabidopsis, and which are directed by numerous classes of endogenous sRNA, including the microRNA (miRNA; Lee & Ambros, 2001), small-interfering RNA (siRNA; Hamilton & Baulcombe, 1999), repeat-associated small-interfering RNA (rasiRNA; Meister & Tuschl, 2004), *trans*-acting small-interfering RNA (tasiRNA; Adenot et al., 2006; Xie et al., 2005) and natural antisense transcript small-interfering RNA (natsiRNA; Borsani et al., 2005) classes of sRNA.

In this chapter we discuss the RNA silencing-related activities of the ten Arabidopsis AGO protein family members, and by comparison with the known functions of characterised animal AGOs, as well as in other plant species, we suggest where future insights may be made.

2. AGO protein domain structure

The crystal structure of plant AGO proteins remains to be determined, therefore most of our current knowledge is based on studies of AGO purified from the bacteria *Thermus thermophilus* (Fig.1). These analyses have revealed that AGOs are large proteins (ca 90-100 kDa) comprised of a single variable N-terminal domain and three conserved C-terminal domains, including the PAZ, MID and PIWI domains (Vaucheret, 2008). The N-terminal domain is thought to facilitate the separation of the sRNA/target transcript duplex post cleavage. The conserved PAZ and MID domains of the C-terminus recognize and anchor the 3' and 5' ends of the bound sRNA to its target mRNA respectively (Wang et al., 2008, Wang et al., 2009; Parker, 2010). The third C-terminal domain, the PIWI domain, specifies the endonuclease or "Slicer" activity of cleavage-competent AGOs. This domain adopts a folded structure that closely resembles the catalytic domain of the *Bacillus holodurans* RNaseH enzyme and which usually carries an Asp-Asp-His (DDH) motif in its active site (Rivas et al., 2005). Mutagenesis studies have demonstrated that altering the amino acid composition of this motif abolishes the Slicer activity of several target transcript-cleaving AGOs (Liu et al., 2004; Rivas et al., 2005). However, presence of the DDH motif does not guarantee cleavage activity. For example, the DDH Slicer motif is present in human AGO2 and AGO3, however only AGO2 is capable of catalysing sRNA-directed target transcript cleavage (Liu et al., 2004; Meister et al., 2004). Conversely, absence of the DDH Slicer motif does not preclude the AGO from cleavage-based RNA silencing. This is demonstrated by the

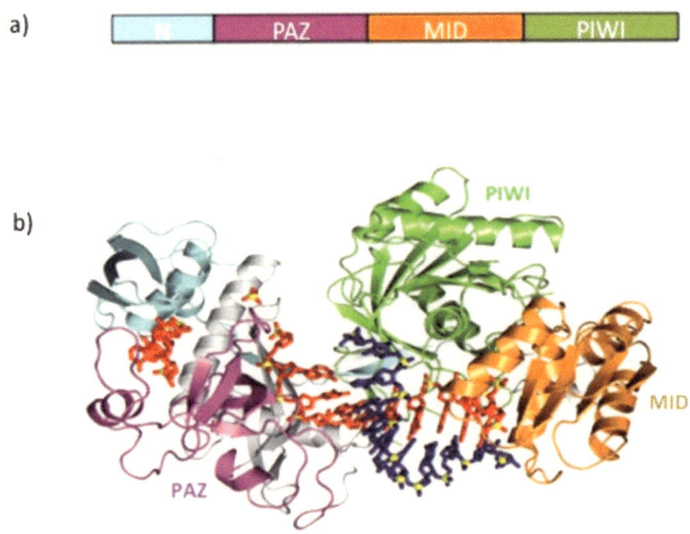

Fig. 1. *Domains and crystal structure of AGO proteins.* (a) AGO consists of a single variable N-terminal domain and three conserved C-terminal domains, the PAZ, MID and PIWI domains. b) Crystal structure of the *Thermus thermophilus* AGO bound to a guide RNA and its target mRNA (Wang et al., 2008)

Drosophila AGO, *Dm*PIWI which instead encodes an Asp-Asp-Lys (DDK) Slicer motif and is cleavage-competent (Saito et al., 2006).

In addition to mediating the Slicer activity of cleavage-competent AGOs, the PIWI domain has been demonstrated to serve as an interface for protein-protein interactions, namely interaction with glycine-tryptophan (GW) repeat proteins. In animals for example, the interaction of AGOs with GW182 has been shown to be essential for translational repression (Liu et al., 2005; Eulalio et al., 2008). To date, no GW182 orthologues have been identified in plants. However, in the RNA-directed DNA methylation (RdDM) RNA silencing pathway of Arabidopsis, AGO4 has been shown to interact with the GW protein NRPD1 to recruit the DNA methylation machinery required for the effector step of this pathway (El-shami et al., 2007). Whether other Arabidopsis AGO family members also interact with GW proteins remains to be determined.

3. The Arabidopsis Argonaute protein family

AGO1 is the founding member of the Arabidopsis AGO protein family. The *ago1* mutant plant was originally identified in a forward genetics screen, exhibiting pleiotropic developmental defects, characterized by tubular shaped leaves that were thought to closely resemble the tentacles of a small squid of the *Argonauta* genus (Bohmert et al., 1998). Subsequent phenotypic and/or molecular studies of plant lines defective for the activity of the miRNA biogenesis machinery proteins SERRATE (*se*), DICER-LIKE1 (*dcl1*) and dsRNA BINDING PROTEIN *(drb1)*, or of transformed plant lines expressing miRNA resistant targets implicated the involvement of AGO1 in miRNA biogenesis (Lobbes et al., Park et al., 2002; Vaucheret et al., 2004). Alleles of *ago1* were also isolated in genetic screens identifying plant lines where the expression of a post-transcriptionally silenced sense transgene (termed S-PTGS in plants) was reactivated (Fagard et al., 2000). Taken together, these studies identified AGO1 as playing an integral, central role in the parallel sRNA-directed RNA silencing pathways of Arabidopsis.

The identification of the Arabidopsis AGO1 protein prompted extensive searches for orthologues in other model organisms. Indeed, AGO proteins were found to be highly conserved across plant and animal kingdoms (Catalanotto et al., 2000; Fagard et al., 2000). In Arabidopsis, the complete annotation of its genome identified nine other AGO family members (termed AGO2 to AGO10 respectively), and phylogenetic analysis of this protein family at the amino acid level identified three distinct clades, namely the AGO1/AGO5/AGO10, AGO2/AGO3/AGO7, and AGO4/AGO6/AGO8/AGO9 clades (Vaucheret, 2008; Fig.2). It is important to note that although the distribution of the 10 Arabidopsis AGO proteins into three distinct clades is purely based on amino acid sequence homology, and does not directly infer similarities in activity or redundancies in function, several examples of functional redundancy have been identified between AGO clade members, namely between AGO1 and AGO10 of the AGO1/5/10 clade (Mallory et al., 2009), and AGO4, AGO6 and AGO9 of the AGO4/6/8/9 clade (Havecker et al., 2010).

In addition to the identification of functional redundancy amongst family members, some Arabidopsis AGO proteins have also been shown to exhibit strong preferences to load sRNA species of a particular size and/or 5' terminal nucleotide (Havecker et al., 2010; Mi et al., 2008; Takeda et al., 2008). For example, AGO1 binds sRNAs that are predominantly of the 21-nt size class with have a 5' terminal uracil, whereas AGO2 preferentially binds 21-nt sRNAs, with a 5' terminal adenine. Unlike AGOs 1 and 2, AGO5 predominantly binds sRNAs of the 24-nt size class and with a cytosine at their 5' terminal residue. AGOs 4, 6 and

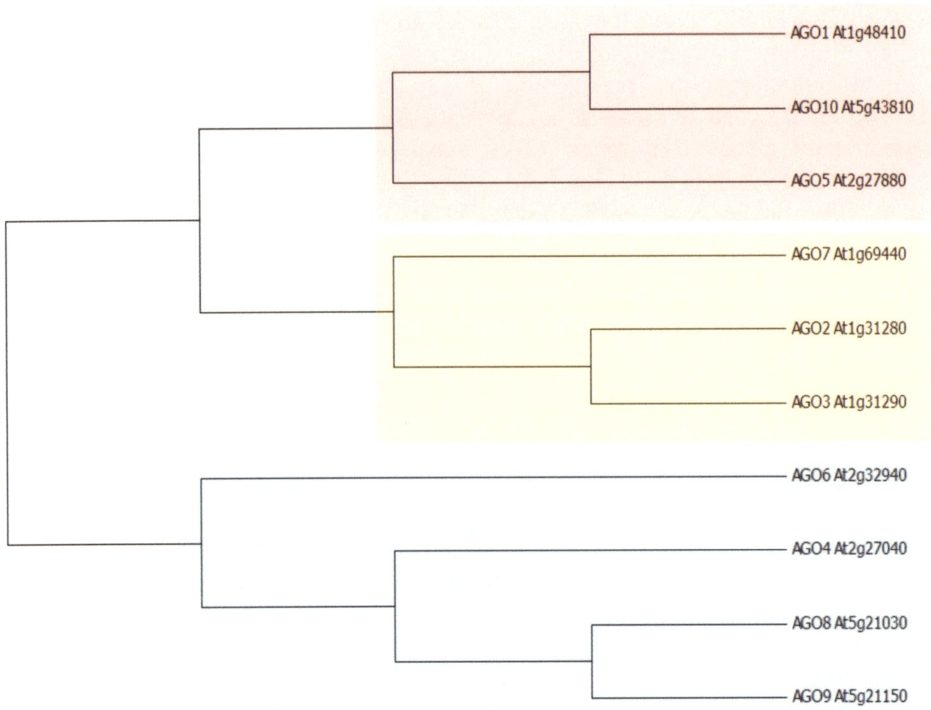

Fig. 2. *Phylogenetic tree constructed from the full-length amino acid sequences of the ten Arabidopsis AGO family members.* The phylogeny clade divisions are marked in different colours. Drawing not to scale.

9 also preferentially associate with 24-nt sRNAs but prefer to bind sRNAs of this size class with 5' adenine residues. The 5' terminal nucleotide preference for AGOs 3, 7, 8 and 10 remain to be determined. All known 5' terminal nucleotide and size class preferences are summarized in Table 1.

Family member	Clade	Protein size (aa)	Molecular Weight	Protein Accession No.	5′ terminal nucleotide preference	sRNA length preference (nt)
AGO1	1/5/10	1048	116190.3	NP_175274	U	21
AGO2	2/3/7	1014	113422.7	NP_174413	A	21
AGO3	2/3/7	1194	129184.1	NP_174414	Unknown	Unknown
AGO4	4/6/8/9	924	102839.7	NP_565633	A	24
AGO5	1/5/10	997	111087.8	NP_850110	C	24
AGO6	4/6/8/9	878	98680.7	NP_180853	A	24
AGO7	2/3/7	990	113395.8	NP_177103	Unknown	Unknown
AGO8	4/6/8/9	850	95506.0	NP_197602	Unknown	Unknown
AGO9	4/6/8/9	896	100523.6	NP_197613	A	24
AGO10	1/5/10	988	110866.7	NP_199194	Unknown	Unknown

Table 1. *Summary of the 5′ terminal nucleotide and size (nt) preferences of Arabidopsis AGOs determined through immunoprecipitation experiments.* The protein size, clade member, molecular weight, 5′ terminal nucleotide and Genbank protein accession number also listed.

3.1 The AGO1/AGO5/AGO10 clade

3.1.1 AGO1

AGO1 has been shown to direct sRNA-mediated gene expression regulation for all currently characterized Arabidopsis miRNAs (Baumberger & Baulcombe, 2005; Vaucheret et al., 2004). Most *ago1* mutants exhibit pleiotropic developmental defects characteristic of perturbed miRNA function. In these plants, the miRNA levels are reduced, and their target transcript expression levels increased. In addition, the majority of plant miRNAs have a 5' terminal uracil residue and are preferentially loaded by AGO1 (Mi et al, 2008). The high level of miRNA/target transcript sequence complementary in plants results in AGO1 repressing target gene expression via miRNA-mediated target transcript cleavage. A recent study has suggested that AGO1 can also repress target gene expression via translational repression (Brodersen et al., 2008), however, it remains unclear whether this is a widespread RNA silencing mechanism in plants. To maintain steady-state expression of AGO1, the expression of the *Ago1* transcript is itself regulated by a miRNA. Regulation of *Ago1* by miR168 ensures that AGO1 levels remain constant, in turn ensuring normal plant development. AGO1 homeostasis is indeed crucial for normal plant development as the expression of a miRNA-resistant AGO1 transgene caused severe developmental defects that led to the eventual death of the plant (Vaucheret et al., 2004, 2006).

In addition to its role in the miRNA biogenesis pathway, AGO1 also performs a dual function in the biogenesis of the closely related endogenous sRNA class, the tasiRNAs. AGO1 uses loaded miRNAs, namely miR173 and miR828 (Allen et al., 2005; Rajagopalan, et al., 2006; Yoshikawa et al., 2005) to target the non-protein-coding transcripts *Tas1*, *Tas2* and *Tas4* for miRNA-mediated cleavage respectively. This initial cleavage event identifies these cleavage products for dsRNA synthesis by the RNA-directed RNA polymerase RDR6 (Peragine et al., 2004). Following dsRNA synthesis and processing of these molecules, the resulting tasiRNAs are loaded by AGO1-catalyzed RISC for sRNA-mediated target transcript cleavage (Yoshikawa, et al. 2005). More recently, AGO1 has also been shown to be involved in the generation of 'secondary' or 'transitive' siRNAs from sRNA cleaved transcripts (Chen et al., 2010; Cuperus et al., 2010). Furthermore, AGO1 also mediates the effector step for siRNA-directed RNA silencing. These siRNAs may be derived from either an infecting virus, or from introduced transgenes (including sense, antisense or hairpin RNA transgenes). AGO1 is the primary AGO family member involved in the antiviral response, and *ago1* plants are hyper-susceptible to several viruses, including *Cucumber mosaic virus* (CMV) (Morel et al., 2002). CMV encodes the silencing suppressor protein (SSP) 2b, which directly impairs the function of AGO1 (Zhang et al., 2006). Members of the Polerovirus family have also been shown to encode SSPs which target the action of AGO1 and Arabidopsis *ago1* plants have also been demonstrated to be hyper-susceptible to these viruses (Baumberger et al., 2007; Bortolamiol et al., 2007).

The central role played by AGO1 in sRNA-directed RNA silencing is mirrored by its expressional domain. Array data reveals that *Ago1* is ubiquitously expressed at high levels throughout development (Schmid et al., 2005). Experiments in Arabidopsis using the AGO1 promoter fused to a GUS reporter gene revealed that the promoter is active in all aerial tissues, but its activity appears to be highest in meristematic and vascular tissue (Vaucheret et al., 2006). In addition to being expressed ubiquitously, AGO1 seems to function in both the cytoplasm and nucleus of the plant cell. It appears to be strictly cytoplasmic when processing viral RNAs but Fang & Spector (2007) and Song et al., (2007) have reported that AGO1 is in the nucleus and is most concentrated around small nuclear bodies termed nuclear dicing bodies or D-bodies. The miRNA biogenesis machinery proteins DCL1, HYL1 and SE are also found in D-bodies, where miRNA precursor transcripts are processed prior to loading of the mature miRNA guide strand into AGO1.

3.1.2 AGO5

To date, no *ago5* mutant alleles have been identified in any forward genetic screens. Furthermore, T-DNA knockout lines are wild-type in appearance and the role of this AGO family member in sRNA-directed RNA silencing remains to be determined. No changes in endogenous or exogenous sRNA classes were detected in an *ago5* mutant (Takeda et al., 2008). In contrast to AGO1, the expression profile for AGO5 is highly specific to reproductive tissues (Schmid et al., 2005), accumulating in the sperm cell cytoplasm in mature pollen and growing pollen tubes (Borges et al., 2011).
Sequencing of the sRNAs bound to AGO5 revealed its preference for species 24-nts in length and with a 5' terminal cytosine residue. However, AGO5 is also able to bind 21-nt sRNAs. MiR169 is one of a small number Arabidopsis miRNAs that do not have uracil as the 5' terminal nucleotide, and this 21-nt miRNA preferentially associates with AGO5 rather than AGO1 (Mi et al., 2008; Takeda et al., 2008). The biological function of miR169 remains to be determined in Arabidopsis, but this highly conserved miRNA is important for floral development in petunia and anthirinum (Cartolano et al., 2007; Combier et al., 2006), to suggest that AGO5/miR169 may be involved in regulating gene expression in Arabidopsis. Furthermore, AGO5 has been shown to bind both 21 and 24-nt viral siRNA size classes (Takeda et al., 2008). However, *ago5* plants do not appear to be hyper-susceptible to plant viruses (Harvey et al., 2011; Wang et al., 2011), suggesting that this AGO family member may only play a minor or subservient role in viral defence under normal conditions (e.g. in the presence of AGO1 activity).

3.1.3 AGO10

The AGO10 mutant alleles, *pinhead* and *zwille* were identified through forward genetic screens (Lynn et al., 1999; Moussian et al., 1998). Both alleles are characterized by abnormal shoot apical meristem (SAM) development, but these mutants do not display any other readily observable developmental defects. Despite the high level of amino acid sequence similarity between AGO10 and AGO1, *ago10* mutants are not impaired in S-PTGS and show no reduction in the accumulation miRNAs, tasiRNAs or any other siRNA class assessed in this mutant background (Morel et al., 2002; Takeda et al., 2008).
As the closest paralogue of AGO1, it had been postulated that AGO10 may have similar activities and function redundantly with AGO1. Indeed, previous studies have shown that the *ago1:ago10* double mutant is embryo lethal, strongly suggesting functional redundancy between AGO10 and AGO1 during post-embryonic development (Lynn et al., 1999). Fusion of the AGO1 promoter and coding sequence to a reporter gene revealed that AGO1 is expressed in whole embryos, with its expression highest in provascular cells from the globular to early torpedo stages. The expression of AGO10 partially overlaps the expressional domain of AGO1. Fusion of the AGO10 promoter and coding sequence to a reporter gene showed that its expression is more restricted in whole embryos than observed for AGO1, becoming limited to provascular strands and the adaxial side of cotyledons at the globular stage (Mallory et al., 2009). Moreover, the expression of the AGO10 coding sequence, fused to the AGO1 promoter, revealed that this family member can partially

compensate for AGO1 activity, to again suggest that AGO10 may be involved in sRNA-mediated gene expression regulation in specific cells and/or tissues.
Consistent with the SAM defects observed in *pinhead* and *zwille* mutants, recent studies have demonstrated that AGO10 acts as a critical regulator of SAM maintenance by specifically interacting with miR165 and miR166 (Liu et al., 2009; Zhu et al., 2011). Members of both miRNA families regulate the expression of class III homeodomain-Leucine Zipper (HD-Zip III) transcription factors, which in turn determine the fate of the SAM (Jung & Park, 2007; Zhou et al., 2007). AGO10 exhibits a higher binding affinity for miR165/166 than AGO1, and when miR165/166 loading to AGO10 is perturbed, plants exhibit a defective SAM. Although the exact mechanism of how AGO10 regulates SAM development via miR165/166 regulation remains elusive, Zhou et al., 2011 demonstrated that the miRNA-binding activity of AGO10, and not its miRNA-directed Slicer activity is the important determinant of this interaction. The authors went on to suggest that AGO10 may in fact be specifically sequestering miR165/166 duplexes to prevent their incorporation into AGO1 and subsequent repression of the HD-Zip III transcription factors.

3.2 The AGO2/AGO3/AGO7 clade

3.2.1 AGO2/AGO3

AGO2 and AGO3 are thought to have arisen from a recent duplication event, as these two family members share a very high level of amino acid sequence similarity and are adjacent to one another in the Arabidopsis genome. Array data reveals that all three family members of the AGO2/3/7 clade have overlapping expression domains (Schmid et al., 2005). AGO2 and 3 are most highly expressed in developing seeds and siliques, and at lower levels in senescing leaves and flowers. Both family members also have dynamic cellular localization, being expressed in both the nucleus and cytoplasm (Takeda et al., 2008). Although, to date, no functional similarity or redundancy has been reported for AGO2 and 3, their high level of sequence similarity, proximal genomic positioning and shared expression patterns strongly suggests that they have the same or similar RNA silencing roles in Arabidopsis. However, no forward genetic mutants have been identified for either family member and T-DNA knockout mutants of AGO2 and AGO3 are wild-type in appearance (Lobbes et al., 2006). Furthermore, northern blotting has shown wild-type accumulation for all sRNA species assessed in *ago2* and *ago3* plants (Katiyar-Agarwal et al., 2007; Takeda et al., 2008).
AGO2 is preferentially loaded with sRNA species, including viral sRNAs, possessing a 5' terminal adenine residue (Mi et al., 2008; Takeda et al., 2008). More recent studies have implicated the involvement of AGO2 in antiviral defence, showing that *ago2* mutants are hyper-susceptible to *Turnip crinkle virus* (TCV) and CMV infection, and that AGO2 expression is induced upon TCV and CMV infection of wild-type plants (Harvey et al., 2011; Wang et al., 2011). Furthermore, AGO2 has been shown to act downstream of the viral secondary siRNA biogenesis together with AGO1 in a non-redundant manner, essential for defence against CMV infection (Wang et al., 2011). Despite AGO2 playing such an important antiviral role in the defence against TCV and CMV, *ago2* mutants are not hyper-susceptible to all plant viruses. For example, *ago2* mutants show wild-type-like symptoms upon *Tobacco mosaic virus* (TMV) infection. Unlike TCV and CMV, TMV does not encode a SSP that impairs the function of AGO1. The induction of AGO2 upon TCV and CMV infection is therefore thought to result from a decreased accumulation of the AGO1-dependent, AGO2-regulating miRNA, miR403 (Harvey et al., 2011). This may also be true for *Ago3* as its transcript is also regulated by miR403. This raises the question: is this a system that has

evolved to provide back-up protection against viruses that target AGO1 with their SSPs (eg 2b of CMV and P38 of TCV) or an unselected for, accidental consequence of reduced miR403 accumulation? Whereas the former seems likely, it is interesting that rice orthologs of Arabidopsis AGOs 2 and 3 do not possess the 3' UTR miR403 target site and would not provide an elevatable back-up system.

3.2.2 AGO7

Alleles of the *ago7* mutant were originally identified in a reverse genetics screen for plant lines exhibiting accelerated juvenile-to-adult phase change (Hunter et al., 2003; Peragine et al., 2004; Yoshikawa et al., 2005). This screen also identified mutant alleles of DCL4, RDR6 and SGS3 (*dcl4, rdr6* and *sgs3* mutant plant lines respectively). Subsequent studies revealed that DCL4, RDR6 and SGS3 are essential players in the biogenesis of tasiRNA sRNAs from the non-protein-coding TAS transcripts, *Tas1, Tas2, Tas3* and *Tas4*. In addition to expressing an accelerated juvenile-to-adult transition, *ago7* plants display floral morphogenesis defects, a phenotypic characteristic subsequently associated with plant lines where TAS3 biogenesis is disrupted (Adenot et al., 2006; Garcia et al., 2006). AGO7 has since been demonstrated to exclusively function in the TAS3 biogenesis pathway (Montgomery et al., 2008). In TAS3 tasiRNA biogenesis, miR390 is specifically loaded to AGO7 to direct AGO7 binding to the two miR390 target sites within the *Tas3* mRNA. AGO7 cleaves the targeted transcript at only the 3' target site and this event identifies the cleaved mRNA for RDR6-directed dsRNA synthesis (Yoshikawa et al., 2005; Montgomery et al., 2008). A subset of the TAS3-specific tasiRNAs are subsequently loaded to AGO1 to target the auxin response factor family members *Arf3* and *Arf4* for cleavage-based repression. ARF3 and ARF4 are required for specification of the adaxial fate of Arabidopsis rosette leaves (Fahlgren et al., 2006; Garcia et al., 2006), therefore, AGO7-mediated, miR390-directed regulation of gene expression is essential for normal plant development in Arabidopsis.

As mentioned above, array data suggests that AGO7 shares an overlapping expressional domain with the two other AGO2/AGO3/AGO7 clade members (Schmid et al., 2005). Fusion of the AGO7 promoter to the GUS reporter gene revealed that AGO7 is predominantly expressed in the vasculature of seedlings and in the cells and tissues immediately surrounding the SAM (Montgomery et al., 2008). GUS expression was also observed in the adaxial-most cells of developing leaf primordial to again demonstrate the importance of AGO7 expression for normal leaf development (Fahlgren et al., 2006; Garcia et al., 2006). As described for *ago2* plants, the *ago7* mutant is hyper-susceptible to TCV infection (Qu et al., 2008). This suggests a possible additional antiviral role for AGO7. However, *ago7* mutants are not hyper-susceptible to any other plant virus, and furthermore, direct association of AGO7 with the accumulation of viral-specific siRNAs remains to be demonstrated.

Besides its preferential association with miR390, the 5' terminal nucleotide preference of AGO7 is unknown. Unlike AGO1, AGO2, AGO4 and AGO5, the AGO7/miR390 association is not based on the 5' terminal nucleotide of the sRNA. Replacing the 5' terminal adenine of miR390 with a cytosine residue does not influence the preferential association of this sRNA with AGO7 (Montgomery et al., 2008), suggesting a specialized association mechanism.

3.3 The AGO4/AGO6/AGO8/AGO9 clade

3.3.1 AGO4

The *ago4* mutant was originally identified in a forward genetics screen for mutants impaired in TGS of the SUPERMAN locus, along with the RdDM machinery proteins

CHROMOMETHYLASE3 (CMT3) and KYPTONITE (KYP; Zilberman et al., 2003). Subsequent research has shown that AGO4 functions in the effector step of RdDM to maintain sRNA-directed DNA methylation of repetitive genomic sequences (e.g. maintains transposons in their epigenetically silent state; Xie et al., 2004; Zilberman et al., 2004). Array data shows that AGO4 is expressed ubiquitously (Schmid et al., 2005). This is consistent with the AGO4 promoter-GUS reporter gene expression pattern observed in transgenic Arabidopsis plants, where GUS was found to be expressed throughout developing embryos, mature leaves and flowers (Havecker et al., 2010).

In correlation with its role in sRNA-directed DNA methylation, AGO4 appears to be exclusively located in the nucleus (Li et al., 2006). In the nucleus, AGO4 co-localizes with RdDM machinery proteins, including the plant specific DNA-dependent RNA polymerases, PolIV and PolV, as well as RDR2, DCL3 and DOMAINS REARRANGED METHYLASE2 (DRM2) in two types of specialized nuclear compartments, namely Cajal-bodies and AB-bodies (Li et al., 2006; Pontes et al., 2006). Co-localization of AGO4 to two specialized nuclear bodies suggests that AGO4 is not only required for sRNA-directed DNA methylation, but also for the maintenance of heterochromatin (Irvine et al., 2006). Accordingly, AGO4 preferentially binds repeat-associated (rasiRNAs) and heterochromatin-specific (hcsiRNAs) siRNAs of the 24-nt size class. Although there is an even distribution of 24-nt rasiRNAs and hcsiRNAs with 5' terminal adenine, cytosine, guanine and uracil residues in Arabidopsis, AGO4 preferentially binds sRNAs of this size class with 5' terminal adenine residues (Mi et al., 2008; Havecker et al., 2010). Curiously, AGO4 does not appear to be involved in either the biogenesis or effector step of another class of endogenous 24-nt sRNA, the natsiRNA class. This class of 24-nt siRNA was demonstrated to accumulate to wild-type levels in the absence of AGO4 activity (Xie et al., 2004). Similar observations were made for plant lines deficient in the activity of a number of other RdDM machinery proteins to suggest that the rasiRNA/hcsiRNA and natsiRNA silencing pathways operate through different AGO-catalysed effector complexes.

In virus-infected wild-type Arabidopsis plants virus-specific 24-nt siRNAs accumulate to readily detectable levels, although at much lower levels than those of virus-specific 21-nt siRNAs. However, *ago4* mutants do not appear to be hyper-susceptible to any plant virus, to suggest that another 24-nt binding AGO family member may be responsible for sRNA-directed methylation of viral transcripts. Intriguingly, *ago4* plants are hyper-susceptibile to the bacterial pathogen *Pseudomonas syringae* (Agorio & Vera, 2007), suggesting that AGO4 may be involved in directing a defence response against only specific pathogens. Alternatively, the epigenetic de-repression of other genes in this mutant background could be causing this hyper-susceptibility effect.

3.3.2 AGO6

AGO6 specifically acts at the transcriptional level in the hcsiRNA-directed RNA silencing pathway (Zheng et al., 2007; Havecker et al., 2010). The *ago6* mutant was originally identified in a forward genetics screen for plant lines where the expression of a transcriptionally-silent transgene was reactivated in the *ros1* mutant background (Zheng et al., 2007). The authors showed that the level of transcriptional reactivation was higher in the *ago4/ros1* double mutant background than in the *ago6/ros1* mutant. This suggests that AGO6 does not play as wide a role in sRNA-directed heterochromatin RNA silencing as that directed by AGO4 in Arabidopsis. However, AGO6 does appear to be partially redundant with AGO4 function as the level of transgene reactivation was demonstrated to be even higher in the *ago4/ago6/ros1* triple mutant, compared to either of the analysed double mutants. Furthermore, array and reporter gene expression data reveal that the expressional domain of AGO6 overlaps that of AGO4 (Schmid et al., 2005; Havecker et al., 2008). Taken together, these analyses suggest that these two AGO family members act on a shared subset of repeat elements, and that their overlapping function occurs in similar tissues and at the same developmental time point.

3.3.3 AGO8/AGO9

As with AGOs 2 and 3, AGO8 and AGO9 are predicted to have arisen from a recent gene duplication event (Vaucheret, 2008). The amino-acid sequences of these two AGOs are very similar (although AGO8 is not annotated in TAIR), and the AGO8 and AGO9 genes are almost adjacent to one another on chromosome 5 of the Arabidopsis genome. According to array data, the tissue-specific expression patterns of *Ago8* and *Ago9* mRNAs are also highly similar (Schmid et al., 2005). However, the *Ago8* transcript is expressed at a much lower level than *Ago9* and contains a splicing-induced frame-shift, which is predicted to render the AGO8 protein non-functional (Takeda et al., 2008).
To date, no forward genetic *ago8* or *ago9* alleles have been identified in any mutant screening population. T-DNA insertion-mutant lines of *AGO8* or *AGO9* are wild-type in appearance and have unchanged miRNA, tasiRNA and siRNA accumulation levels. However, a recent study has implicated the involvement of AGO9 in the siRNA-directed maintenance of the silencing state of several classes of repetitive DNA element (Havecker et al., 2010), and closer examination of the *ago9* mutant has revealed a previously overlooked apomixes-like fertilization-independent seed production phenotype (Olmedo-Monfil, 2010).

4. Function of mammalian AGO proteins

The four AGO proteins (AGOs 1 to 4) encoded by the mouse and human genomes perform key effector roles directed by the three endogenous sRNA classes of these respective species, namely the miRNA (Lee & Ambros, 2001), siRNA (Meister & Tuschl, 2004) and PIWI-interacting RNA (piRNA) classes (Vagin et al., 2006). Unlike members of the Arabidopsis AGO family, mammalian AGOs do not exhibit 5' terminal nucleotide preferences for either the loading or sorting of sRNAs. The four mammalian AGOs appear to bind sRNAs with little discrimination, except for sense piRNAs which have been shown to specifically incorporate into AGO4 (Arvin et al., 2008). In *Drosophila* and *C. elegans* however, the degree of complementarity between sRNA duplex strands and/or the structure of the sRNA has been demonstrated to strongly influence the sorting of sRNAs into their respective AGO protein family members (Tomari et al., 2007; Forstemann et al., 2007; Steiner et al., 2007). Taken together, these studies suggest that in contrast to Arabidopsis, *Drosophila* and *C. elegans,* mammals lack specific rules for sRNA/AGO sorting.
Although all four mammalian AGOs exhibit similar siRNA binding affinities and each appear to specify a role in posttranscriptional regulation of miRNA expression, only AGO2 performs the effector function of siRNA-directed RNA silencing (Liu et al., 2004; Meister et al., 2004; Rivas et al., 2005). SiRNAs delivered into mammalian cells direct AGO2-mediated RNA silencing through target transcript cleavage and require a high degree of sRNA/target

RNA complementarity (Liu et al., 2004). In contrast, mammalian miRNAs have a low level of complementarity to their targets with the predominant mode of miRNA-directed gene expression regulation mediated via translational repression mechanisms. All four AGOs, including the Slicer efficient AGO2, direct translational repression through their shared partnership with GW182. With the assistance of GW182, miRNA-loaded mammalian AGOs typically target their regulated mRNAs in the 3′ UTR. Translational repression is thought to occur through disruption of crucial interactions between the 5' Cap and the 3' poly-A tail of the regulated transcript, leading to a reduction in translational initiation and/or transcript destabilization (Liu et al., 2005; Eulalio et al., 2008).

In addition to performing the sRNA effector function, there is growing evidence to support important roles for mammalian AGOs in sRNA processing. For example, AGO2 has been implicated in miRNA biogenesis through direct binding of the precursor miRNA (pre-miRNA) molecule (Cheloufi et al., 2010; Cifuentes et al., 2010; Diderichs & Haber, 2007; Tan et al., 2009). In the canonical miRNA biogenesis pathway (Fig.3), the DNA-dependent RNA polymerase II (Pol II)-transcribed primary miRNA (pri-miRNA) transcript is recognized and bound by the dsRNA binding domain (dsRBD) protein Pasha. Pasha in turn recruits the RNase III-like endonuclease Drosha to form a multi-protein complex, the Microprocessor. Within the Microprocessor, and with the assistance of Pasha, Drosha cleaves the pri-miRNA to liberate a shorter precursor molecule of 60 to 70-nt in length, the pre-miRNA. The pre-miRNA is subsequently transported to the cytoplasm and further processed by Dicer and its dsRNA binding domain partner protein Laquacious to release a 22 to 23-nt mature miRNA duplex. Following the unwinding of duplex strands, the mature miRNA sRNA is then loaded by one of the four mammalian AGOs to form miRNA-loaded RISC (miRISC). However, and as mentioned above, recent studies have revealed that the direct binding of AGO2 to the pre-miRNA dsRNA and not the mature miRNA itself, can also form an active miRISC, capable of either; i) cleaving miRNA targets *in vitro* in the absence of Dicer activity (Tan et al., 2009), or; ii) processing of the pre-miRNA dsRNA into a shorter intermediate known as the AGO2-cleaved pre-miRNA (ac-pre-miRNA) (Diderichs & Haber, 2007). The significance of the AGO2-generated pre-miRNA remains to be determined, however, in mice and zebrafish the biogenesis of a conserved vertebrate miRNA, miR451, has been shown to also require the endonucleatic activity of AGO2, and that its biogenesis occurs independently of Dicer (Cheloufi et al., 2010; Cifuentes et al., 2010). In this non-canonical biogenesis pathway (Figure-3), AGO2 directly binds pre-miR451 and trims this molecule to produce the mature miR451 sRNA. The resulting mature sRNA can then be directly loaded by AGO2 to form an active miRISC.

The exact mechanism of how AGO2-mediated "trimming" occurs remains to be determined. Examination of the pre-miR451 sequence reveals two differences to most mammalian miRNA precursor transcriptss, and Cheloufi et al. (2010) proposed that these differences may identify the miR451 precursor molecule for entry into the AGO2-mediated miRNA biogenesis pathway. Firstly, the pre-miR451 is 17-nt shorter than most pre-miRNAs. This marks pre-miR451 as an unlikely Dicer substrate since it has been shown in mice extracts that Dicer cannot process shorter pre-miRNA efficiently (Siolas et al., 2005). Secondly, the mature miR451 sequence includes some of the loop region and complementary arm of the stem-loop of the precursor molecule. This unique precursor structure, and mature miRNA position within the precursor, may interfere with Dicer's ability to recognize this open-looped molecule for processing.

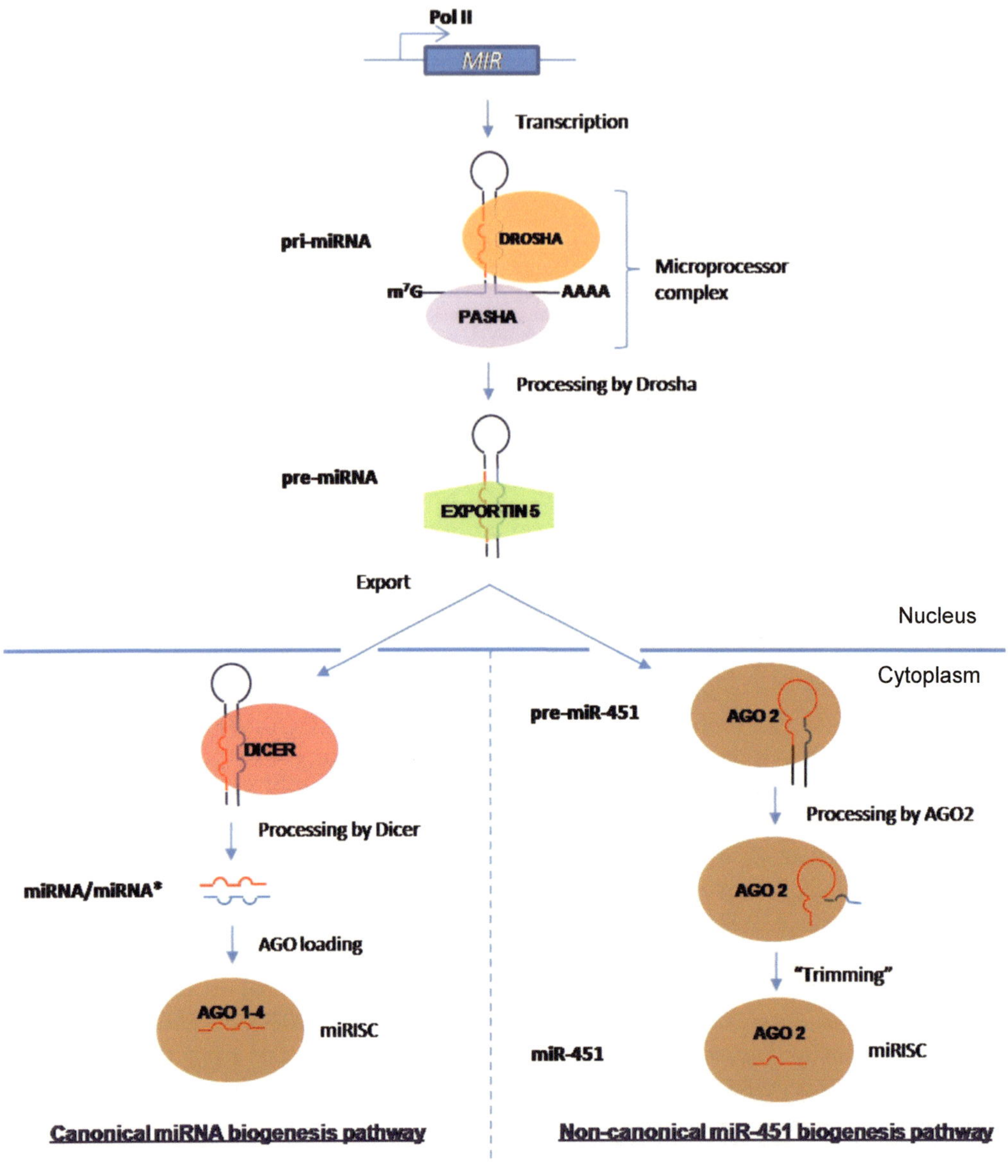

Fig. 3. *The canonical miRNA and non-canonical miR451 biogenesis pathways in mammals.*

5. Conclusions

The availability of the Arabidopsis genome sequence and insertion mutants for the majority of its genes has been invaluable in advancing the understanding of plant cell and developmental biology. Knowing exactly how many Dicer-, Agonaute-, DRB-, and RDR-like genes are present in the genome, coupled with insertion and point mutants of these and associated genes (including those identified from forward and reverse genetic screens) have allowed plant biologists to generate an in depth picture of the parallel RNA silencing pathways in Arabidopsis. It is tempting to conclude that we now have a close-to-full picture of AGO-mediated sRNA-directed regulation in plants. Some broad simplifications that can be made are:

1. AGO1 is the most important AGO, without which a plant cannot survive, regulate its development, or defend itself against viral infection.
2. The 10 members of the Arabidopsis AGO protein family can be divided into 3 functional groups:
   i. RNA slicers
   ii. RNA binders, and
   iii. chromatin modifiers
3. The above functional groupings largely follow the sequence-based phylogenetic clades described above. Members of the AGO1/5/10 clade are Slicers, AGOs 2, 3 and 7 bind sRNAs (however AGO7 has been demonstrated to direct *Tas3* cleavage), and the four remaining family members of the AGO4/6/8/9 clade are modifiers
   i. AGO 1/5/10 - slicers
   ii. AGO 2/3/7 - binders (AGO7 also cuts)
   iii. AGO 4/6/8/9 - modifiers
4. Each clade has a main player with ubiquitous and high level expression (AGO1, AGO7 and AGO4) and a pair of important reproductive-specific (flower/embryo-specific) players (AGO5/10, AGO2/3 and AGO8/9). See Figure 4.
5. Arabidopsis AGO1 has similarities in Slicer activity with mammalian AGO2.

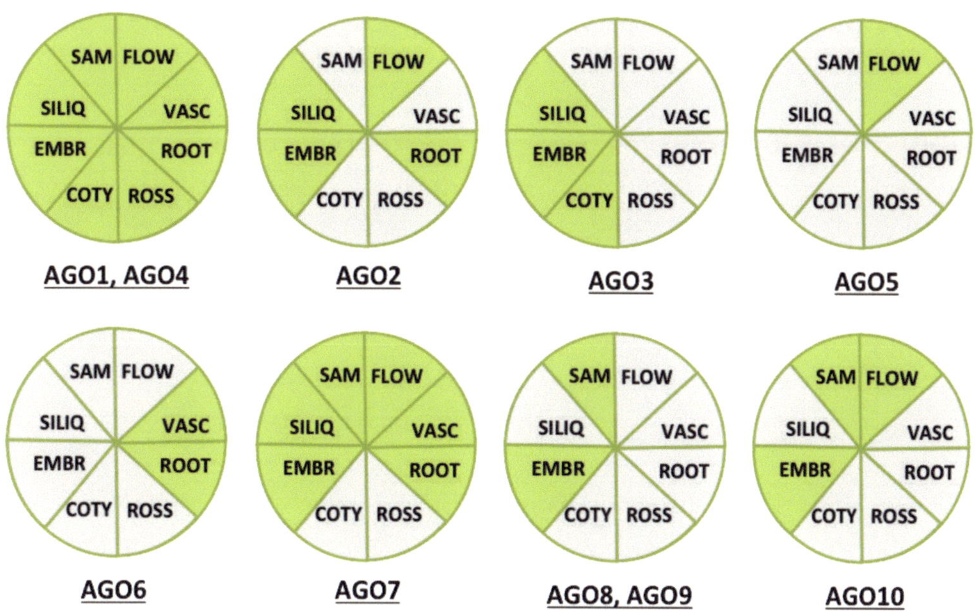

Fig. 4. *Tissue expression domains of Arabidopsis AGO proteins.* The expression of the ten Arabidopsis AGO family members was divided into tissue types, namely the flowers (FLOW), vasculature (VASC), roots (ROOT), rosette leaves (ROSS), cotyledons (COTY), embryos (EMBR), siliques (SILIQ) and shoot apical meristem (SAM). Segments shaded green represent expression, whereas grey shaded segments represent no expression.

However, there are many important questions, both in Arabidopsis and other plant species, yet to be answered before a full picture can be realised. No structural features have been directly determined for any eukaryotic AGO protein. Inferences about their structure/function relationships have been made from the crystal structure of a prokaryotic AGO-related protein and sequence-based structural predictions. Therefore:

i. are the structures of the Arabidopsis AGO proteins similar within a clade but divergent between clades?
ii. Are the structural differences between family members reflective of their different modes of action?
iii. Which Arabidopsis AGOs are responsible for translational repression of mRNAs and viral RNAs?
iv. Which family member(s) use the RDR6/DCL2-generated 22-nt secondary transitivity-inducing siRNAs?
v. What are the 5′ nucleotide preferences for AGOs 3,7,8 and 10?
vi. Is there an AGO that is preferentially loaded with sRNAs possessing a 5′ terminal guanine residue?
vii. How are different AGOs loaded with the appropriate sRNA and the "correct" dsRNA duplex strand chosen?
viii. Is there a non-canonical miRNA biogenesis pathway in Arabidopsis similar to the mammalian AGO2 system?

All of these and many other basic questions remain to be answered. There is also a broader question: are the Arabidopsis sRNA/AGO-mediated processes representative of those in other plant species? For example, rice has 18 AGOs (Fig.5). While the Arabidopsis AGO2/3/7 and AGO4/6/8/9 clades appear to have almost exactly the same number of

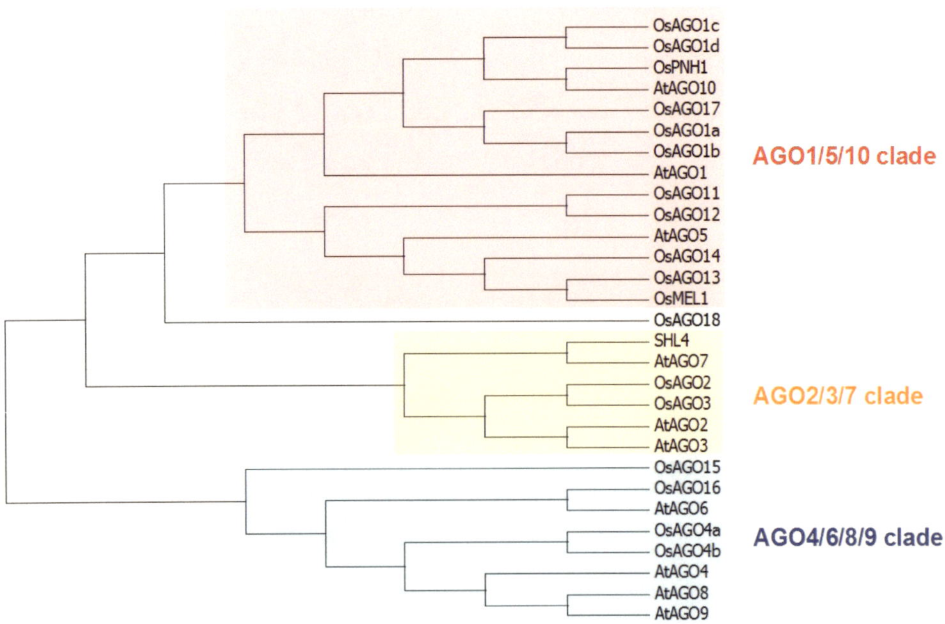

Fig. 5. *Phylogenetic tree constructed from the full-length amino acid sequences of the ten Arabidopsis AGO family members and nineteen Rice AGO family members.* The phylogeny clade divisions marked using different colour shades and labelled adjacently. Drawing not to scale.

counterpart rice genes, there are four AGO1 homologues in rice. Perhaps this expansion will be common in different plant species, reflective of the importance of the AGO1 function, as well as providing functional redundancy or tissue/cell-specific activities. As the sequences of completely assembled genomes of different plant species become known over the next few years, many of these questions will be answered. It is also possible that the different rice AGO1s have a spectrum of functions, and it is intriguing that the rice AGO5 family seems to be expanded and that AGO17 and especially AGO18 are orphans. It will be interesting to see whether these genes have functions absent in Arabidopsis, what roles they play, and whether these roles are monocot specific.

In conclusion, the study of *Ago* genes in Arabidopsis has revealed a family of proteins with elegant and complex activities that are essential for the normal development, genome stability and viral protection of the plant. However, it is clear that we still have much to learn about their mechanisms, actions and diversity across the plant kingdom.

6. References

Adenot, X., Elmayan, T., Lauressergues, D., et al. (2006). DRB4-Dependent TAS3 trans-Acting siRNAs Control Leaf Morphology through AGO7. *Current Biology,* Vol.16, No.9, (May 2006), pp. 927-932, ISSN 0960-9822

Agorio, A. & Vera, P. (2007) ARGONAUTE4 is required for resistance to *Pseudomonas syringae* in *Arabidopsis. Plant cell,* Vol.19, No.11, (November 2007), pp. 3778-3790, ISSN 1532-298X

Allen, E., Xie, Z., Gustafson, AM., et al. (2005) microRNA-directed phasing during trans-acting siRNA biogenesis in plants. *Cell,* Vol.121, No.2, (April 2005), pp. 207-221, ISSN 0092-8674

Aravin, AA., Sachidanandam, R., Bourc'his, D., et al. (2008) A piRNA pathway primed by individual transposons is linked to de novo DNA methylation in mice. *Molecular Cell,* Vol.31, No.6, (September 2008), pp. 785-799, ISSN 1097-2765

Baumberger, N., & Baulcombe, DC. (2005). Arabidopsis ARGONAUTE1 is an RNA Slicer that selectively recruits microRNAs and short interfering RNAs. *Proceedings of the National Academy of Sciences of the United States of America,* Vol.102, No.33, (August 2005), pp. 11928-11933, ISSN 1091-6490

Baumberger, N., Tsai, CH., Lie, M., et al. (2007) The Polerovirus silencing suppressor P0 targets ARGONAUTE proteins for degradation. *Current Biology,* Vol.17, No.18, (September 2007), pp. 1609-1614, ISSN 0960-9822

Bernstein, E., Caudy, AA., Hammond, SM., et al. (2001). Role for a bidentate ribonuclease in the intiation step of RNA interference. *Nature,* Vol.409, No.6818, (January 2001), pp. 363-366, ISSN 0028-0836

Bohmert, K., Camus, I., Bellini, C., et al. (1998). AGO1 defines a novel locus of Arabidopsis controlling leaf development. *EMBO Journal,* Vol.17, No.1, (January 1998), pp. 170-180, ISSN 0261-4189

Borges, F., Pereira, PA., Slotkin, RK., et al. (2011) MicroRNA activity in the *Arabidopsis* male germline. *Journal of Experimental Botany,* Vol.62, No.5, pp. 1611-1620, ISSN 1460-2431

Borsani, O., Zhu, J., Verslues, PE., et al. (2005). Endogenous siRNAs Derived from a Pair of Natural cis-Antisense Transcripts Regulate Salt Tolerance in Arabidopsis. *Cell,* Vol.123, No.7, (December 2005), pp. 1279-1291, ISSN 0092-8674

Bortolamiol, D., Pazhouhandeh, M., Marrocco, K., et al. (2007) The Polerovirus F box protein P0 targets ARGONAUTE1 to suppress RNA silencing. *Current Biology,* Vol.17, No.18, (September 2007), pp. 1615-1621, ISSN 0960-9822

Brodersen, P., Sakvarelidze-Achard, L., Bruun-Rasmussen, M., et al. (2008) Widespread translational inhibition by plant miRNAs and siRNAs. *Science,* Vol.320, No.5880, (May 2008), pp. 1185-1190, ISSN 1095-9203

Cartolano, M., Castillo, R., Efremova, N., et al. (2007) A conserved microRNA module exerts homeotic control over *Petunia hybrid* and *Antirrhinum majus* floral organ identity. *Nature Genetics,* Vol.39, No.7, (July 2007), pp. 901-905, ISSN 1061-4036

Catalanotto, C., Azzalin, G., Macino. G., et al. (2000). Gene silencing in worms and fungi. *Nature,* Vol.404, No.6775, (March 2000), pp. 245-245, ISSN 0028-0836

Chen, HM., Chen, LT., Patel, K., et al. (2010) 22-Nucleotide RNAs trigger secondary siRNA biogenesis in plants. *Proceedings of the National Academy of Sciences of the United States of America,* Vol.107, No.34, (July 2010), pp. 15269-15274, ISSN 1091-6490

Cheloufi, S., Dos Santos, CO., Chong, MM., et al. (2010) A dicer-independent miRNA biogenesis pathway that requires Ago catalysis. *Nature,* Vol.465, No.7298, (June 2010), pp. 584-589, ISSN 0028-0836

Cifuentes, D., Xue, H., Taylor, DW., et al. (2010) A novel miRNA processing pathway independent of Dicer requires Argonaute2 catalytic activity. *Science,* Vol.328, No.5986, (June 2010), pp. 1694-1698, ISSN 1095-9203

Combier, JP., Frugier, F., Billy, F., et al. (2006) MtHAP2-1 is a key transcriptional regulator of symbiotic nodule development regulated by microRNA169 in *Medicago truncatula. Genes and Development,* Vol.20, No.22, (November 2006), pp. 3084-3088, ISSN 1549-5477

Cuperus, JT., Carbonell, A., Fahlgren, N., et al. (2010) Unique functionality of 22-nt miRNAs in triggering RDR6-dependent siRNA biogenesis from target transcripts in Arabidopsis. *Nature Structural Molecular Biology,* Vol.17, No.8, (August 2010), pp. 997-1003, ISSN 1545-9993

Diederichs, S. & Haber, DA. (2007) Dual role for argonautes in microRNA processing and posttranscriptional regulation of microRNA expression. *Cell,* Vol.131, No.6, (December 2007), pp. 1097-1108, ISSN 0092-8674

El-Shami, M., Pontier, D., Lahmy, S., et al. (2007) Reiterated WG/GW motifs form functionally and evolutionarily conserved ARGONAUTE-binding platforms in RNAi-related components. *Genes and Development,* Vol. 21, No. 20, (October 2007), pp. 2539-2544, ISSN 2539-2544

Eulalio, A., Huntzinger, E. & Izaurralde, E. (2008) GW182 interaction with Argonaute is essential for miRNA-mediated translational repression and mRNA decay. *Nature Structural Molecular Biology,* Vol. 15, No.4, (April 2008), pp. 346-353, ISSN 1545-9993

Fagard, M., Boutet, S., Morel, JB., et al. (2000). AGO1, QDE-2, and RDE-1 are related proteins required for post-transcriptional gene silencing in plants, quelling in fungi, and RNA interference in animals. *Proceedings of the National Academy of Sciences of the United States of America,* Vol.97, No.21, (October 2000), pp. 11650-11654, ISSN 1091-6490

Fahlgren, N., Montgomery, TA., Howell, MD., et al. (2006) Regulation of AUXIN RESPONSE FACTOR3 by TAS3 ta-siRNA affects developmental timing and patterning in Arabidopsis. *Current Biology,* Vol.16, No.9, (May 2006), pp. 939-944, ISSN 0960-9822

Fang, Y. & Spector, DL. (2007) Identification of nuclear dicing bodies containing proteins for microRNA biogenesis in living *Arabidopsis* plants. *Current Biology,* Vol.17, No.9, (May 2007), pp. 818-823, ISSN 0960-9822

Forstemann, K., Horwich, MD., Wee, L., et al. (2007) Drosophila microRNAs are sorted into functionally distinct argonaute complexes after production by dicer-1. *Cell,* Vol.130, No.2, (July 2007), pp. 287-297, ISSN 0092-8674

Garcia, D., Collier, SA., Byrne, ME., et al. (2006) Specification of leaf polarity in Arabidopsis via the trans-acting siRNA pathway. *Current Biology,* Vol.16, No.9, (May 2006), pp. 933-938, ISSN 0960-9822

Gregory, RI., Chendrimada, TC., Cooch, N. et al. (2005). Human RISC couple microRNA biogenesis and post-transcriptional gene silencing. *Cell,* Vol.123, No.4, (November 2005), pp. 631-640, ISSN 0092-8674

Hamilton, AJ., & Baulcombe, DC. (1999). A species of small antisense RNA in post-transcriptional gene silencing in plants. *Science,* Vol.286, No.5441, (October 1999), pp. 950-952, ISSN 1095-9203

Harvey, JJ., Lewsey, MG., Patel, K., et al. (2011) An antiviral defense role of AGO2 in plants. *PLos ONE,* Vol.6, No.1, (January 2011), e14639, ISSN 1932-6203

Havecker, ER., Wallbridge, LM., Hardcastle, TJ., et al. (2010) The *Arabidopsis* RNA-directed DNA methylation argonautes functionally diverge based on their expression and interaction with target loci. *Plant Cell,* Vol.22, No.2, (February 2010), pp. 321-334, ISSN 1532-298X

Hunter, C., Sun, H. & Poethig, RS. (2003) The *Arabidopsis* heterochronic gene ZIPPY is an ARGONAUTE family member. *Current Biology,* Vol.13, No.19, (September 2003), pp. 1734-1739, ISSN 0960-9822

Hutvagner, G., & Simard, MJ. (2008). Argonaute proteins: Key players in RNA silencing. *Nature Reviews Molecular Cell Biology,* Vol.9, No.1, (January 2008), pp. 22-32, ISSN 1471-0072

Irvine, DV., Zaratiegui, M., Tolia, NH., et al. (2006) Argonaute slicing is required for heterochromatic silencing and spreading. *Science,* Vol.313, No.5790, (August 2006), pp. 1134-1137, ISSN 1095-9203

Jung, J. & Park, CM. (2007) *MIR166/165* genes exhibit dynamic expression patterns in regulating shoot apical meristem and floral development in *Arabidopsis. Planta,* Vol.225, No.6, (May 2007), pp. 1327-1338, ISSN 0032-0935

Katiyar-Agarwal, S., Gao, S., Vivian-Smith, A., et al. (2007) A novel class of bacteria-induced small RNAs in *Arabidopsis. Genes and Development,* Vol.21, No.23, (November 2007), pp. 3123-3134, ISSN 1549-5477

Kidner, CA., & Martienssen, RA. (2004). Spatially restricted microRNA directs leaf polarity through ARGONAUTE1. *Nature,* Vol.428, No.6978, (March 2004), pp. 81-84, ISSN 0028-0836

Lee, RC., & Ambros, V. (2001). An Extensive Class of Small RNAs in Caenorhabditis elegans. *Science,* Vol.294, No.5543, (October 2001), pp. 862-864, ISSN 1095-9203

Li, CF., Pontes, O., El-shami, M., et al. (2006) An ARGONAUTE4-containing nuclear processing center colocalized with Cajal bodies in *Arabidopsis thaliana. Cell,* Vol.126, No.1, (July 2006), pp. 93-106, ISSN 0092-8674

Liu, J., Carmell, MA., Rivas, F., et al. (2004) Argonaute2 is the catalytic engine of mammalian RNAi. *Science,* Vol.305, No.5689, (July 2004), pp. 1437-1441, ISSN 1095-9203

Liu, J., Rivas, FV., Wohlschlegel, J., et al. (2005) A role for the P-body component GW182 in microRNA function. *Nature Cell Biology,* Vol.7, No.12, (December 2005), pp. 1261-1266, ISSN 1465-7392

Liu, Q., Yao, X., Pi, L., et al. (2009) The *ARGONAUTE10* gene modulates shoot apical meristem maintenance and establishment of leaf polarity by repressing miR165/166 in Arabidopsis. *The Plant Journal,* Vol.58, No.1, (April 2009), pp. 27-40, ISSN 0960-7412

Liu, X., Park, JK., Jiang, F. et al. (2007) Dicer-1, but not Loquacious, is critical for assembly of miRNA-induced silencing complexes. *RNA*, Vol.13, No.12, (December 2007), pp. 2324-2329, ISSN 1469-9001

Lobbes, D., Rallapalli, G., Schmidt, DD., et al. (2006) SERRATE: a new player on the plant microRNA scene. *EMBO Reports,* Vol. 7, No. 10, (October 2006), pp. 1052-1058, ISSN 1469-221X

Lynn, K., Fernandez, A., Aida, M., et al. (1999) The PINHEAD/ZWILLE gene acts pleiotropically in *Arabidopsis* development and has overlapping functions with the *ARGONAUTE1* gene. *Development,* Vol.126, No.3, (February 1999), pp. 469-481, ISSN 1461-7072

Mallory, AC., Hinze, A., Tucker, MR., et al. (2009) Redundant and specific roles of the ARGONAUTE proteins AGO1 and ZLL in development: importance of pairing to the microRNA 5′ region. *PLoS Genetics,* Vol.5, No.9, (September 2009), e1000646, ISSN 1553-7404

Meister, G., Landthaler, M., Patkaniowska, A., et al. (2004) Human Argonaute2 mediates RNA cleavage targeted by miRNAs and siRNAs. *Molecular Cell,* Vol.15, No.2, (July 2004), pp. 185-197, ISSN 1097-2765

Meister, G., & Tuschl, T. (2004). Mechanisms of gene silencing by double-stranded RNA. *Nature,* Vol.431, No.7006, (September 2004), pp. 343-349, ISSN 0028-0836

Mi, S., Cai, T., Hu, Y., et al. (2008) Sorting of small RNAs into *Arabidopsis* argonaute complexes is directed by the 5′ terminal nucleotide. *Cell,* Vol. 133, No. 1, (April 2008), pp. 116-127, ISSN 0092-8674

Montgomery, TA., Howell, MD., Cuperus, JT., et al. (2008) Specificity of ARGONAUTE7-miR390 interaction and dual functionality in TAS3 *trans*-acting siRNA formation. *Cell,* Vol.133, No.1, (March 2008), pp. 128-141, ISSN 0092-8674

Morel, JB., Gordon, C., Mourrain, P., et al. (2002) Fertile hypomorphic ARGONAUTE (ago1) mutants impaired in post-transcriptional gene silencing and virus resistance. *Plant Cell,* Vol.14, No.3, (March 2002), pp. 629-639, ISSN 1532-298X

Moussian, B., (1998) Role of the ZWILLE gene in the regulation of central shoot meristem cell fate during *Arabidopsis* embryogenesis. *EMBO Journal,* Vol.17, No.6, (March 1998), pp. 1799-1809, ISSN 0261-4189

Nowotny, M., Sergei, A., Gaidamakov, RJC., et al. (2005). Crystal structures of RNase H bound to an RNA/DNA hybrid: substrate specificity and metal-dependent catalysis. *Cell,* Vol.121, No.7, (July 2005), pp. 1005-1016, ISSN 0092-8674

Olmedo-Monfil, V., Duran-Figueroa, N., Arteaga-Vazquez, M., et al. (2010) Control of female gamete formation by a small RNA pathway in Arabidopsis. *Nature,* Vol.464, No.7288, (March 2010), pp. 628-632, ISSN 0028-0836

Park, W., Li, J., Song, R., et al. (2002) CARPEL FACTORY, a Dicer homolog, and HEN1, a novel protein, act in microRNA metabolism in *Arabidopsis thaliana. Current Biology,* Vol. 12, No. 17, (September 2002), pp. 1484-1495, ISSN 0960-9822

Parker, JS. (2010). How to slice: snapshots of Argonaute in action. *Silence,* Vol.1, No.3, (January 2010), pp. 1-10, ISSN 1758-907X

Peragine, A., Yoshikawa, M., Wu, G., et al. (2004) SGS3 and SGS2/SDE1/RDR6 are required for juvenile development and the production of trans-acting siRNAs in Arabidopsis. *Gene and Development,* Vol.18, No.19, (October 2004), pp. 2368-2379, ISSN 1549-5477

Pontes, O., Li, CF., Nunes, PC., et al. (2006) The *Arabidopsis* chromatin-modifying nuclear siRNA pathway involves a nucleolar RNA processing center. *Cell,* Vol.126, No.1, (July 2006), pp. 79-92, ISSN 0092-8674

Qu, F., Ye, X. & Morris, TJ. (2008) Arabidopsis DRB4, AGO1, AGO7 and RDR6 participate in a DCL4-initiated antiviral RNA silencing pathway negatively regulated by DCL1. *Proceedings of the National Academy of Sciences of the United States of America,* Vol.105, No.38, (September 2008), pp. 14732-14737, ISSN 1091-6490

Rajagopalan, R., Vaucheret, H., Trejo, J., et al. (2006) A diverse and evolutionarily fluid set of microRNAs in *Arabidopsis thaliana. Genes and Development,* Vol.20, No.24, (December 2006), pp. 3407-3425, ISSN 1549-5477

Rand, TA., Petersen, S., Du, F. et al. (2005). Argonaute2 cleaves the anti-guide strand of siRNA during RISC activation. *Cell,* Vol.123, No.4, (November 2005), pp. 621-629, ISSN 0092-8674

Rivas, FV., Tolia, NH., Song, JJ., et al. (2005). Purified Argonaute2 and an siRNA form recombinant human RISC. *Nature Structural Molecular Biology,* Vol.12, No.4, (April 2005), pp. 340-349, ISSN 1545-9993

Saito, K., Kazumichi, M., Nishida, TM., et al. (2006). Specific association of Piwi with rasiRNAs derived from retrotransposon and heterochromatic regions in the *Drosophila* genome. *Genes and Development,* Vol.20, No.16, (August 2006), pp. 2214-2222, ISSN 1549-5477

Schmid, M., Davison, TS., Henz, SR., et al. (2005) A gene expression map of *Arabidopsis thaliana* development. *Nature Genetics,* Vol.37, No.5, (May 2005), pp. 501-506, ISSN 1061-4036

Siolas, D., Lerner, C., Burchard, J., et al. (2005) Synthetic shRNAs as potent RNAi triggers. *Nature Biotechnology,* Vol.23, No.2, (February 2005), pp. 227-231, ISSN 1087-0156

Song, L., Han, MH., Lesicka, J., et al. (2007) *Arabidopsis* primary microRNA processing proteins HYL1 and DCL1 define a nuclear body distinct from the Cajal body. *Proceedings of the National Academy of Sciences of the United States of America,* Vol.104, No.13, (March 2007), pp. 5437-5442, ISSN 1091-6490

Steiner, FA., Hoogstrate, SW., Okihara, KL., et al. (2007) Structural features of small RNA precursors determine Argonaute loading in Caenorhabditis elegans. *Nature Structural Molecular Biology,* Vol.14, No.10, (October 2007), pp. 927-933, ISSN 1545-9993

Takeda, A., Iwasaki, S., Watanabe, T., et al. (2008) The mechanism selecting the guide strand from small RNA duplexes is different among Argonaute proteins. *Plant and Cell Physiology,* Vol.49, No.4, (March 2008), pp. 493-500, ISSN 1471-9053

Tan, GS., Garchow, BG., Liu, X., et al. (2009) Expanded RNA-binding activities of mammalian Argonaute 2. *Nucleic Acids Research,* Vol.37, No.22, (December 2009), pp. 7533-7545, ISSN 1362-4962

Tolia, NH., & Joshua-Tor, L. (2007). Slicer and the argonautes. *Nature Chemical Biology,* Vol.3, No.1, (January 2007), pp. 36-43, ISSN 1552-4450

Tomari, Y., Du, T. & Zamore, PD. (2007) Sorting of Drosophila small silencing RNAs. *Cell,* Vol.130, No.2, (July 2007), pp. 299-308, ISSN 1097-2765

Vaucheret H., Vazquez, F., Crété, P., et al. (2004) The action of ARGONAUTE1 in the miRNA pathway and its regulation by the miRNA pathway are crucial for plant development. *Genes & Development,* Vol. 18, No. 10, (May 2004), pp. 1187-1197, ISSN 1549-5477

Vaucheret, H., Mallory, AC., Bartel, DP. (2006) AGO1 homeostasis entails coexpression of MIR168 and AGO1 and preferential stabilization of miR168 by AGO1. *Molecular Cell,* Vol.22, No.1, (April 2006), pp. 129–136, ISSN 1097-2765

Vaucheret, H. (2008). Plant ARGONAUTES. *Trends in Plant Science,* Vol.13, No.7, (July 2008), pp. 350-358, ISSN 1360-1385

Vagin, VV., Sigova, A., Li, C., et al. (2006) A distinct small RNA pathway silences selfish genetic elements in the germline. *Science,* Vol.313, No.5785, (July 2006), pp. 320-324, ISSN 1095-9203

Wang, Y., Juranek, S., Li, H., et al. (2009). Nucleation, propagation and cleavage of target RNAs in Ago silencing complexes. *Nature,* Vol.461, No.7265, (October 2009), pp. 754-761, ISSN 0028-0836

Wang, Y., Juranek, S., Li, H., et al. (2008). Structure of an argonaute silencing complex with a seed-containing guide DNA and target RNA duplex. *Nature,* Vol.456, No.7224, (December 2008), pp. 921-926, ISSN 0028-0836

Wang, XB., Jovel, J., Udomporn, P., et al. (2011) The 21-Nucleotide, but Not 22-Nucleotide, Viral Secondary Small Interfering RNAs Direct Potent Antiviral Defense by Two Cooperative Argonautes in Arabidopsis thaliana. *Plant Cell,* (April 2011), ISSN 1532-298X

Winter, D., Vinegar, B., Nahal, H., et al. (2007) An "Electronic Fluorescent Pictograph" Browser for Exploring and Analyzing Large-Scale Biological Data Sets. *PLoS ONE,* Vol.2, No.8, (August 2007), e718, ISSN 1932-6203

Xie, Z., Johansen, LK., Gustafson, AM., et al. (2004) Genetic and functional diversification of small RNA pathways in plants. *PLoS Biology,* Vol.2, No.5, (May 2004), e104, ISSN 1544-9173

Xie, Z., Allen, E., Wilken, A., et al. (2005). DICER-LIKE4 functions in trans-acting siRNA biogenesis and vegetative phase change. *Proceedings of the National Academy of Sciences of the United States of America,* Vol.102, No.36, (August 2005), pp. 12984-12989, ISSN 1091-6490

Yoshikawa, M., Peragine, A., Park, MY., et al. (2005) A pathway for the biogenesis of trans-acting siRNAs in Arabidopsis. *Genes and Development,* Vol.19, No.18, (September 2005), pp. 2164-2175, ISSN 1549-5477

Zilberman, D., Cao, X. & Jacobsen, SE. (2003) ARGONAUTE4 control of locus-specific siRNA accumulation and DNA and histone methylation. *Science,* Vol.299. No.5607, (January 2003), pp. 716-719, ISSN 1095-9203

Zilberman, D., Cao, X., Johansen, LK., et al. (2004) Role of *Arabidopsis* ARGONAUTE4 in RNA-directed DNA methylation triggered by inverted repeats. *Current Biology,* Vol.14, No.13, (July 2004), pp. 1214-1220, ISSN 0960-9822

Zhang, X., Yuan, YR., Pei, Y., et al. (2006) Cucumber mosaic virus-encoded 2b suppressor inhibits *Arabidopsis* Argonaute1 cleavage activity to counter plant defense. *Genes and Development,* Vol.20, No.23, (December 2006), pp. 3255-3268, ISSN 1549-547.

Zhou, G., Kubo, M., Zhong, R., et al. (2007) Overexpression of miR165 affects apical meristem formation, organ polarity establishment and vascular development in *Arabidopsis. Plant and Cell Physiology,* Vol.48, No.3, (March 2007), pp. 391-404, ISSN 1471-9053

Zhu, H., Hu, F., Wang, R., et al. (2011) Arabidopsis Argonaute10 specifically Sequesters miR166/165 to Regulate Shoot Apical Meristem Development. *Cell,* Vol.145, No.2, (April 2011), pp. 242-256, ISSN 0092-8674

8

RNAi in Agriculturally-Important Arthropods

Katherine Aronstein[1], Brenda Oppert[2] and Marcé D. Lorenzen[3]
[1]*Honey Bee Research Unit, USDA-ARS, Weslaco, TX 78596,*
[2]*USDA ARS Center for Grain and Animal Health Research, Manhattan, KS 66502, Raleigh, NC 27695*
[3]*Department of Entomology, North Carolina State University, USA*

1. Introduction

This chapter was inspired by rapid developments in the field of RNA interference (RNAi), an evolutionarily-conserved cellular mechanism that directs protection against nucleic-acid invaders (e.g., viruses and repetitive DNA sequences including transposable elements) in plants, animals, protozoans and fungi. It is now evident that prokaryotes also possess an RNA-based defense system, though completely distinct from that in eukaryotes. The recent discovery of post-transcriptional gene silencing (PTGS) has generated tremendous interest in basic and applied research, including the development of *in vitro* and *in vivo* therapeutic approaches to reduce expression of disease-associated genes. This cutting-edge technology has already been successfully used in genomic manipulations of insect disease vectors, such as development of Dengue-resistant mosquitoes (Blair et al., 2006; Franz et al., 2006 ; Mathur et al., 2010).

Our aim in this chapter is to provide an overview of the profound knowledge accumulated in recent years from invertebrate RNAi studies, but with a focus on agriculturally important arthropods. We start with a brief discussion of the RNAi mechanism to introduce readers to key concepts that underlie the practical application of RNAi discussed in the remainder of the chapter. Our discussion will include a number of important issues that should be carefully considered when working with multi-cellular organisms, including bidirectional transport of silencing signals, processing of dsRNA, homology-driven mRNA degradation and subsequent gene silencing.

We will look at examples of gene silencing in different arthropod systems to illustrate commonalities and differences found in their silencing machinery. Arthropods are a diverse group of organisms, including ticks, mites, spiders, crabs, and insects, many of which are economically significant pests of agricultural crops, parasites of commercially managed pollinators and vectors of livestock diseases.

Considering the huge economic impact of honey bees on crop production, and particularly on pollination of specialty crops, a substantial part of this chapter will be dedicated to honey bee research. Recently, catastrophic losses of honey bee colonies drew national media attention and ignited a renewed interest in basic and applied bee research (Aronstein et al., 2006; Campbell et al., 2010; Dearden et al., 2009; Maori et al., 2009a, 2009b; Nelson et al., 2007). The latest achievements in basic honey bee research provide a better understanding of bee physiology and behavior. Analysis of gene function by selective gene silencing has been a powerful tool to dissect the complex mechanisms regulating biological processes involved in bee development, immunity, olfaction, learning and memory. Applied studies have focused on practical implementation of RNAi for control of honey bee diseases and parasites that cannot be achieved using conventional management techniques (Liu et al., 2010; Maori et al., 2009a, 2009b; Paldi et al., 2010). Examples will include: 1) development of RNAi-based control for *Nosema ceranae,* an intracellular parasite infecting adult bees, and 2) development of an antiviral treatment to protect bees against Israeli Acute Paralysis Virus (IAPV) and Chinese Sacbrood Virus (CSBV).

The success of RNAi technology as a control method for agricultural pests depends heavily on target specificity, gene-silencing efficiency and systemic spread of silencing. Originally, systemic RNAi was thought to be unique to plants and nematodes, however recent research revealed that systemic transfer of a silencing signal occurs in many arthropods. The first commercial use of RNAi in agriculture was demonstrated via oral RNAi in transgenic plants (*in planta* RNAi) toward several economically-important coleopteran pests, including the Western corn rootworm, *Diabrotica virgifera virgifera* and Colorado potato beetle, *Leptinotarsa decemlineata* (Baum et al., 2007). Oral RNAi has also been reported in Diptera, Hemiptera, Hymenoptera and Lepidoptera (Araujo et al., 2006; Aronstein et al., 2006; Lehane et al., 2008; Turner et al., 2006; Walshe et al., 2009). Our discussion will focus on the successful use of this strategy, as well as the challenges encountered by researchers seeking to use this sensitive, targeted approach to pest control.

We include an overview of the development of RNAi in the coleopteran model and stored product pest, the red flour beetle, *Tribolium castaneum*. The fact that the *T. castaneum* genome has been sequenced, coupled with the beetle's ability to mount a robust, systemic RNAi response to injected dsRNAs, makes it an excellent model for RNAi. Of particular interest is the discovery of new pest control targets through a candidate gene approach to RNAi. While much can be learned from small-scale RNAi studies, we will also discuss a large-scale RNAi-based screen in this beetle.

The first high-throughput RNAi screens in insects were performed in *D. melanogaster* cell lines (Bellés, 2010; Boutros & Ahringer, 2008; D'Ambrosio & Vale, 2010). Since then, genome-wide screens have revealed the function of genes involved in phenotype (physiology/morphology), neurobiology, signal transduction, ion transport, pathogen response, as well as metabolic and gene-processing pathways, among others (Mummery-Widmer et al., 2009). Currently efforts are underway to apply whole-genome RNAi screens in economically important arthropods, such as the cattle tick, *Rhipicephalus microplus* (Kurscheid et al., 2009) and *T. castaneum* (Angelini et al., 2009; Lynch et al., 2009). These and other RNAi-based studies will enable functional analysis of homologous genes in different arthropod species, as well as provide insight into the function of vertebrate homologs that could possibly aid in the identification and validation of drug targets.

2. RNAi mechanisms in arthropods

Like other organisms, arthropods, have evolved efficient homology-driven gene silencing mechanisms for protection against nucleic acid invaders (Deddouche et al., 2008; Gaines et al., 1996; Lu et al., 2004; Olson et al., 1996). Since its discovery, significant efforts have been made to unravel the molecular mechanisms of RNAi. While the core components of RNAi appear to be well conserved across phyla, molecular mechanisms underlying signal amplification and systemic spread of silencing are highly diverged. Improvements in dsRNA design algorithms and delivery methods triggered an avalanche of new research projects in over 30 insect species (Orthoptera, Dictyoptera, Isoptera, Hemiptera, Coleoptera, Neuroptera, Hymenoptera, Lepidoptera, and Diptera). The most extensive work has been facilitated by sequenced genomes and performed in model insects, including *D. melanogaster*, *T. castaneum* and the silkworm, *Bombyx mori*. The use of RNAi in honey bee research has attracted enormous interest, driven by their economic importance and the sharp increase in colony losses in recent years. Below, we'll discuss some of these issues in attempt to decipher the ambiguities in research findings that, in some cases, generate more questions than answers. Understanding the critical steps in the RNAi process will facilitate the transfer of this technology to additional arthropod species.

2.1 Core RNAi components

The post-transcriptional silencing of gene function is a very rapid process where double-stranded RNA (dsRNA) directs sequence-specific degradation of mRNA. In general, this complicated chain of reactions can be viewed as a two-step process. First, a long dsRNA is cleaved into small interfering RNAs (siRNA), and second, siRNAs are incorporated into silencing complexes (RISC). Following RISC assembly, siRNAs guide degradation of homologous mRNAs (Hammond et al., 2000).

The core components of the RNAi machinery have been thoroughly studied using a combination of biochemical, genetic, and bioinformatic approaches (Hamilton et al., 2002; Hammond et al., 2000; Rolff & Reynolds, 2009; Tomoyasu et al., 2008; Zamore et al., 2000). When dsRNA is introduced into insect cells, it is recognized by a dsRNA-specific RNase-III type ribonuclease called Dicer and cleaved into siRNAs that are 21–23 nt in length. Unlike most animals, insect genomes encode two Dicer-like proteins. One of them, Dcr-2 is involved in RNA interference in *Drosophila*, whereas Dcr-1 recognizes precursors of miRNAs. With the assistance of dsRNA-binding motif proteins (dsRBM), the next phase in the RNAi pathway involves the loading of siRNAs into RISCs. Most evidence indicates that RISCs contain only one siRNA strand, specifically the "guide ssRNA". Therefore, careful selection of siRNA sequences that favor incorporation of the antisense strand into the RISC may improve efficacy and specificity of RNAi. Another essential member of the RISC complex is the RNase H enzyme Argonaute (AGO) that mediates recognition of the target mRNA. Using the siRNAs as a guide, AGO finds complimentary sequences and cleaves homologous mRNA, consequently leading to its degradation.

While most core RNAi components were characterized in *D. melanogaster*, many have been identified in other insects, nematodes and chelicerates. Recently analyzed genomes of the honey bee, red flour beetle, and silkworm (Consortium, 2008; Consortium, 2006; Richards & Consortium, 2008) indicate they each encode the core components of the RNAi machinery, including Dicer enzymes, Ago1 and 2, dsRBMs and other members of the cell-autonomous RNAi machinery.

2.2 Mechanism of dsRNA up-take

In the model nematode, *Caenorhabditis elegans*, systemic RNAi can be induced by dsRNA injection, ingestion or immersion. However, microinjection of dsRNA in *Drosophila* failed to induce systemic RNAi, resulting in the erroneous conclusion that RNAi is a cell-autonomous process in insects (Boutla et al., 2001; Kennerdell & Carthew, 1998, 2000; Roignant et al., 2003). Since then systemic gene silencing has been demonstrated in many insect species (Amdam et al., 2003; Aronstein et al., 2006; Bucher et al., 2002; Hughes & Kaufman, 2000; Miller et al., 2008; Posnien et al., 2009).

Injection, and in some cases ingestion of long dsRNA, produces very robust silencing effects both locally and in tissues distant from the site of introduction in arthropods, suggesting that the systemic nature of RNAi is conserved among the Arthropoda. This discovery promoted the use of RNAi technology in chelicerates and in a wider range of insect species, especially those for which transgenic protocols have not been developed. However, questions remain about the longevity of this effect in different arthropod species. Most studies report a time or stage when gene silencing was confirmed, but the effect was short-lived and did not necessarily coincide with the observed phenotypic change. In general, RNAi in arthropods is transient. However, in some cases the trans-developmental effects can persist long enough to be observed over several developmental stages (e.g., embryonic, larval and pupal) (Grossmann et al., 2009; Liu & Kaufman, 2004; Ronco et al., 2008; Tomoyasu & Denell, 2004).

In the honey bee, injections of *vitellogenin* (*Vg*) dsRNA into newly emerged workers knocked-down *Vg* expression and dramatically affected the behavior of aged bees, causing a premature shift from nesting tasks to those of foraging (Amdam et al., 2003; Nelson et al., 2007). Injection or oral administration of *Am18w* dsRNA into 5-day-old bee larvae resulted in silencing of this Toll-like receptor transcript and produced significant morphological defects (Fig. 1) in both pupae and adults (Aronstein et al., 2006; Aronstein & Saldivar, 2005).

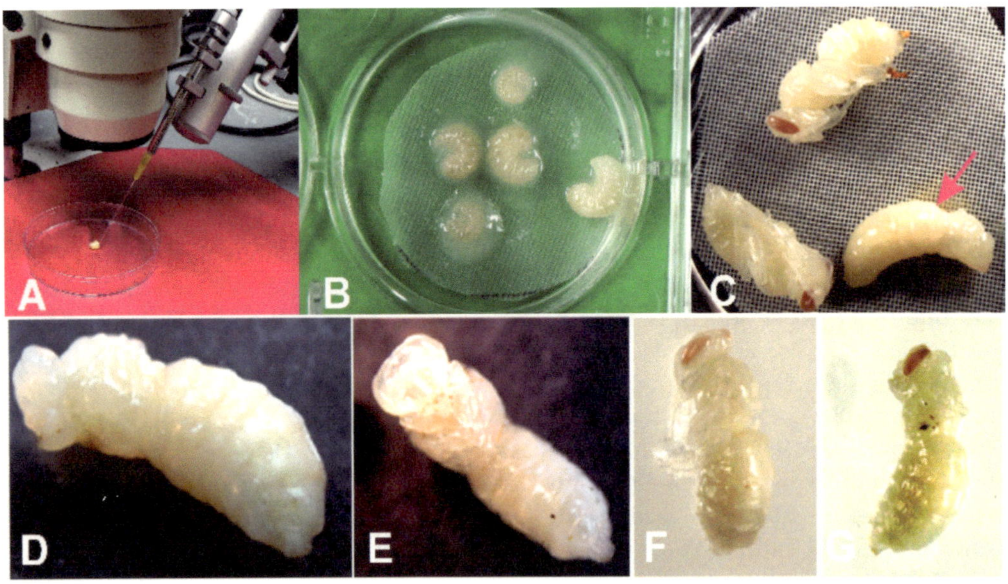

Fig. 1. RNAi-mediated silencing of the honey bee (*Apis mellifera*) *Am18w* encoding Toll-like receptor: 5-day-old-larvae were injected A) or fed/soaked B) with *Am18w* dsRNA as described by Aronstein and Saldivar (2005) and Aronstein et al. (2006). Silencing of *Am18w* resulted in severe morphological defects observed in pupae (C - E) and adult bees (F - G). The abnormalities were most evident in the thorax and head of pupae (C, red arrow), such as complete absence of or shortened appendages, as well as fused body segments.

In the Indian mealmoth, *Plodia interpunctella*, and *T. castaneum*, silencing of a gene encoding tryptophan oxygenase in embryos resulted in loss of eye-color pigmentation in 1st instar larvae (Fabrick et al., 2004; Lorenzen et al., 2002). Interestingly, the loss-of-function phenotype persisted until pupation in the beetle, approximately four weeks, while the phenotypic changes were not tracked past the initial larval stage in the mealmoth.

In addition to trans-developmental effects, trans-generational RNAi has also been observed in insects. For example, zygotic expression of multiple target genes has been silenced by injecting dsRNA into female pupae or adults (i.e., parental RNAi) in *T. castaneum*, a parasitic wasp, *Nasonia vitripennis*, crickets, *Gryllus bimaculatus* or milkweed bugs, *Oncopeltus fasciatus* (Bucher et al., 2002; Lynch & Desplan, 2006; Mito et al., 2011; Ronco et al., 2008; Tomoyasu et al., 2008; Werren & Loehlin, 2009). Recent *Drosophila* studies demonstrated that flies too have the ability to activate systemic RNAi, albeit in response to viral infection (Saleh et al., 2009).

The ability of RNAi signals to move cell-to-cell within the organism suggests the existence of molecular mechanisms for transporting signals bidirectionally across cell membranes, and from the site of introduction to distant tissues. Moreover, to support the long lasting effect of silencing, there may be an additional mechanism for RNAi amplification. It appears that arthropods can efficiently import and export silencing signals, although molecular mechanisms underlying these processes are still debated. Below we discuss recently proposed models explaining mechanisms of import and export of silencing signals in different arthropod systems.

2.2.1 Sid-dependent up-take

Organisms exhibit substantial differences in their ability to take up and distribute dsRNA. Some are capable of both up-take and systemic spread (Araujo et al., 2006; Dong & Friedrich, 2005; Saleh et al., 2006; Soares et al., 2005; Walshe et al., 2009), while others apparently readily take up dsRNA, but have significant difficulties with systemic distribution (Dietz et al., 2007; Roignant et al., 2003; Van Roessel et al., 2002). However, the inability of an organism to foster systemic effects of dsRNA could be due to shortcomings in methodology which may be mitigated by improved applications, such as extended hairpin RNA-based transgenic RNAi (Artymovich, 2009; Carthew, 2003; Kennerdell et al., 2002), as well as other improvements in RNAi protocols discussed in Section 4.

In nematodes, a two-step model has been proposed to explain the complex mechanism of large (~500 bp) dsRNA transport (Winston et al., 2007). According to this model, ingested dsRNA does not require Sid-1 (a systemic-interference-defective) to pass through the gut lumen in *C. elegans*. Instead, endocytosis of dsRNA by Sid-2, an intestinal luminal transmembrane protein, is proposed for the import of dsRNA across the midgut lining. Vesicles containing dsRNA bud off from the gut lumen and release their content into the body cavity, where they are taken up by cells in different tissues via Sid-1-assisted passive diffusion in a concentration dependent manner (Feinberg & Hunter, 2003; Jose & Hunter, 2007). Several other genes (*Rsd-2*, *Rsd-3* and *Rsd-6*) are involved in the systemic spread of dsRNA in *C. elegans*, which was previously attributed to endocytosis, suggesting that transport of dsRNA in *C. elegans* can also use a Sid-1-independent mechanism.

While some core processes remain common among different arthropod phyla, it appears that mechanisms of dsRNA up-take and transport are largely diverged. A single *sid-1* gene has been identified in most sequenced insect genomes, with the exception of three *sid-1* homologs found in *T. castaneum* and *B. mori* genomes (Aronstein et al., 2006; Aronstein & Saldivar, 2005; Huvenne & Smagghe, 2010; Tomoyasu et al., 2008). However, the correlation between the presence of *sid-1,* or *sid-1-like* (*sil*), in insect genomes and systemic RNAi is uncertain (Tomoyasu et al., 2008). One reason for this uncertainty is the lack of one-to-one orthology between the *sil* genes and *sid-1*. It has been proposed that the three *sil* genes in *T. castaneum* are orthologus to *C. elegans tag-130,* rather than *sid-1* (Tomoyasu et al., 2008). While *tag-130* is not required for systemic RNAi in nematodes, it is possible that the *sil* genes in *T. castaneum* are orthologous to *tag-130*, but still function in systemic RNAi. On the other hand, it is also possible that the *sil* genes are orthologous to *sid-1,* but play no role in systemic RNAi. However, the most satisfying explanation to date is that the *sil* genes are functional *sid-1* orthologs. This observation correlated with the fact that flour beetles and honey bees are proficient in systemic RNAi, and dipterans (which lack *sil* genes) are extremely poor. The existence of a Sid-2-mediated mechanism is also questionable, as *sid-2* orthologs have not been found in any animal genomes other than *C. elegans*, but this may be due to the rapid evolution of *sid-2* homologs.

2.2.2 Sid-independent transport

While substantial progress has been made towards understanding dsRNA up-take in nematodes, the molecular mechanisms for the transport of silencing signals in other arthropods are still mostly unknown. A new model explaining dsRNA entry and initiation of RNAi silencing in arthropods has been proposed (Saleh et al., 2006; Ulvila et al., 2006). According to this model, dsRNA up-take relies on receptor-mediated endocytosis followed by an active spread of the silencing signal by vesicle-mediated intracellular trafficking (Tomoyasu et al., 2008; Ulvila et al., 2006). The role of SR-CI and Eater in the up-take of dsRNA has been recently tested in *Drosophila* S2 cells, demonstrating that more than 90% of dsRNA up-take depends on these two receptors (Ulvila et al., 2006). However, silencing of 8 Toll and 19 scavenger receptors did not significantly affect the inhibition of RNAi, indicating that other members of pattern recognition receptors must be tested to evaluate the receptor-mediated endocytosis model (Saleh et al., 2006). Furthermore, systemic transport of endogenous silencing signals may be stimulated by specific physiological conditions, such as exposure to viruses. Saleh et al. (2009) demonstrated that receptor-mediated endocytosis is involved in an antiviral response in *Drosophila*. Nevertheless, specific mechanisms associated with dsRNA up-take and transport throughout the body in other insects continues to be the subject of ongoing research.

2.2.3 Mechanism of signal amplification

To sustain silencing, some organisms may employ a strategy for signal amplification. In *C. elegans,* primary siRNAs are amplified through an RNA-directed RNA polymerase (RdRP)-dependent mechanism leading to generation of secondary siRNAs and amplification of silencing (Hamilton et al., 2002). While RdRP activity has not been demonstrated in other organisms, molecular components of this amplification mechanism have recently been identified in the cattle tick genome (Kurscheid et al., 2009). Although insect genomes do not encode a canonical invertebrate RdRP homologue, there is a possibility that RdRP-like activity may occur via other enzymes (Lipardi & Paterson, 2009). The existence of the amplification mechanism in nematodes and possibly in the chelicerate arthropods provides an interesting perspective on the existence of alternative RNAi mechanisms in evolutionarily-diverged groups of animals.

3. Applied research projects using RNAi

Understanding the mechanisms involved in the different phases of gene silencing is absolutely essential for the development of effective RNAi-based applications to control pests of agricultural crops, vectors of livestock disease, and predators and parasites of beneficial insects. RNAi also holds considerable potential as a therapeutic approach to silence disease-causing genes in beneficial insects, particularly important in arthropods deficient in protein-based adaptive immune responses. The identification and utilization of these new approaches in different insect systems may provide more effective control applications. For example, receptor-mediated endocytotic machinery could offer a starting point for novel dsRNA delivery strategies. Below, we describe some of the most recent research findings that harness RNAi technology and hold promise for the development of a new class of therapeutic drugs and pest-control applications.

3.1 RNAi in beneficial arthropods and other non-pests

As honey bees are primary pollinators for most agricultural crops, substantial resources have been devoted to solving recent problems with honey bee health. Therefore, we begin our discussion of RNAi as it relates to agriculture with an overview of the success of the technology related to applications in honey bee research.

3.1.1 Disease control in Honey Bee colonies

The unprecedented loss of honey bee colonies over the past several years has endangered not only the honey bee industry, but also threatens to wipe out agricultural production of crops dependent on pollination. Since 2006, significant colony losses have been reported in many countries around the world, challenging the beekeeping industry to meet pollination demands. The worldwide economic value of the pollination service mainly provided by bees is estimated at $217 billion USD, particularly in added value of specialty crops such as nuts, berries, fruits, and vegetables (Gallai et al., 2009). Among numerous threats, honey bees face diverse parasites and pathogens, some of which are implicated in the massive colony losses, termed Colony Collapse Disorder (CCD) (Genersch, 2010).
Microbial pathogens and parasites in the honey bee colonies are traditionally controlled by antimicrobial drugs and pesticides. Although necessary, these activities, often result in the over exposure of bees to synthetic chemicals that ultimately affect the bee's health and behavior. Misuse of chemicals has also been suspected in some colony losses reported by beekeepers. Therefore, development and implementation of RNAi technology holds great potential for new non-toxic applications for disease control in bee hives. This approach has rapidly emerged as a genetic tool for combating microsporidial and viral diseases in bees. Some bee pathogens, such as *Nosema ceranae* (Higes et al., 2008; Higes et al., 2009) and Israeli Acute Paralysis Virus (IAPV) or a combination of the two (Bromenshenk et al., 2010) , were recently implicated in world-wide losses of bee colonies. Analysis of the *N. ceranae* genome demonstrated the presence of RNA silencing machinery in this species, suggesting that RNAi can be exploited for control of infection within the host (Cornman et al., 2009). Indeed, *in vivo* experiments targeting expression of *N. ceranae* ADP/ATP transporter genes demonstrated inhibiting effects on *Nosema* development, as well as the level of pathogen in the host when fed dsRNA (Paldi et al., 2010). However, activity against *Nosema* in these experimental treatments declined sharply within two to three weeks post treatment.

RNAi has also emerged as an important antiviral defense in insects. Since most honey bee viruses are positive-stranded RNA viruses that generate dsRNA in the process of viral replication, they are particularly vulnerable to the insect's silencing machinery. RNAi applications based on silencing the internal ribosome entry site (IRES) of IAPV were recently tested and showed great potential for developing a novel antiviral drug for use in bee colonies (Maori et al., 2009a, 2009b). One dsRNA product, "Remebee," is currently being tested in a large-scale field trial (Hunter et al., 2010). This product is delivered to bees during routine feeding and is recommended for multiple applications in bee colonies, subject to FDA approval. To control another bee virus, Chinese Sacbrood Virus (CSBV), second instar *Apis. cerana* larvae were fed dsRNA targeting VP1 structural protein (Liu et al., 2010). Silencing of the target gene (*VP1)* was observed 12 h post feeding, but long-term effects of this treatment on the level of CSBV in *A. cerana* have not been evaluated.

We are currently assessing an RNAi-based approach for the control of sexual reproduction in the most prevalent bee fungal pathogen, *Ascosphaera apis* (Aronstein, unpublished). In this study, dsRNAs target newly identified *A. apis* mating type transcription factors (MAT-1 and MAT-2) (Aronstein et al., 2007). If successful, RNAi-based control methods could potentially fill the current void (i.e. no chemical treatments are available for the prevention and/or control of chalkbrood disease in bee colonies).

3.1.2 Silkworm and other beneficials

In *B. mori*, RNAi has been used primarily as a tool to investigate gene function at different developmental stages (Goldsmith et al., 2005). Specifically, RNAi has been used to delineate a number of physiological processes in silkworm, including cocoon pigmentation (Tabunoki et al., 2004), the sex pheromone biosynthetic pathway (Ohnishi et al., 2006), segmentation and appendage formation (Masumoto et al., 2009), and programmed cell death (Lee et al., 2009). Transgenic *B. mori* have been developed with a heat shock inducible and inheritable RNAi system to further probe gene function (Dai et al., 2007). RNAi is also being used to address problems in silkworm culture. For example, transgenic *B. mori* larvae expressing dsRNA targeting a baculovirus gene, *baculoviral immediate early-1* (*ie-1*), induced strong protection against infection by the *B. mori* nucleopolyhedrovirus (Kanginakudru et al., 2007).

Another beneficial, *Nasonia* wasps, primarily parasitize large pest flies, making these four closely related parasitoid species a useful tool for biocontrol. After the honey bee genome, *N. vitripennis* is only the second species of Hymenoptera with a sequenced genome (Rütten et al., 2004; Werren et al., 2010), and is rapidly emerging as a powerful model organism for functional studies. Rapid advances in *Nasonia* genomics have already helped to delineate basic mechanisms of embryonic development (Lynch & Desplan, 2010) and sex determination (Verhulst et al., 2010) in this species, and will help to further improve our understanding of the systemic nature (Werren & Loehlin, 2009) and trans-generational effects of gene silencing (Lynch & Desplan, 2006).

3.2 Using RNAi for pest control

RNAi applications have already demonstrated great success in silencing essential biological functions of many arthropod-pests (Price & Gatehouse, 2008). However, current *in vivo* applications will require substantial improvements in silencing efficiency, stabilization of dsRNAs and improved formulations to be implemented in the field.

3.2.1 Red flour beetle

The red flour beetle has been associated with human agriculture for at least four thousand years. It is a major pest of stored grains worldwide, causing millions of dollars in damage annually. However, *Tribolium* also has become one of the best understood model organisms in biology in the past few decades, and is the first beetle to have a sequenced genome (Richards & Consortium, 2008). As previously mentioned, injection of dsRNA elicits a robust systemic RNAi response in *T. castaneum*, and can be performed during any life stage (Fig. 2).

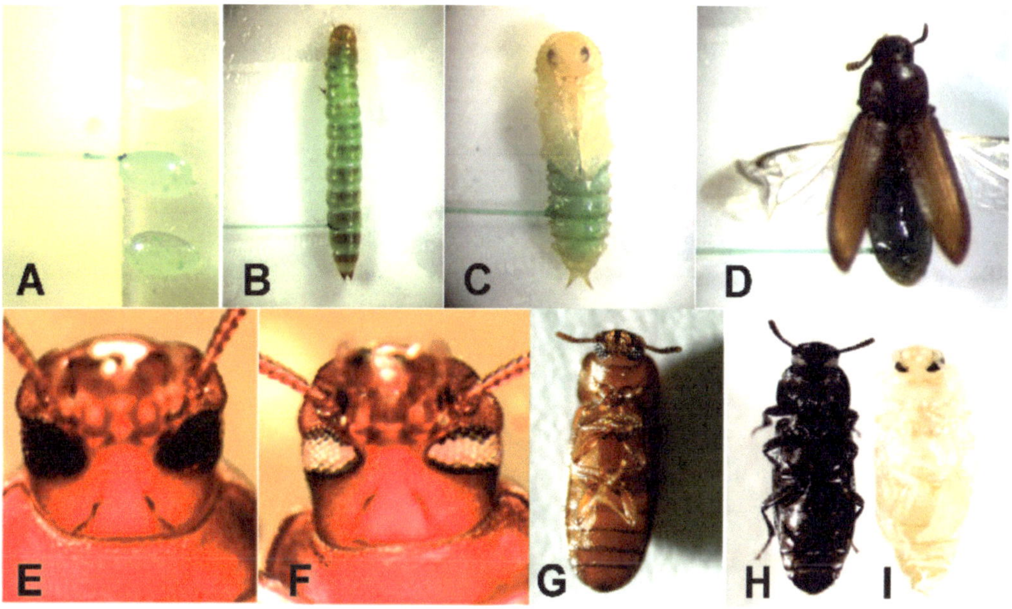

Fig. 2. RNAi-mediated gene silencing in the red flour beetle, *Tribolium castaneum*. RNAi can be performed at any life stage in flour beetles by injecting dsRNAs into A) embryos, B) larvae, C) pupae or D) adults. Injected dsRNAs are generally dyed to provide confirmation of injection (in this case a green dye was used). Effect of *T. castaneum scarlet* (*Tcst*) dsRNA on eye pigmentation. Last-instar larvae were injected with *Tcst* dsRNA and observed as adults; E) uninjected individual with wild-type eye color, F) wild-type individual that was injected with *Tcst* dsRNA during last larval stage. Note absence of eye pigmentation in the ommatidia (black "mascara" around eye is from a different pigment pathway). Effect of *T. castaneum laccase-2* (*TcLac2*) dsRNA on body color. G) wild-type body color, H) "black" body color mutant, I) "black" mutant that was injected with *TcLac2* during last larval stage.

From its initial use in 1999 to phenocopy null mutations of the *T. castaneum Deformed* gene (Brown et al., 1999), to its wide use in functional genomic screens, RNAi has become an extremely valuable tool both to elucidate gene function and to identify potential pest control targets. Here we will discuss key *Tribolium*-based RNAi studies with significance to pest control.

Arthropods are known for their hard chitinous exoskeleton. The chitin/cuticle pathway that gives rise to this arthropod-specific structure has been the object of much interest due to its relevance as a pest control target. While researchers have studied this pathway for many years, RNAi has revolutionized studies in this field. For example, a group in Manhattan, Kansas (USDA-ARS and Kansas State University) has been using RNAi to identify *T. castaneum* genes that encode proteins responsible for exoskeleton biosynthesis and degradation. Candidate genes from other insects have been selected and orthologs identified via blast analysis of the *T. castaneum* genome database, BeetleBase (http://beetlebase.org/). Prior to RNAi analysis, the spatiotemporal pattern of gene expression is determined via RT-PCR to ensure RNAi is performed at appropriate time points. Chitin/cuticle pathway genes, including those required for chitin synthesis (Arakane et al., 2005b; Arakane et al., 2008), molting, survival and fecundity (Arakane et al., 2010b; Arakane et al., 2009; Arakane et al., 2008; Broehan et al., 2010; Hogenkamp et al., 2007; Zhu et al., 2008) and tanning of the epidermal cuticle (Arakane et al., 2010a; Arakane et al., 2009; Arakane et al., 2005a) have been functionally characterized, revealing a wealth of potential biotargets for arthropod-specific pest control.

While the candidate gene approach has been of enormous value in *T. castaneum*, it imposes limitations due to reliance on sequence conservation. Therefore a genome-wide RNAi screen is underway (Lynch et al., 2009). This project, known as iBeetle, targets all genes (identification based on gene predictions, as well as expression data) at two life stages. Specifically, dsRNAs are injected into 5th-instar larvae (analysis of injected animal), as well as into female pupae (analysis of offspring). Alterations in cuticular phenotypes, fluorescently marked muscles, melanotic stink glands, metamorphosis control and fertility are being scored (G. Bucher, personal communication). Approximately 5,500 genes will be screened by fall 2011, with completion of the project scheduled for fall 2014. The genome-wide collection of PCR templates for dsRNA synthesis in the iBeetle-Library will be made available to the community (http://ibeetle.uni-goettingen.de/resources.html). This invaluable resource will facilitate subsequent RNAi screens for additional processes.

3.2.2 Plant-mediated RNAi in crop pests

Although a comprehensive review of RNAi in plants is beyond the scope of this chapter, it is important to highlight transgenic approaches for generating RNAi-based insect-resistant plants (Artymovich, 2009; Baum et al., 2007; Mao et al., 2007). RNAi applications have been effective in silencing target genes in some insects upon oral administration of dsRNA. Our examples detail how this approach has enhanced plant resistance to economically important agricultural pests, such as the cotton bollworm, *Helicoverpa armigera*, and Western corn rootworm (WCR), *D. v. virgifera*, in commercially produced crops (e.g., corn, cotton, and tobacco).

The key to successful *in planta* RNAi depends not only on the identification of suitable gene targets, but also on the expression and delivery of sufficient amounts of intact dsRNA for up-take by the insects. Examples of successful gene silencing by oral delivery have been described in insect species from different orders (Table 1). With few exceptions, most oral RNAi assays in insects have targeted mRNAs in the gut. The first report of oral RNAi in an insect was in a lepidopteran, the light brown apple moth, *Epiphyas postvittana*, with temporary knockdown of a gut target, carboxylesterase 1, and an adult antennae target, pheromone binding protein 1 (Turner et al., 2006). Since then, additional reports of ingested dsRNA leading to knockdowns in Lepidoptera (Bautista et al., 2009; Mao et al., 2007; Whyard et al., 2009), Coleoptera (Baum et al., 2007; Whyard et al., 2009) , Diptera (Walshe et al., 2009; Whyard et al., 2009), Hemiptera (Price & Gatehouse, 2008), and Isoptera (Zhou et al., 2008) , suggest that knockdown of specific targets may be feasible in most insects.

Order	Insect	Gene Target	LC_{50}	Percent Mortality[1]	Reference
Coleoptera	*Diabrotica virgifera virgifera*	subunits of vacuolar ATPase and others	2-5 ng/cm^2	80-95	Baum et al., 2007
Coleoptera	*Diabrotica undecimpunctata howardii*	subunits of vacuolar ATPase	780 ng/cm^2	45	Baum et al., 2007
Coleoptera	*Leptinotarsa decemlineata*	subunits of vacuolar ATPase	52 ng/cm^2	90	Baum et al., 2007
Coleoptera	*Tribolium castaneum*	vacuolar ATPase E	0.003 mg/g diet	70	Whyard et al., 2009
Diptera	*Drosophila* spp.	vacuolar ATPase E and tubulin γ	0.2-0.6 mg/ml	40-70	Whyard et al., 2009
Diptera	*Glossina morsitans morsitans*	tsetse-EP, a major midgut protein	435 ng/µl	40	Walshe et al., 2009
Hemiptera	*Acyrthosiphon Pisum*	vacuolar ATPase E	0.003 mg/g diet	60	Whyard et al., 2009
Hemiptera	*Rhodnius prolixus*	nitroporin 2	1 µg/µl	not reported	Price & Gatehouse, 2008
Isoptera	*Reticulitermes flavipes*	cellulase hexamerin[2]	15.3 µg/cm^2 6.6 µg/cm^2	75 45	Zhou et al., 2008
Lepidoptera	*Epiphyas postvittana*	carboxylesterase 1 pheromone binding protein 1	1 µg	not reported	Turner et al., 2006
Lepidoptera	*Helicoverpa armigera*	cytochrome P450 (CYP6AE14)	3 mg/g diet	not reported	Mao et al., 2007
Lepidoptera	*Manduca sexta*	vacuolar ATPase E	0.01 mg/g diet	50	Whyard et al., 2009
Lepidoptera	*Plutella xylostella*	cytochrome P450 (CYP6BG1)	662-824 µg/µl	90[3]	Bautista et al., 2009

[1]Values are the maximum observed mortality and are approximate (exact values were not given).
[2]Administered in combination with juvenile hormone.
[3]Decrease in resistance to permethrin was 1-2.6-fold in dsRNA fed larvae compared to control.

Table 1. Reports of oral delivery of dsRNA that reduce the levels of target RNA in insects.

RNAi directed against a number of gene targets (e.g., *b-tubulin*, *v-ATPase A* and *v-ATPase E*) was effective in several economically important coleopteran pests (Baum et al., 2007). Oral RNAi targeting *v-ATPase* subunits and others resulted in significant larval mortality in perhaps the most economically important pest in the U.S., *D. v. virgifera*. It was further demonstrated that *D. v. virgifera* is highly sensitive to knockdown of a gene encoding the delta subunit of the coatomer complex (COPI) that is involved in intracellular protein trafficking. Similar results were obtained with orthologs for *v-ATPase* in Southern corn rootworm, *D. undecimpunctata howardii*, and Colorado potato beetle, *Leptinotarsa decemlineata*, but not in the cotton boll weevil, *Anthonomus grandis*. However, increased sensitivity to the cotton metabolite gossypol was reported in a lepidopteran, the cotton bollworm, *Helicoverpa armigera*, with a silenced cytochrome P450 gene, CYP6AE14 (Mao et al., 2007).

Accordingly, transgenic plants are being engineered to express a variety of dsRNAs to silence important biological functions in insects (Artymovich, 2009). Transgenic corn expressing a *v-ATPase* subunit A hairpin RNA demonstrated significant protection to damage by WCR larvae (Baum et al., 2007), while cotton engineered to express dsRNA targeting cytochrome P450 *CYP6AE14* caused knockdown of the transcript in the *H. armigera* gut and reduced larval growth (Mao et al., 2007). Thus far, initial laboratory tests of transgenic RNAi approaches to plant protection appear to be as successful as those based on the expression of insecticidal toxins against coleopteran and lepidopteran herbivores. However, further development and refinement of this technology, as well as large-scale field tests will likely be required to know the true potential of *in planta* RNAi.

3.2.3 Chelicerates (ticks, mites, spiders)

Double-stranded RNA has been successfully delivered to ticks via injection (various developmental stages and tissues), infection (viral vector), ingestion (oral), and incubation (whole body soaking) (de la Fuente et al., 2007). Oral RNAi was used to knockdown an anticomplement gene (*isac*) in the blacklegged tick, *Ixodes scapularis*. Affected nymphs weighed less than those fed a control dsRNA (*lacZ*) and had lower spirochete loads when infected with *Borrelia burgdorferi* (Soares et al., 2005). Another medically relevant study demonstrated that dsRNA can be transmitted through the blood-brain barrier in *I. scapularis* (Karim et al., 2008). Cy3-labeled dsRNA specific for either *β-actin* or *Na+-K+-ATPase* was injected into the abdomen of unfed adult females, and β-actin protein or Na+-K+-ATPase activity was measured after supplying a partial blood meal. Labeled dsRNAs were detected in the synganglia (CNS), and effective knockdown was confirmed via tissue-specific RT-PCR.
R. microplus is an economically significant tick ectoparasite that transmits a variety of pathogens, such as *Anaplasma marginale*, thereby increasing cattle exposure to vector-borne infectious diseases. Silencing of a defensin gene, *varisin*, by injection of dsRNA into male ticks reduced their ability to infect calves with *A. marginale* (Kocan et al., 2008). Additional RNAi targets, such as those affecting tick mortality and fecundity, have been identified through RNAi screens in *R. microplus* (Kurscheid et al., 2009).
Parental RNAi was used to knock-down expression of a homeobox gene, *Distal-less* (*Dll*), in the two-spotted spider mite, *Tetranychus urticae* (Khila & Grbic, 2007). Injection of either *Tu-Dll*-specific dsRNA or siRNA into adult female mites resulted in offspring with truncated and fused leg segments. This experiment demonstrated the conserved nature of Dll function and illustrates the power of RNAi in mites.
Efforts to use RNAi to control a major mite parasite of the honey bee are underway. The gene encoding glutathione S-transferase, involved in detoxification of pesticides used to control mites in the hive, was targeted successfully in *Varroa destructor* with dsRNA (Campbell et al., 2010). Two different dsRNA delivery methods were evaluated, microinjection and soaking mites in dsRNA solution. Although injection of dsRNA produced up to 96% silencing of the target (*VdGST-mu1)* gene for over 72 h, there were problems with high mortality in controls. However, encouraging results were obtained by soaking mites in a solution of dsRNA in 0.9% NaCl. The method enables high-throughput screening to identify the best targets for control of this devastating pest of honey bees, even though the exact mechanism of dsRNA up-take is unknown.

3.2.4 Improvements to other insect control methods

Current insect control methods benefit from RNAi studies. For example, the symbionts *Heterorhabditis bacteriophora* (a nematode) and, *Photorhabdus luminescens* (a bacterium) are a lethal combination in some insects. Using genes described in *C. elegans* as a model, various phenotypes were disrupted in *H. bacteriophora* soaked in dsRNA (Ciche & Sternberg, 2007). These studies facilitate the discovery of genes involved in symbiosis and/or insect pathogenesis.

RNAi has also been used to explore host-pathogen interactions in mosquitoes. One study explored the role of an antibacterial peptide encoded by a defensin family member (DEF) in *Anopheles gambiae* (Blandin et al., 2002). Targeting this *A. gambiae* defensin with gene-specific dsRNA resulted in *DEF* knock down (up to 12 days) and increased the mosquito's vulnerability to Gram-positive bacteria (Blandin et al., 2002). However, *DEF* knock down had no effect on the malaria parasite, *Plasmodium berghei*. To identify genes involved in mosquito immunity to *P. berghei*, researchers (Michel et al., 2005; Osta et al., 2004) targeted a number of candidate genes in *A. gambiae*. They discovered that reduction of transcripts encoding a type-C lectin, a leucine-rich protein or a serpin (SRPN2) were sufficient to make the mosquito refractory to infection by *P. berghei* in the midgut. Such studies may inspire the development of new methods to control protozoan infections in humans (Lehane et al., 2008; Solis et al., 2009; Walshe et al., 2009).

Researchers are also using RNAi to create mosquitoes that are resistant to dengue fever. Franz and colleagues made transgenic *A. aegypti* that express an inverted-repeat specific for the dengue type 2 (DEN-2) virus (Franz et al., 2006). Careful promoter selection resulted in transgenic *A. aegypti* that mount an RNAi response to DEN-2 virus in midgut epithelial cells immediately after a bloodmeal. Moreover, the authors demonstrated that after viral infection, transgenic mosquitoes expressing the hairpin RNA had reduced viral loads and DEN-2 virus-derived siRNAs in the midgut compared to control insects.

In agriculture, RNAi applications are being developed as control strategies for the *Asian citrus psyllid* which vectors Citrus Greening disease (Hunter et al., 2008), the Colorado potato beetle (Zhu et al., 2011), and *Varroa* mites as described above in section 3.2.3. Results such as these bode well for the future of RNAi in pest control strategies.

4. Future studies for practical implementation of RNAi technology

The success of RNAi depends both on the biology of the organism, and the method of dsRNA delivery. Intrinsic factors, such as the efficiency of dsRNA up-take, relative turnover of target mRNA/protein, signal amplification and systemic spread are important for robust RNAi. Extrinsic factors amenable to manipulation include dsRNA concentration, target gene selection, transcript localization, dsRNA synthesis and route of introduction. One of the most important considerations is determining if the observed phenotype is gene-specific or an "off target" effect. Another critical requirement is the stability and intracellular availability of the RNAi signal. Often such requirements can be met by improved delivery systems, such as stable, transgenic expression of hairpin RNAs (Kennerdell & Carthew, 2000; Tavernarakis et al., 2000), or alternatively, by expression of dsRNA in non-pathogenic bacteria that can be fed directly to the target organism, as demonstrated in nematodes (Timmons & Fire, 1998) and arthropods (Tian et al., 2009; Zhu et al., 2011).

Injection of dsRNA can elicit a stress response in some insects and potentially compromise the study. Moreover, mechanical damage to the cuticle and underlying tissue can stimulate innate immunity (Aronstein et al., 2006; Aronstein & Saldivar, 2005; Brey et al., 1993; Han et al., 1999), complicating interpretation of gene expression data. While appropriate controls (buffer and/or "control" dsRNA) can address some of these issues, alternative approaches for non-viral and virus-mediated dsRNA delivery have demonstrated great potential (Leng et al., 2009; Yuan et al., 2011). Direct delivery of dsRNA (soaking and/or feeding) is particularly popular in arthropod studies and appears to be feasible in at least some hemipteran, coleopteran, lepidopteran, and hymenopteran insects (Araujo et al., 2006; Aronstein et al., 2006; Baum et al., 2007; Eaton et al., 2002; Mao et al., 2007; Turner et al., 2006). However, most currently used methods reveal significant impediments preventing their application in large-scale *in vivo* trials.

To increase the efficiency of RNAi, current and future studies are directed at improving existing methodologies and adapting innovative technologies. A new bacterially-expressed dsRNA delivery technology, TransKingdom RNAi (*tk*RNAi) (Keates et al., 2008; Tian et al., 2009; Xiang et al., 2006; Xiang et al., 2009), recently emerged as a powerful tool for the control of parasites and disease agents in mammalian systems. This method utilizes attenuated, non-pathogenic bacteria that are safe, effective, and inexpensive vectors for delivering RNAi to target cells. Similar methods have been used successfully in nematodes (Newmark et al., 2003; Timmons & Fire, 1998), trophozoites (*Entamoeba histolytica*) (Solis et al., 2009) and other organisms (Keates et al., 2008; Nguyen & Fruehauf, 2008). Bacteria-based RNAi is technically suitable for production of large quantities of dsRNA, and therefore opens interesting perspectives for mass screening of novel gene targets and development of environmentally-safe pest control applications.

The application of RNAi to pest control, while still at a formative stage, is already taking different forms; 1) *in planta* dsRNA expression for the direct protection of crops; 2) bacteria-based dsRNA expression for the indirect control of parasites and pathogens of beneficial organisms; and 3) *in vivo* dsRNA expression for generating disease refractoriness in arthropod vectors of disease. Unlike *in planta* and bacteria-based RNAi, the use of RNAi for the spread of disease refractoriness requires genetic drive to push inheritance of the effecter gene (i.e. hairpin RNA) through target populations.

Among the most promising gene-drive candidates is a synthetic "*Medea*" element (Chen et al., 2007) which is based on the genetic principles observed in the Maternal-Effect Dominant Embryonic Arrest (*Medea*) factors found in *Tribolium* (Beeman et al., 1992; Lorenzen et al., 2008). Heterozygous (*M*/+) females transmit dominant-lethal activity to hatchlings by maternal action, but the lethal effect is manifested only in those progeny that fail to inherit an *M* allele from either parent. Thus, each *M* allele is bifunctional, encoding both a maternally loaded "poison" and a zygoticly expressed "antidote". Current and future efforts need to focus on both the development of improved RNAi effecter genes, as well as on improved methods for driving population replacement if the goal of controlling arthropod vectors of disease by *in vivo* dsRNA expression is to be realized.

5. Acknowledgment

We thank Eduardo Saldivar (USDA-ARS; Weslaco, TX), William Klobasa (North Carolina State University, Raleigh, NC) and Yasuyuki Arakane (Chonnam National University, Korea) for providing photographs of honey bee microinjection, *Tribolium* microinjection and *laccase2* RNAi phenotypes, respectively. We are also grateful to Gregor Bucher for providing information about the iBeetle project.

6. Disclaimer

Mention of trade names or commercial products in this (article) (publication) is solely for the purpose of providing specific information and does not imply recommendation or endorsement by the U.S. Department of Agriculture.
USDA is an equal opportunity provider and employer.

7. References

Amdam, G.V.; Simoes, Z.L.; Guidugli, K.R.; Norberg, K. & Omholt, S.W. (2003). Disruption of vitellogenin gene function in adult honeybees by intra-abdominal injection of double-stranded RNA. *BMC biotechnology*, Vol. 3, No. Journal Article, pp. 1 ISSN 1472-6750; 1472-6750

Angelini, D.R.; Kikuchi, M. & Jockusch, E.L. (2009). Genetic patterning in the adult capitate antenna of the beetle *Tribolium castaneum*. *Developmental biology*, Vol. 327, pp. 240-251

Arakane, Y.; Muthukrishnan, S.; Beeman, R.W.; Kanost, M.R. & Kramer, K.J. (2005a). *Laccase 2* is the phenoloxidase gene required for beetle cuticle tanning. *Proceedings of the National Academy of Sciences of the United States of America*, Vol. 102, pp. 11337-11342

Arakane, Y.; Specht, C.A.; Kramer, K.J.; Muthukrishnan, S. & Beeman, R.W. (2008). Chitin synthases are required for survival, fecundity and egg hatch in the red flour beetle, *Tribolium castaneum*. *Insect Biochemistry and Molecular Biology*, Vol. 38, No. 10, pp. 959-962 ISSN 0965-1748; 0965-1748

Arakane, Y.; Lomakin, J.; Beeman, R.W.; Muthukrishnan, S.; Gehrke, S.H.; Kanost, M.R. & Kramer, K.J. (2009). Molecular and functional analyses of amino acid decarboxylases involved in cuticle tanning in *Tribolium castaneum*. *Journal of Biological Chemistry*, Vol. 284, No. 24, (2009 Jun 12), pp. 16584-16594

Arakane, Y.; Dittmer, N.T.; Tomoyasu, Y.; Kramer, K.J.; Muthukrishnan, S.; Beeman, R.W. & Kanost, M.R. (2010b). Identification, mRNA expression and functional analysis of several *yellow* family genes in *Tribolium castaneum*. *Insect Biochemistry and Molecular Biology*, Vol. 40, No. 3, (2010 Mar), pp. 259-266

Arakane, Y.; Muthukrishnan, S.; Kramer, K.J.; Specht, C.A.; Tomoyasu, Y.; Lorenzen, M.D.; Kanost, M. & Beeman, R.W. (2005b). The *Tribolium chitin synthase* genes *TcCHS1* and *TcCHS2* are specialized for synthesis of epidermal cuticle and midgut peritrophic matrix. *Insect molecular biology*, Vol. 14, No. 5, pp. 453-463 ISSN 0962-1075; 0962-1075

Arakane, Y.; Baguinon, M.C.; Jasrapuria, S.; Chaudhari, S.; Doyungan, A.; Kramer, K.J.; Muthukrishnan, S. & Beeman, R.W. (2010a). Both UDP N-acetylglucosamine pyrophosphorylases of *Tribolium castaneum* are critical for molting, survival and fecundity. *Insect Biochemistry and Molecular Biology*, Vol. 41, No. 1, (2011 Jan), pp. 42-50

Arakane, Y.; Dixit, R.; Begum, K.; Park, Y.; Specht, C.A.; Merzendorfer, H.; Kramer, K.J.; Muthukrishnan, S. & Beeman, R.W. (2009). Analysis of functions of the chitin deacetylase gene family in *Tribolium castaneum*. *Insect Biochemistry and Molecular Biology*, Vol. 39, No. 5-6, (2009 May-Jun), pp. 355-365

Araujo, R.N.; Santos, A.; Pinto, F.S.; Gontijo, N.F.; Lehane, M.J. & Pereira, M.H. (2006). RNA interference of the salivary gland nitrophorin 2 in the triatomine bug *Rhodnius prolixus* (Hemiptera: Reduviidae) by dsRNA ingestion or injection. *Insect Biochemistry and Molecular Biology*, Vol. 36, No. 9, pp. 683-693 ISSN 0965-1748; 0965-1748

Aronstein, K. & Saldivar, E. (2005). Characterization of a honey bee Toll related receptor gene *Am18w* and its potential involvement in antimicrobial immune defense. *Apidologie*, Vol. 36, pp. 3-14

Aronstein, K.; Pankew, T. & Saldivar, E. (2006). SID-1 is implicated in systemic gene silencing in the honey bee. *Journal of Apicultural Research*, Vol. 45, No. 1, pp. 20-24.

Aronstein, K.A.; Murray, K.D.; de Leon, J.; Qin, X. & Weinstock, G. (2007). High mobility group (HMG-box) genes in the honey bee fungal pathogen *Ascosphaera apis*. *Mycologia*, Vol. 99, No. 4, pp. 553-561

Artymovich, K.A. (2009). Using RNA interference to increase crop yield and decrease pest damage. *MMG 445 Basic Biotechnology eJournal*, Vol. 5, pp. 7-12

Baum, J.A.; Bogaert, T.; Clinton, W.; Heck, G.R.; Feldmann, P.; Ilagan, O.; Johnson, S.; Plaetinck, G.; Munyikwa, T.; Pleau, M.; Vaughn, T. & Roberts, J. (2007). Control of coleopteran insect pests through RNA interference. *Nature biotechnology*, Vol. 25, No. 11, pp. 1322-1326 ISSN 1087-0156; 1087-0156

Bautista, M.A.; Miyata, T.; Miura, K. & Tanaka, T. (2009). RNA interference-mediated knockdown of a cytochrome P450, *CYP6BG1*, from the diamondback moth, *Plutella xylostella*, reduces larval resistance to permethrin. *Insect Biochemistry and Molecular Biology*, Vol. 39, No. 1, pp. 38-46 ISSN 1879-0240; 0965-1748

Beeman, R.W.; Friesen, K.S. & Denell, R.E. (1992). Maternal-effect selfish genes in flour beetles. *Science*, Vol. 256, pp. 89-92

Bellés, X. (2010). Beyond *Drosophila*: RNAi in vivo and functional genomics in insects. *The Annual Review of Entomology*, Vol. 55, pp. 111-128

Blair, C.D.; Sanchez-Vargas, I.; Franz, A.W.E. & Olson, K.E. (2006). Rendering Mosquitoes Resistant to Arboviruses through RNA Interference. *Microbe*, Vol. 1, No. 10, pp. 466-470

Blandin, S.; Moita, L.F. & Kocher, T. (2002). Reverse genetics in the mosquito *Anopheles gambiae*: targeted disruption of the *Defensin* gene. *EMBO Reports*, Vol. 3 No. 9, pp. 852-856

Boutla, A.; Delidakis, C.; Livadaras, I.; Tsagris, M. & Tabler, M. (2001). Short 59-phosphorylated double-stranded RNAs induce RNA interference in *Drosophila*. *Current biology*, Vol. 11, pp. 1776-1780

Boutros, M. & Ahringer, J. (2008). The art and design of genetic screens: RNA interference. *Nature Reviews Genetics*, Vol. 9, pp. 554-566

Brey, P.T.; Lee, W.-J.; Yamakawa, M.; Koizumi, Y.; Perrot, S.; Francois, M. & Ashida, M. (1993). Role of the integument in insect immunity: Epicuticular abrasion and induction of cecropin synthesis in cuticular epithelial cells. *Proceedings of the National Academy of Sciences of the United States of America*, Vol. 90, pp. 6275-6279

Broehan, G.; Arakane, Y.; Beeman, R.W.; Kramer, K.J.; Muthukrishnan, S. & Merzendorfer, H. (2010). Chymotrypsin-like peptidases from *Tribolium castaneum*: a role in molting revealed by RNA interference. *Insect Biochemistry and Molecular Biology*, Vol. 40, No. 3, pp. 274-283 ISSN 1879-0240; 0965-1748

Bromenshenk, J.J.; Henderson, C.B.; Wick, C.H.; Stanford, M.F.; Zulich, A.W.; Jabbour, R.E.; Deshpande, S.V.; McCubbin, P.E.; Seccomb, R.A.; Welch, P.M.; Williams, T.; Firth, D.R.; Skowronski, E.; Lehmann, M.M.; Bilimoria, S.L.; Gress, J.; Wanner, K.W. & Cramer Jr., R.A. (2010). Iridovirus and Microsporidian Linked to Honey Bee Colony Decline. *PLoS One*, Vol. 5, No. 10, pp. 1-11

Brown, S.J.; Mahaffey, J.P.; Lorenzen, M.D.; Denell, R.E. & Mahaffey, J.W. (1999). Using RNAi to investigate orthologous homeotic gene function during development of distantly related insects. *Evolution & Development*, Vol. 1, pp. 11-15

Bucher, G.; Scholten, J. & Klingler, M. (2002). Parental RNAi in *Tribolium* (Coleoptera). *Current biology : CB*, Vol. 12, No. 3, pp. R85-86 ISSN 0960-9822; 0960-9822

Campbell, E.M.; Budge, G.E. & Bowman, A.S. (2010). Gene-knockdown in the honey bee mite *Varroa destructor* by a non-invasive approach: studies on a glutathione S-transferase. *Parasites & Vectors*, Vol. 3, pp. 73

Carthew, R.W. (2003). RNAi Applications in *Drosophila melanogaster*, in *RNAi: a guide to gene silencing*, H. Gregory, (Ed) Cold Spring Harbor Press, Cold Spring Harbor

Chen, C.H.; Huang, H.; Ward, C.M.; Su, J.T.; Schaeffer, L.V.; Guo, M. & Hay, B. (2007). A synthetic maternal-effect selfish genetic element drives population replacement in *Drosophila*. *Science*, Vol. 316, pp. 597-600

Ciche, T.A. & Sternberg, P.W. (2007). Postembryonic RNAi in *Heterorhabditis bacteriophora*: a nematode insect parasite and host for insect pathogenic symbionts. *BMC developmental biology*, Vol. 7, No. Journal Article, pp. 101 ISSN 1471-213X; 1471-213X

Consortium, I.S.G. (2008). The genome of a lepidopteran model insect, the silkworm *Bombyx mori*. *Insect Biochemistry and Molecular Biology*, Vol. 38, No. 12, pp. 1036-1045

Consortium, T.H.G.S. (2006). Insights into social insects from the genome of the honeybee *Apis mellifera*. *Nature*, Vol. 443, pp. 931-949

Cornman, R.S.; Chen, Y.P.; Schatz, M.C.; Street, C.; Zhao, Y.; Desany, B.; Egholm, M.; Hutchison, S.; Pettis, J.S.; Lipkin, W.I. & Evans, J.D. (2009). Genomic Analyses of the Microsporidian *Nosema ceranae*, an Emergent Pathogen of Honey Bees. *PLoS pathogens*, Vol. 5, No. 6, (June 2009), pp. 1-14

D'Ambrosio, M.V. & Vale, R.D. (2010). A whole genome RNAi screen of *Drosophila* S2 cell spreading performed using automated computational image analysis. *The Journal of Cell Biology*, Vol. 191 No. 3, pp. 471-478

Dai, H.; Jiang, R.; Wang, J.; Xu, G.; Cao, M.; Wang, Z. & Fei, J. (2007). Development of a heat shock inducible and inheritable RNAi system in silkworm. *Biomolecular Engineering*, Vol. 24, No. 6, pp. 625-630

de la Fuente, J.; Kocan, K.M.; Almazan, C. & Blouin, E.F. (2007). RNA interference for the study and genetic manipulation of ticks. . *Trends in Parasitology*, Vol. 23, pp. 427-433

Dearden, P.K.; Duncan, E.J. & Wilson, M.J. (2009). RNA interference (RNAi) in honeybee (*Apis mellifera*) embryos. *Cold Spring Harbor protocols*, Vol. 2009, No. 6, pp. pdb.prot5228 ISSN 1559-6095

Deddouche, S.; Matt, N.; Budd, A.; Mueller, S.; Kemp, C.; Galiana-Arnoux, D.; Dostert, C.; Antoniewski, C.; Hoffmann, J.A. & Imler, J.-L. (2008). The DExD/H-box helicase

Dicer-2 mediates the induction of antiviral activity in *Drosophila. Nature Immunology*, Vol. 9, pp. 1425-1432

Dietz, G.; Chen, D.; Schnorrer, F.; Su, K.-C.; Barinova, Y.; Fellner, M.; Gasser, B.; Kinsey, K.; Oppel, S.; Scheiblauer, S.; Couto, A.; Marra, V.; Keleman, K. & Dickson, B.J. (2007). A genome-wide transgenic RNAi library for conditional gene inactivation in *Drosophila. Nature*, Vol. 448, pp. 151-156

Dong, Y. & Friedrich, M. (2005). Nymphal RNAi: systemic RNAi mediated gene knockdown in juvenile grasshoppers. *BMC biotechnology*, Vol. 5, No. 25, pp. 1-7

Eaton, B.A.; Fetter, R.D. & Davis, G.W. (2002). Dynactin is necessary for synapse stabilization. *Neuron*, Vol. 34, pp. 729-741

Fabrick, J.A.; Kanost, M.R. & Baker, J.E. (2004). RNAi-induced silencing of embryonic tryptophan oxygenase in the Pyralid moth, *Plodia interpunctella. Journal of Insect Science*, Vol. 4, No. 15, pp. 9

Feinberg, E.H. & Hunter, C.P. (2003). Transport of dsRNA into cells by the transmembrane protein SID-1. *Science*, Vol. 301 No. 5639, pp. 1545-1547

Franz, A.W.E.; Sanchez-Vargas, I.; Adelman, Z.N.; Blair, C.D.; Beaty, B.J.; James, A.A. & Olson, K.E. (2006). Engineering RNA interference-based resistance to dengue virus type 2 in genetically modified *Aedes aegypti. Proceedings of the National Academy of Sciences of the United States of America*, Vol. 103, No. 11, (Mar 14), pp. 4198-4203

Gaines, P.J.; Olson, K.E.; Higgs, S.; Powers, A.M.; Beaty, B.J. & Blair, C.D. (1996). Pathogen-derived resistance to dengue type 2 virus in mosquito cells by expression of the premembrane coding region of the viral genome. *Journal of virology*, Vol. 70, pp. 2132-2137

Gallai, N.; Salles, J.-M.; Settele, J. & Vaissière, B.E. (2009). Economic valuation of the vulnerability of world agriculture confronted with pollinator decline. *Ecological economics*, Vol. 68, pp. 810-821

Genersch, E. (2010). Honey bee pathology: current threats to honey bees and beekeeping. *Mini-Review Applied Microbiology and Biotechnology*, Vol. 87, No. 1, pp. 87-97

Goldsmith, M.R.; Shimada, T. & Abe, H. (2005). The genetics and genomics of the silkworm, *Bombyx mori. Annual Review of Entomology*, Vol. 50, pp. 71-100

Grossmann, D.; Scholten, J. & Prpic, N.M. (2009). Separable functions of *wingless* in distal and ventral patterning of the *Tribolium* leg. *Development genes and evolution*, Vol. 219, pp. 469-479

Hamilton, A.; Voinnet, O.; Chappell, L. & Baulcombe, D. (2002). Two classes of short interfering RNA in RNA silencing. *The EMBO Journal*, Vol. 21, No. 17, (September 2002), pp. 4671-4679

Hammond, S.M.; Bernstein, E.; Beach, D. & Hannon, G.J. (2000). An RNA-directed nuclease mediates posttranscriptional gene silencing in *Drosophila* cells. *Nature*, Vol. 404, pp. 293-296

Han, Y.S.; Chun, J.S.; Schwartz, A.; Nelson, S. & Paskewitz, S.M. (1999). Induction of mosquito hemolymph proteins in response to immune challenge and wounding. *Developmental & Comparative Immunology*, Vol. 23, pp. 553-562

Higes, M.; Martin-Hernandez, R.; Garrido-Bailon, E.; Gonzalez-Porto, A.V.; García-Palencia, P.; Meana, A.; Nozal, M.J.d.; Mayo, R. & Bernal, J.L. (2009). Honeybee colony collapse due to *Nosema ceranae* in professional apiaries. *Environmental Microbiology Reports*, Vol. 1, No. 2, pp. 110-113

Higes, M.; Martín-Hernández, R.; Botías, C.; Bailón, E.G.; González-Porto, A.V.; Barrios, L.; Nozal, M.J.d.; Bernal, J.L.; Jiménez, J.J.; Palencia, P.G. & Mañes, A.M. (2008). How natural infection by *Nosema ceranae* causes honeybee colony collapse. *Environmental microbiology*, Vol. 10, No. 10, pp. 2659-2669

Hogenkamp, D.; Arakane, Y.; Kramer, K.J.; Muthukrishnan, S. & Beeman, R.W. (2007). Characterization and expression of the *ß-N*-acetylhexosaminidase gene family of *Tribolium castaneum*. *Insect Biochemistry and Molecular Biology*, Vol. 38, No. 4, (2008 Apr), pp. 478-489

Hughes, C.L. & Kaufman, T.C. (2000). RNAi analysis of *Deformed, proboscipedia* and *Sex combs reduced* in the milkweed bug *Oncopeltus fasciatus*: novel roles for Hox genes in the hemipteran head. *Development*, Vol. 127, pp. 3683-3694

Hunter, W.; Ellis, J.; vanEngelsdorp, D.; Hayes, J.; Westervelt, D.; Glick, E.; Williams, M.; Sela, I.; Maori, E.; Pettis, J.; Cox-Foster, D. & Paldi, N. (2010). Large-scale field application of RNA interference (RNAi) technology to reduce impact of Israeli Acute Paralysis Virus (IAPV) induced disease in honey bees (*Apis mellifera*), Hymenoptera: Apidae. *PLoS pathogens*, Vol. 6, No. 12, pp. e1001160

Hunter, W.B.; Shelby, K.; Dowd, S.; McKenzie, C. & Shatters Jr, R. (2008). Gene Expression in Asian Citrus Psyllid Adults Feeding from Florida Citrus: Application to biology and vector control. *IRCHLB Proceedings*, (December), pp. 233-237

Huvenne, H. & Smagghe, G. (2010). Mechanisms of dsRNA uptake in insects and potential of RNAi for pest control: a review. *Journal of insect physiology*, Vol. 56, No. 3, pp. 227-235 ISSN 1879-1611; 0022-1910

Jose, A.M. & Hunter, C.P. (2007). Transport of sequence-specific RNA interference information between cells. *Annual Review of Genetics*, Vol. 41, pp. 305-330

Kanginakudru, S.; Royer, C.; Edupalli, S.V.; Jalabert, A.; Mauchamp, B.; Chandrashekaraiah; Prasad, S.V.; Chavancy, G.; Couble, P. & Nagaraju, J. (2007). Targeting *ie-1* gene by RNAi induces baculoviral resistance in lepidopteran cell lines and in transgenic silkworms. *Insect molecular biology*, Vol. 16, No. 5, pp. 635-644 ISSN 0962-1075; 0962-1075

Karim, S.; Kenny, B.; Troiano, E. & Mather, T.N. (2008). RNAi-mediated gene silencing in tick synganglia: a proof of concept study. *BMC biotechnology*, Vol. 8, pp. 30

Keates, A.C.; Fruehauf, J.; Xiang, S. & Li, C.J. (2008). TransKingdom RNA interference: a bacterial approach to challenges in RNAi therapy and delivery. *Biotechnology and Genetic Engineering Reviews*, Vol. 25, pp. 113-128

Kennerdell, J.R. & Carthew, R.W. (1998). Use of dsRNA-mediated genetic interference to demonstrate that *frizzled* and *frizzled 2* act in the wingless pathway. *Cell*, Vol. 95, pp. 1017-1026

Kennerdell, J.R. & Carthew, R.W. (2000). Heritable gene silencing in *Drosophila* using double-stranded RNA. *Nature biotechnology*, Vol. 18, No. 8, pp. 896-898

Kennerdell, J.R.; Yamaguchi, S. & Carthew, R.W. (2002). *Genes & Development*, Vol. 16, pp. 1884-1889

Khila, A. & Grbic, M. (2007). Gene silencing in the spider mite *Tetranychus urticae*: dsRNA and siRNA parental silencing of the *Distal-less* gene. *Development genes and evolution*, Vol. 217, pp. 241-251

Kocan, K.M.; Fuente, J.d.l.; Manzano-Roman, R.; Naranjo, V.; Hynes, W.L. & Sonenshine, D.E. (2008). Silencing expression of the *defensin*, *varisin*, in male *Dermacentor variabilis* by RNA interference results in reduced *Anaplasma marginale* infections *Experimental & applied acarology*, Vol. 46, pp. 17-28

Kurscheid, S.; Lew-Tabor, A.E.; Valle, M.R.; Bruyeres, A.G.; Doogan, V.J.; Munderloh, U.G.; Guerrero, F.D.; Barrero, R.A. & Bellgard, M.I. (2009). Evidence of a tick RNAi pathway by comparative genomics and reverse genetics screen of targets with known loss-of-function phenotypes in *Drosophila*. *BMC molecular biology*, Vol. 10, (26 March), pp. 26

Lee, K.S.; Kim, B.Y.; Choo, Y.M.; Yoon, H.J.; Kang, P.D.; Woo, S.D.; Sohn, H.D.; Roh, J.Y.; Gui, Z.Z.; Je, Y.H. & Jin, B.R. (2009). Expression profile of cathepsin B in the fat body of *Bombyx mori* during metamorphosis. *Comparative biochemistry and physiology Part B, Biochemistry & molecular biology*, Vol. 154, No. 2, pp. 188-194 ISSN 1879-1107; 1096-4959

Lehane, M.J.; Gibson, W. & Lehane, S.M. (2008). Differential expression of fat body genes in *Glossina morsitans morsitans* following infection with *Trypanosoma brucei brucei*. *International journal for parasitology*, Vol. 38, No. 1, pp. 93-101 ISSN 0020-7519; 0020-7519

Leng, Q.; Woodle, M.C.; Lu, P.Y. & Mixson, A.J. (2009). Advances in Systemic siRNA Delivery. *Drugs Future*, Vol. 34, No. 9, pp. 721

Lipardi, C. & Paterson, B.M. (2009). Identification of an RNA-dependent RNA polymerase in *Drosophila* involved in RNAi and transposon suppression. *Proceedings of the National Academy of Sciences of the United States of America*, Vol. 106, pp. 15645-15650

Liu, P.Z. & Kaufman, T.C. (2004). *Hunchback* is required for suppression of abdominal identity, and for proper germband growth and segmentation in the intermediate germband insect *Oncopeltus fasciatus*. *Development*, Vol. 131, pp. 1515-1527

Liu, X.; Zhang, Y.; Yan, X. & Han, R. (2010). Prevention of Chinese Sacbrood Virus Infection in *Apis cerana* using RNA Interference. *Current microbiology*, Vol. 61, No. 5, pp. 422-428

Lorenzen, M.D.; Brown, S.J.; Denell, R.E. & Beeman, R.W. (2002). Cloning and characterization of the *Tribolium castaneum* eye-color genes encoding tryptophan oxygenase and kynurenine 3-monooxygenase. *Genetics*, Vol. 160, No. 1, pp. 225-234

Lorenzen, M.D.; Gnirke, A.; Margolis, J.; Garnes, J.; Campbell, M.; Stuart, J.; Aggarwal, R.; Richards, S.; Park, Y. & Beeman, R.W. (2008). The maternal-effect, selfish genetic element *Medea* is associated with a composite *Tc1* transposon. *Proceedings of the National Academy of Sciences of the United States of America*, Vol. 105, pp. 10085-10089

Lu, R.; Li, H.; Li, W.-X. & Ding, S.-W. (2004). RNA-based immunity in insects, S. H. Gillespie, G. L. Smith, A. Osbourn, (Eds), Cambridge University Press, ISBN 0 521 84312 X,

Lynch, J.A. & Desplan, C. (2006). A method for parental RNA interference in the wasp *Nasonia vitripennis*. *Nature Protocols*, Vol. 1, pp. 486-494

Lynch, J.A. & Desplan, C. (2010). Novel modes of localization and function of *nanos* in the wasp *Nasonia*. *Development*, Vol. 137, pp. 3813-3821

Lynch, J.A.; Panfilio, K.A. & Fonseca, R.N.d. (2009). As *Tribolium* matures as a model insect, coleopteran community congregates in Cologne. *Development genes and evolution*, Vol. 219, No. 9-10, pp. 531-533

Mao, Y.B.; Cai, W.J.; Wang, J.W.; Hong, G.J.; Tao, X.Y.; Wang, L.J.; Huang, Y.P. & Chen, X.Y. (2007). Silencing a cotton bollworm P450 monooxygenase gene by plant-mediated RNAi impairs larval tolerance of gossypol. *Nature biotechnology*, Vol. 25, No. 11, pp. 1307-1313 ISSN 1087-0156; 1087-0156

Maori, E.; Paldi, N.; Shafir, S.; Kalev, H.; Tsur, E.; Glick, E. & Sela, I. (2009a). IAPV, a bee-affecting virus associated with Colony Collapse Disorder can be silenced by dsRNA ingestion. *Insect molecular biology*, Vol. 18, No. 1, pp. 55-60 ISSN 1365-2583; 0962-1075

Maori, E.; Paldi, N.; Shafir, S.; Kalev, H.; Tsur, E.; Glick, E. & Sela, I. (2009b). A bee-affecting virus associated with colony collapse disorder can be silenced by dsRNA ingestion. *Insect molecular biology*, Vol. 18, pp. 55-60

Masumoto, M.; Yaginuma, T. & Niimi, T. (2009). Functional analysis of Ultrabithorax in the silkworm, *Bombyx mori*, using RNAi. *Development genes and evolution*, Vol. 219, No. 9-10, pp. 437-444 ISSN 1432-041X; 0949-944X

Mathur, G.; Sanchez-Vargas, I.; Alvarez, D.; Olson, K.E.; Marinotti, O. & James, A.A. (2010). Transgene-mediated suppression of dengue viruses in the salivary glands of the yellow fever mosquito, *Aedes aegypti*. *Insect molecular biology*, Vol. 19, No. 6, pp. 753-763

Michel, K.; Pinto, S.; Budd, A. & Kafatos, F. (2005). *Anopheles gambiae* SRPN2 facilitates midgut invasion by the malaria parasite *Plasmodium berghei*. *EMBO Reports*, Vol. 6, No. 9, pp. 891-897

Miller, S.C.; Brown, S.J. & Tomoyasu, Y. (2008). Larval RNAi in *Drosophila*? *Development genes and evolution*, Vol. 218, pp. 505-510

Mito, T.; Nakamura, T.; Bando, T.; Ohuchi, H. & Noji, S. (2011). The advent of RNA interference in Entomology. *Entomological Science*, Vol. 14, pp. 1-8

Mummery-Widmer, J.L.; Yamazaki, M.; Stoeger, T.; Novatchkova, M.; Bhalerao, S.; Chen, D.; Dietzl, G.; Dickson, B.J. & Knoblich, J.A. (2009). Genome-wide analysis of Notch signalling in *Drosophila* by transgenic RNAi. *Nature*, Vol. 458, No. 7241, (Apr 23), pp. 987-992

Nelson, C.M.; Ihle, K.E.; Fondrk, M.K.; Page, R.E. & Amdam, G.V. (2007). The gene *vitellogenin* has multiple coordinating effects on social organization. *PLoS biology*, Vol. 5, No. 3, pp. e62 ISSN 1545-7885; 1544-9173

Newmark, P.A.; Reddien, P.W.; Cebria, F. & Alvarado, A.S. (2003). Ingestion of bacterially expressed double-stranded RNA inhibits gene expression in planarians. *Proceedings of the National Academy of Sciences of the United States of America*, Vol. 100, No. 1, (September 30, 2003), pp. 11861-11865

Nguyen, T. & Fruehauf, J.H. (2008). Bacterial Vectors for RNAi Delivery, in *Patho-Biotechnology*, R. Sleator, C. Hill, (Eds), Landes Bioscience,

Ohnishi, A.; Hull, J.J. & Matsumoto, S. (2006). Targeted disruption of genes in the *Bombyx mori* sex pheromone biosynthetic pathway. *Proceedings of the National Academy of Sciences of the United States of America*, Vol. 103, pp. 4398-4403

Olson, K.E.; Higgs, S.; Gaines, P.J.; Powers, A.M.; Davis, B.S.; Kamrud, K.I.; Carlson, J.O.; Blair, C.D. & Beaty, B.J. (1996). Genetically engineered resistance to dengue-2 virus transmission in mosquitoes. *Science*, Vol. 272, pp. 884-886

Osta, M.A.; Christophides, G.K. & Kafatos, F.C. (2004). Effects of Mosquito Genes on *Plasmodium* Development. *Science*, Vol. 303 No. 5666 (26 March), pp. 2030-2032

Paldi, N.; Glick, E.; Oliva, M.; Zilberberg, Y.; Aubin, L.; Pettis, J.; Chen, Y. & Evans, J.D. (2010). Effective gene silencing in a microsporidian parasite associated with honeybee (*Apis mellifera*) colony declines. *Applied and Environmental Microbiology*, Vol. 76, No. 17, pp. 5960-5964

Posnien, N.; Schinko, J.; Grossmann, D.; Shippy, T.D.; Konopova, B. & Bucher, G. (2009). RNAi in the red flour beetle (*Tribolium*). *Cold Spring Harbor protocols*, Vol. 2009, No. 8, pp. pdb.prot5256 ISSN 1559-6095

Price, D.R.G. & Gatehouse, J.A. (2008). RNAi-mediated crop protection against insects. *Trends in biotechnology*, Vol. 26 No. 7, pp. 393-400

Richards, S. & Consortium, T.G.S. (2008). The genome of the model beetle and pest *Tribolium castaneum*. *Nature*, Vol. 452, pp. 949-955

Roignant, J.Y.; Carré, C.; Mugat, B.; Szymczak, D.; Lepesant, J.A. & Antoniewski, C. (2003). Absence of transitive and systemic pathways allows cell-specific and isoform-specific RNAi in *Drosophila*. *RNA*, Vol. 9, No. 3, pp. 299-308

Rolff, J. & Reynolds, S. (Eds.) (2009). *Insect Infection and Immunity. Evolution, Ecology, and Mechanisms*, Oxford University Press,ISBN 978-0-19-955135-4, New York

Ronco, M.; Uda, T.; Mito, T.; Minelli, A.; Noji, S. & Klingler, M. (2008). Antenna and all gnathal appendages are similarly transformed by *homothorax* knock-down in the cricket *Gryllus bimaculatus*. *Developmental biology*, Vol. 313, pp. 80-92

Rütten, K.B.; Pietsch, C.; Olek, K.; Neusser, M.; Beukeboom, L.W. & Gadau, J. (2004). Chromosomal anchoring of linkage groups and identification of wing size QTL using markers and FISH probes derived from microdissected chromosomes in *Nasonia* (Pteromalidae: Hymenoptera). *Cytogenetics and Genome Research*, Vol. 105, No. 1, pp. 126-133

Saleh, M.C.; van Rij, R.P.; Hekele, A.; Gillis, A.; Foley, E.; O'Farrell, P.H. & Andino, R. (2006). The endocytic pathway mediates cell entry of dsRNA to induce RNAi silencing. *Nature Cell Biology*, Vol. 8, No. 8, pp. 793-802

Saleh, M.C.; Tassetto, M.; van Rij, R.P.; Goic, B.; Gausson, V.; Berry, B.; Jacquier, C.; Antoniewski, C. & Andino, R. (2009). Antiviral immunity in *Drosophila* requires systemic RNA interference spread. *Nature*, Vol. 458, (Feb 8), pp. 346–351

Soares, C.A.G.; Lima, C.M.R.; Dolan, M.C.; Piesman, J.; Beard, C.B. & Zeidner, N.S. (2005). Capillary feeding of specific dsRNA induces silencing of the *isac* gene in nymphal *Ixodes scapularis* ticks. *Insect molecular biology*, Vol. 14, pp. 443-452

Solis, C.F.; Santi-Rocca, J.; Perdomo, D.; Weber, C. & Guillén, N. (2009). Use of Bacterially Expressed dsRNA to Downregulate *Entamoeba histolytica* Gene Expression. *PLoS One*, Vol. 4, No. 12, pp. e8424

Tabunoki, H.; Higurashi, S.; Ninagi, O.; Fujii, H.; Banno, Y. & Nozaki, M. (2004). A carotenoid-binding protein (CBP) plays a crucial role in cocoon pigmentation of silkworm (*Bombyx mori*) larvae. *FEBS letters*, Vol. 567 pp. 175-178

Tavernarakis, N.; Wang, S.L.; Dorovkov, M.; Ryazanov, A. & Driscoll, M. (2000). Heritable and inducible genetic interference by double-stranded RNA encoded by transgenes. *Nature Genetics*, Vol. 24, pp. 180-183

Tian, H.; Peng, H.; Yao, Q.; Chen, H.; Xie, Q.; Tang, B. & Zhang, W. (2009). Developmental Control of a Lepidopteran Pest *Spodoptera exigua* by Ingestion of Bacteria Expressing dsRNA of a Non-Midgut Gene. *PLoS One*, Vol. 4, No. 7, pp. e6225

Timmons, L. & Fire, A. (1998). Specific interference by ingested dsRNA. *Nature*, Vol. 395, pp. 854

Tomoyasu, Y. & Denell, R.E. (2004). Larval RNAi in *Tribolium* (Coleoptera) for analyzing adult development. *Development genes and evolution*, Vol. 214, pp. 575-578

Tomoyasu, Y.; Miller, S.C.; Shuichiro, T.; Schoppmeier, M.; Grossmann, D. & Bucher, G. (2008). Exploring systemic RNA interference in insects: a genome-wide survey for RNAi genes in *Tribolium*. *Genome Biology*, Vol. 9, No. 1, pp. R10

Turner, C.T.; Davy, M.W.; MacDiarmid, R.M.; Plummer, K.M.; Birch, N.P. & Newcomb, R.D. (2006). RNA interference in the light brown apple moth, *Epiphyas postvittana* (Walker) induced by double-stranded RNA feeding. *Insect molecular biology*, Vol. 15, No. 3, pp. 383-391 ISSN 0962-1075; 0962-1075

Ulvila, J.; Parikka, M.; Kleino, A.; Sormunen, R.; Ezekowitz, R.A.; Kocks, C. & Rämet, M. (2006). Double-stranded RNA is internalized by scavenger receptor-mediated endocytosis in *Drosophila* S2 cells. *Journal of Biological Chemistry*, Vol. 281, No. 20, (2006 May 19), pp. 14370-14375

Van Roessel, P.; Hayward, N.M.; Barros, C.S. & Brand, A.H. (2002). Two-color GFP imaging demonstrates cell-autonomy of GAL4-driven RNA interference in *Drosophila*. *Genesis*, Vol. 34, pp. 170-173

Verhulst, E.C.; Beukeboom, L.W. & Zande, L.v.d. (2010). Maternal Control of Haplodiploid Sex Determination in the Wasp *Nasonia*. *Science*, Vol. 328 No. 5978 (30 April 2010), pp. 620-623

Walshe, D.P.; Lehane, S.M.; Lehane, M.J. & Haines, L.R. (2009). Prolonged gene knockdown in the tsetse fly *Glossina* by feeding double stranded RNA. *Insect molecular biology*, Vol. 18, No. 1, pp. 11-19 ISSN 1365-2583; 0962-1075

Werren, J. & Loehlin, D. (2009). Larval RNAi in *Nasonia* (Parasitoid Wasp). *Cold Spring Harbor protocols*, Vol. 10,

Werren, J.H.; Richards, S.; Desjardins, C.A.; Niehuis, O.; Gadau, J.; Colbourne, J.K. & Group, N.G.W. (2010). Functional and evolutionary insights from the genomes of three parasitoid *Nasonia* species. *Science*, Vol. 327, No. 5963, (Jan 15), pp. 343-348

Whyard, S.; Singh, A.D. & Wong, S. (2009). Ingested double-stranded RNAs can act as species-specific insecticides. *Insect Biochemistry and Molecular Biology*, Vol. 39, No. 11, pp. 824-832 ISSN 1879-0240; 0965-1748

Winston, W.M.; Sutherlin, M.; Wright, A.J.; Feinberg, E.H. & Hunter, C.P. (2007). *Caenorhabditis elegans* SID-2 is required for environmental RNA interference. *Proceedings of the National Academy of Sciences of the United States of America*, Vol. 104, No. 25, (June 19, 2007), pp. 10565-10570

Xiang, S.; Fruehauf, J. & Li, C.J. (2006). Short hairpin RNA-expressing bacteria elicit RNA interference in mammals. *Nature biotechnology*, Vol. 24, pp. 697-702

Xiang, S.; Keates, A.C.; Fruehauf, J.; Yang, Y.; Guo, H.; Nguyen, T. & Li, C.J. (2009). In vitro and in vivo gene silencing by TransKingdom RNAi (tkRNAi). *Methods in molecular biology*, Vol. 487, pp. 147-160

Yuan, X.; Naguib, S. & Wu, Z. (2011). Recent advances of siRNA delivery by nanoparticles. *Expert Opinion on Drug Delivery*, Vol. 8, No. 4, pp. 521-536

Zamore, P.D.; Tuschl, T.; Sharp, P.A. & Bartel, D.P. (2000). RNAi: double-stranded RNA directs the ATP-dependent cleavage of mRNA at 21 to 23 nucleotide intervals. *Cell*, Vol. 101, pp. 25-33

Zhou, X.; Wheeler, M.M.; Oi, F.M. & Scharf, M.E. (2008). RNA interference in the termite *Reticulitermes flavipes* through ingestion of double-stranded RNA. *Insect Biochemistry and Molecular Biology*, Vol. 38, No. 8, pp. 805-815 ISSN 0965-1748; 0965-1748

Zhu, F.; Xu, J.; Palli, R.; Ferguson, J. & Palli, S.R. (2011). Ingested RNA interference for managing the populations of the Colorado potato beetle, *Leptinotarsa decemlineata*. *Pest management science*, Vol. 67, No. 2, pp. 175-182

Zhu, Q.; Arakane, Y.; Banerjee, D.; Beeman, R.W.; Kramer, K.J. & Muthukrishnan, S. (2008). Functional specialization among insect chitinase family genes revealed by RNA interference. *Proc Natl Acad Sci USA*, Vol. 105, No. 18, pp. 6650-6655

9

RNA Processing During Early Embryogenesis: Managing Storage, Utilisation and Destruction

Angus Macaulay*, Sara Scantland* and Claude Robert
Laboratory of Functional Genomics of Early Embryonic Development.
Centre de recherche en biologie de la reproduction, Institut des nutraceutiques et des aliments fonctionnels, Faculté des sciences de l'agriculture et de l'alimentation, Université Laval (Québec)
Canada

1. Introduction

The classical model of the life of a messenger RNA (mRNA) is generally depicted as a cascade of typical cellular events initiated with the transcription of the genomic sequence followed by the usual maturation of the produced transcript through splicing of the intronic regions, addition of the cap structure on its 5' end and polyadenylation of the 3' end. The mature mRNA is then exported out of the nucleus and sent for translation in the endoplasmic reticulum where it will serve as template/blueprint for the production of the encoded protein. The typical life cycle of an mRNA is then concluded by its decay in cellular structures that take the shape of granules called processing bodies. These well accepted steps offer a general perspective of the life and death of most mRNAs in most cellular contexts. Nonetheless, this general model does not fit well with embryogenesis mainly due to the presence of transcriptionnaly impaired cells composing the early stage embryos. In fact, the stage at which the embryo acquires the potential to transcribe its genome is widely variable between species. For instance, the mouse genome is readily activated following fertilization while in Human; transcription is initiated between the 6 and 8-cell stage. Other non-mammalian species provide more extreme situations amongst which Xenopus leavis represents a prime example of non-classical RNA management as the early embryogenesis is accomplished through 12 cell cycles conducted in the absence of transcriptional activity. In this model organism, the first embryonic cells become transcriptionally active once the embryo is composed of roughly 4,000-8,000 cells.

In the absence of transcription, the embryonic cell sustains its protein production using mRNAs found in the stocks that were stored during oogenesis. These stockpiles of transcripts are accumulated during the oocyte growth that took place in the ovary, and are generally accepted as a large component of the maternal legacy that is associated with developmental competence of the resulting embryo once the egg is fertilized. The mechanisms by which the oocyte stores these transcripts are still only partly understood.

*These authors contributed equally to this work.

Since some of these transcripts are destined to be used several days or even weeks later, the cytoplasmic storage inevitably involves their stabilization and protection from degradation. Several important proteins that play key roles in mRNA stabilization have been identified, mostly from studies performed on non-mammalian model organisms. Knowledge transfer has allowed identifying orthologs in mouse and Human.

To sustain protein synthesis, the stored transcripts must be released from their stabilized state and appropriately allowed to proceed to translation by the recruitment of the initiating factors that will facilitate the binding and progression of ribosomes. On this aspect also, the mechanisms by which the mRNAs are specifically recruited to fulfill the protein requirements of the cell are still poorly understood. The involvement of several key proteins has been highlighted; however, the current model only provides a partial perspective of the recruitment processes that must involve some elements to target specific transcripts from storage that must be governed in a temporarily regulated manner.

One of the main considerations pertaining to how this spatio-temporal management may occur relies on the information encoded in the untranslated regions of the mRNAs. Indeed, elegant studies performed in model organisms have shown the importance of these non-coding regions to regulate the location of the mRNAs within the cell. So far, the mammalian oocyte and the early blastomeres have yet to show clear partitioning of the cell's cytoplasm as it is the case for other non-mammalian species. Recent evidence suggest the involvement of small non-coding RNAs namely microRNAs in the regulation of the stored maternal RNA reserve. Currently, our knowledge is based upon evidence of the complex nature of maternal RNA management, regulation of which occurs at different levels.

Once translated, the mRNAs are typically destined for decay in the processing bodies. The classical string of events includes mRNA decapping, poly(A) tail removal and complete transcript degradation by the action of nucleases. Within the early embryonic context, a large proportion of stored maternal mRNAs are believed to be destroyed without ever being translated. This apparent waste of resources is still unexplained however recent evidence suggests maternal stores must be depleted for successful embryonic genome activation. This situation stresses the importance of the decay pathway as an active aspect of early embryogenesis. Following embryonic genome activation, the blastomeres gradually adopt a more classical RNA processing strategy where, for example, environmental stimulus could drive cellular response through signal transduction leading to nuclear transcriptional events resulting in novel mRNA production to be translated.

Herein are discussed the species related similarities and divergence in transcriptional silencing during oogenesis which account for the accumulation of the maternal RNA stores. A perspective of the embryonic program that is driven by these stored transcripts will also be presented by contrasting the different strategies adopted across species. Finally, the current mechanisms regarding the management of these transcripts in a space and time dependant manner will be addressed through the presentation of known key proteins in addition to the action of small non-coding RNAs.

2. The oocyte's legacy to early development is accumulated in the ovary

Successful zygote formation begins with the fusion of a male and female gamete. Although equal contributions of nuclear material are combined from each parent resulting in transmission of half their genetic information to their offspring, the structural composition of the resulting embryo originates almost entirely from the oocyte. The oocyte endowment includes the future zygotic cytoplasm with all the organelles and various components e.g. proteins, stocks of RNA or calcium. In fact, compared to the oocyte, the sperm transfers little cytoplasm, and even though many mitochondria exist in the sperm, those that are transferred to the oocyte's cytoplasm do not persist in development past about the 4 cell stage in rodents and in cattle (Shalgi et al. 1994; Sutovsky et al. 1996). Amongst the known spermatic contributions to zygotic composition aside from the haplotype, the spermatozoon donates a centriole that leads to the sperm aster that mediates pronuclei fusion (Sutovsky et al. 1996). More recently, protein and additional nucleic acid material originating from the spermatic micro-cytoplasm have been identified to be passed to the oocyte's cytoplasm. It is the case for phospholipase C zeta that has been shown to induce the calcium release after fertilization as part of the mechanism driving the block to polyspermy (Swann 2004) and RNA molecules either messengers or small non-coding Review: (Lalancette et al. 2008). So far the functional relevance of these RNA molecules to perform specific and essential tasks in support of early embryonic development still remains unclear. As it will be discussed later, the oocyte's cytoplasm represents a rich source of messenger (Schultz and Wassarman 1977; Gilbert et al. 2009) and small non-coding RNAs Review: (Krawetz 2005). Although some reports indicate a potential role of the spermatic RNA molecules, early embryonic development is undisputedly supported by the resources accumulated during oogenesis. As discussed below, the accumulated RNA stores support early development until the embryonic genome is activated which occurs, in most species, after several cell cycles.

Oogenesis leads to the production of the largest cells of the body enabling the accumulation of large amount of resources. Depending upon the species, the mammalian oocyte ranges from 70 to 140 μm in diameter and is much larger in reptiles, fish and birds by the time of ovulation. The description of the neuroendocrine regulation of oogenesis is far beyond the scope of the current objective. However, it is important to position the accumulation of RNA in the oocyte during oogenesis which takes place in the ovary. Briefly, upon recruitment from the ovarian reserves, a cohort of follicles each bearing an immature oocyte initiates growth which is heavily mediated by gonadotrophins secreted from the hypophysis. The follicles are composed of mainly two types of somatic cells which are granulosa and theca cells. These cells structurally form the individual unit that is a follicle within which an oocyte is found. The somatic cells work in tandem to support oogenesis by modifying hormones (progestins to androgens to estrogens in response to gonadotrophins).

As folliculogenesis progresses, the enclosed oocytes undergo oogenesis. The follicle was long believed to support the gamete's growth by communicating from the outer cell compartment towards the inside where the gamete would passively benefit (Biggers et al. 1967). The growth of both the follicle and the gamete is now known to be governed by bi-directional communication mainly between the oocyte and the granulosa cells. So far, outside towards the inside communication has been reported through direct contact through gap junctions between the somatic cells and to the oocyte. A subset of granulosa cells in close proximity to the oocyte, the cumulus cells, are further differentiated and have direct contact with the oocyte's plasma membrane through transzonal projections. The cumulus cells play a large role regulating the level of cyclic nucleotides in the oocyte which in turn prevent meiosis resumption (Conti et al. 2002). The oocyte signals back by secreting factors such as BMP15 and GDF9 that stimulates granulosa cell growth and differentiation (Hussein et al. 2006). This communication is essential to maintain a certain level of synchrony between the follicle and the gamete especially during early folliculogenesis when the gamete is still growing in size. Typically, a mammalian oocyte reaches it's full diameter before the follicle has reached full size. The follicle will continue to grow, filling with follicular fluid, and increasing in surrounding granulosa cell population (Pedersen and Peters 1968). The relationship between the size of the follicle and of the enclosed oocyte in several mammalian species can be found in Table 1. Oocyte growth is accompanied with the accumulation of large amounts of RNA observable in the early growth phase. In mice, by about 65% of growth to full size, 95% of the RNA has accumulated, the remaining 5% occurs over the final stages of growth (Pedersen and Peters 1968).

Specie	Size of full grown oocyte	Follicular size at which full grown oocytes are found	Size of pre-ovulatory follicle	References
Human	> 105 μm	5 - 7 mm	> 20 mm	(Gougeon 1986)
Mouse	70 μm	> 2 mm	4 mm	(Rose et al. 1999)
Sheep	> 120 μm	~1.5 mm	> 5 mm	(Turnbull et al. 1977)
Bovine	> 130 μm	> 2 mm	20 - 25 mm	(Fair et al. 1995)
Pig	144 μm	> 3 mm	> 10 mm	(Knox 2005)
Rabbit	80-90 μm	650-700 μm	> 1.6 mm	(Žitný et al. 2004) (Osteen and Mills 1980) (Hulot and Mariana 1985)

Table 1. Relationship between follicular and oocyte size across different mammalian species

The build-up of maternal RNA stores is driven by heavy transcriptional activity of the gamete's genome (Tomek et al. 2002). In most mammalian species, this transcriptional activity is however, greatly reduced or completely shutdown once the oocyte reaches its full size (Table 2). Some studies show clear patterns of transcription shutdown like in the pig and in cattle (Motlik J 1984; Fair et al. 1995) By measuring the rate of ^{3}H-uridine incorporation it was shown RNA synthesis is fully active during early oogenesis, but as the oocyte grows, this activity shuts down, and by the time the oocyte is full size, activity that remains is limited to the nucleolus (Moore and Lintern-Moore 1978). In the mouse, however, the shutdown of transcription is very brief and occurs just before meiosis resumption (Rodman and Bachvarova 1976; Wassarman and Letourneau 1976).

Aside from endogenous transcription, accumulation of maternal RNA is also known to be occurring through RNA transfer from the surrounding somatic cells in non-mammalian species. In *c. elegans* or drosophila and other insects like notonecta, maternal mRNAs are transferred to the oocytes through translocation channels or cell–cell bridges that connect nurse cells and the oocytes (Hurst et al. 1999). As germ cells divide to become oocytes in the drosophila, they remain directly connected to each other by connections termed ring canals (Deng and Lin 1997). Aggregates of RNA move from the other germ cells, or from supporting cells to the oocyte in an ordered method (Hurst et al. 1999). The transfer of mRNA between cells may be motor protein mediated as mRNA can associate to form a ribo-nucleo-particle (RNP) with motor-like proteins, or proteins that associate with dyneins (Hurst et al. 1999; Schnorrer et al. 2000). This RNA accumulation through endogenous transcription and/or transfer from surrounding somatic cells and oocytes makes the immature oocyte the most RNA rich cell of the body. Although numbers differ between studies, total RNA content differs importantly between species (Table 2).

Specie	Immature oocyte (GV stage) total RNA content	Detectable period of RNA polymerase II activity
Human	330 pg (Kocabas et al. 2006)	Growth until large diameter oocytes with condensed chromatin (Miyara et al. 2003)
Mouse	0.35 ng (Piko and Clegg 1982) 0.35-0.43 ng (Bachvarova et al. 1985) 0.45 ng (Olszańska and Borgul 1993) 0.6 ng (Sternlicht and Schultz 1981)	Arrested in full size SN phase oocytes (Bouniol-Baly et al. 1999)
Sheep	0.76 ng (Olszańska and Borgul 1993)	Oocyte size of 110 μm with Surrounded Nucleus Configuration (Russo et al. 2007)
Bovine	0.35 ng (Gilbert et al. 2009) 0.98 ng (Olszańska and Borgul 1993) 2.0 ng (Lequarre 2004) 2.4 ng (Bilodeau-Goeseels and Schultz 1997)	Arrested in full size GV3 configuration oocytes (Lodde et al. 2008)
Pig	0.65 ng (Olszańska and Borgul 1993)	Arrested in full size GV3/4 stage oocytes (Sun et al. 2004)
Rabbit	15 ng (Olszańska and Borgul 1993)	Arrested in oocytes with "Tight Chromatin" (TC) configuration (Wang et al. 2006)
Birds	1.0 μg (Japanese quail), 2.1 μg (hen) (Olszańska and Borgul 1993)	N/A

Table 2. Total RNA content in immature oocytes

In some species, transcriptional arrest is observed by the presence of a non-permissive state of chromatin and/or the depletion of RNA polymerase. The decrease in transcriptional activity is mediated by gonadotropin influence on the supporting granulosa cells (De La Fuente and Eppig 2001). Chromatin state changes are indicative of transcriptional arrest when the chromatin becomes condensed. Concurrently, there is a depletion of RNA polymerases in oocytes that have undergone DNA condensation (Bouniol-Baly et al. 1999; Miyara et al. 2003). Most pre-ovulatory oocytes in the mouse exhibit a chromatin configuration termed "surrounded nucleus" (SN). Alternatively, non-surrounded nucleus (NSN) configuration can also exist. Condensed DNA associating closely with the nucleolus characterizes SN configuration (Miyara et al. 2003). SN configuration is also related to RNA polymerase I and II activity. In SN chromatin configuration, polymerase activity is arrested

(Bouniol-Baly et al. 1999). When other species are taken into account, the conformation change in chromatin is not the same as in mice. In rabbits, sheep, humans, and cows, conformation changes are significant, but not characterized solely by SN or NSN charactersistics. The DNA still typically condenses, and can be labeled as surrounding or non-surrounding, but more descriptive stages that take into account related morphological changes have been described (Tan et al. 2009).

In rabbits, there are more terms to describe oocyte chromatin configuration as the oocyte matures. As described by Wang et al. (2006) the progression observed in the rabbit oocyte is as follows: net-like (NL), loosely condensed (LC), tightly condensed (TC), and singly condensed (SC) chromatin configurations. Transcription shuts down at the tightly condensed stage.

In human oocytes, Combelles and colleagues describe four states of chromatin related to maturation and the ability to fertilize. In the first class, class A, the oocyte is smaller in diameter and has a partially surrounded nucleolus and fibrillar chromatin distributed in the nucleoplasm. The three other classes (B, C and D) have peri-nuclear condensed chromatin and resemble the surrounded nucleolus conformation of the mouse, the difference being that oocyte diameter is larger and the chromatin is less widely distributed in the nucleoplasm. Class B has very compact chromatin and no distribution of chromatin in the nucleoplasm. Class C is the largest in oocyte diameter, and large masses of chromatin surround the nucleolus. In class D there are threads of chromatin extending in the nucleoplasm (Combelles et al. 2002). These reports are similar to Miyara and colleagues who propose a size dependant chromatin configuration change in oocytes and a subsequent decrease in polymerase activity to none in pre-ovulatory oocytes with condensed configuration.

In bovine oocyte maturation, the terms GV0-GV3 are predominantly used (Lodde et al. 2008) though SN and Non SN configurations are also referred to in literature (Tan et al. 2009). In GV0 oocytes, there is much transcription in the nucleolus and a number of morphological differences exist that distinguish the bovine oocyte from later GV stages that include erected microvilli, small clusters of immature mitochondria, few ooplasmic vesicles, the presence of a golgi apparatus, and scattered cortical granules (Lodde et al. 2008). In the later GV stages, the nucleus becomes peripheral, microvilli become bent, mitochondria become hooded, there are increasing numbers of ooplasmic vesicles, and the gogli begins to disassociate and the cortical granules become clustered before moving to the periphery of the oocyte. Intense transcriptional activity is seen in the GV0 oocyte, and then in the GV1 oocyte the activity is sparsely detected by H^3-Uridine such that by GV3 stage no transcriptional activity exists (Lodde et al. 2008). In porcine oocytes similar chromatin configuration nomenclature exists, with the exception that there is a GV4 stage, and that the later stages (GV3 and GV4) are associated with more atretic follicles (Sun et al. 2004). Overall, preovulatory oocytes largely exhibit, some form of condensed transcriptionally inactive chromatin status and a lack of polymerase activity (Bouniol-Baly et al. 1999).

3. RNA is used to sustain protein synthesis during early development before the activation of the embryonic genome

The reduction in transcriptional activity in the mature oocyte, which may even be complete transcriptional silencing, occurs during oocyte growth, and lasts until embryonic genome activation (EGA). The developmental period which occurs in the absence of transcription is referred to as the embryonic program. During this transcriptionnaly repressed period, control over gene expression involves post-translational modifications that regulate protein activity and permit for the compensation of protein turnover or synthesis of stage specific proteins that also rely on the maternal RNA stores.

A classic example of gene expression control operating at both the translational and post-translational levels involves the action of the M-phase promoting factor (MPF). This complex regulating meiosis resumption, is composed of two subunits, a cyclin-dependant kinase (CDK1) and a regulatory cyclin unit (CCNB1) (Masui 2001). The complex has to be activated in a two step process to allow dissolution of the germinal vesicle, the first step of meiosis resumption. To begin, CDK1 and CCNB1 have to be present or have to be synthesised if they are not. Second, the complex must be activated. Depending on the species, one of the two proteins is usually present in the cytoplasm whereas the other has to be translated in a time-specific manner to allow meiosis resumption (Chesnel and Eppig 1995; Robert et al. 2002). The presence of the components of the MPF is necessary but not sufficient to grant meiotic competence. Post-translational regulation is compulsory to allow MPF activation through the dephosphorylation of the CDK1 subunit. This kind of tight recruitment regulation of both stockpiled mRNAs and proteins is ubiquitous and allows early development progression given that no transcription occurs until the embryonic genome activates.

4. The duration of transcriptional silencing is species specific

The duration of the period of transcriptional silence varies between species. While being short in the mouse oocyte, the silent period can last several days in many other species. Indeed, the mouse genome is activated as early as the end of the zygotic stage. According to previous work (Schultz 1993), while a period of minor gene activation occurs during G2 in the 1-cell embryo, the major activation occurs during the 2-cell stage. Thus, in the mouse, the maternal contribution is only required to support a single cell cycle. This is an important difference with other mammals like humans, pigs, rabbits, cattle and sheep where the embryonic genome activation occurs later, at the end of the third or fourth cell cycle (Table 3).

In other model organisms, the maternal stores can support up to 16 cell cycles, which corresponds to approximately 65,536 cells. There is an important difference between mammals and non-mammal species such as fish, amphibians, insects and birds. In zebrafish, the activation of transcription begins at cell cycle 10 (512 to 1,024 cells). The first nine cycles are controlled by a 15 minute oscillator that allows perfectly synchronous cleavage (Kane and Kimmel 1993). In Xenopus, the embryo undergoes 12 rapid 35 minutes long synchronous cleavages (4,096-8,192 cells) before detectable transcription is observed (Newport and Kirschner 1982). In drosophila, the bulk of embryo transcription begins during the 14th cell cycle (8,192-16,384 cells) (McCleland et al. 2009). Finally, the chicken represents an extreme model of embryonic program with it first transcriptional activity detected in the 16th cell cycle, when the embryo consists of about 30 to 50 thousand cells. The large variability in the number of cell cycles and the number of cells required to achieve the maternal to embryo transition in different animal species is remarkable and is a tribute to the vast amount of resources that can be stably accumulated during oogenesis.

The total time elapsed (in hours) before the EGA is also impressive in its own right. Even though the mouse reaches the point of EGA (also referred to as the maternal to zygotic transition (MZT), due to the stage during which it occurs) early, it still transpires 23 hours after fertilization (Schultz 1993). By adding the time from meiosis resumption and the MII stage arrest, which lasts around 10 hours, the total period of transcriptional silence lasts more than 30 hours. In large mammals, the duration of RNA storage may be extended when considering that in the bovine, fully grown oocytes are typically found in follicles of 3 mm and a proportion of those oocytes already harbor transcriptionally inactive, highly condensed chromatin (GV3 stage) (Akhtar and Veenstra 2009). Oocyte growth to full size involves transcriptional silencing and includes the time for the 3 mm follicle to reach preovulatory size which requires 4 to 8 days depending on a two or three wave cycle. In addition there is the time taken to reach the other key developmental steps that are, the duration from the LH surge up to ovulation (1 day), the time for fertilization to occur, and the time for the zygote to reach the EGA 3-4 days later. Considering this timeline and that some of the maternal RNA present in these oocytes may have been stored during early stages of oocyte recruitment, and will not be enlisted for translation until the time of EGA, these RNAs will have necessitated storage for more than two weeks before they are used.

Interestingly, the number of cell cycles undergone before EGA and the duration of the transcriptional silence are two uncorrelated factors. Indeed, the number of cells at EGA may be several thousand in Drosophila and Xenopus, but transcriptional silence only lasts 3 and 7 hours in each of these species respectively, as the first cell cycles are extremely rapid (Newport and Kirschner 1982; Schultz 1993). Similarly, the chicken embryo reaches the 16th cell cycle (30,000-50,000 cells) a mere 24 hours post-fertilization (Elis et al. 2008).

Specie	Developmental stage	Number of cell cycles	References
Mouse	1-cell	0	(Schultz 1993)
Pig	4-6 cells	2-3	(Anderson et al. 2001)
Human	4-8 cells	2-3	(Braude et al. 1988)
Bovine	8-16 cells	3-4	(Memili et al. 1998)
Rabbit	8-16 cells	3-4	(Henrion et al. 1997)
Sheep	8-16 cells	3-4	(Crosby et al. 1988)
Zebrafish	512-1,024 cells	9-10	(Kane and Kimmel 1993)
Xenopus	4,096-8,192 cells	12-13	(Newport and Kirschner 1982)
Drosophila	8,192-16,384 cells	13-14	(McCleland et al. 2009)
Chicken	30,000-50,000 cells	15-16	(Elis et al. 2008)

Table 3. Developmental stage at which the embryonic genome gets activated

5. Storing RNA for later

As mentioned, the oocyte contains all the materials needed to carry out early embryo development up to the stage at which the genome activates. This is exemplified by the fact that the duration of the embryonic program is determined by the stage at which the developmental block occurs when in the presence of alpha-amanitin, an RNA polymerase II specific inhibitor. Distinctly from the textbook processes through which mRNAs are matured in the nucleus and exported, capped, and polyadenylated, to the cytoplasm where they are readily translated and then sent for destruction, these essential maternal RNA molecules involve additional steps for transcript stabilization to render them physiologically inert, a state from which they will be recruited in a time orderly fashion to be either translated or simply sent directly for decay (Figure 1).

However, several aspects have been known for some time and parallels can be drawn from the knowledge gathered in other cell types known to store mRNAs. Additionally, it seems that a close relationship exists between factors involved in RNA storage and in RNA decay. For instance, it has been reported in numerous species that stored mRNAs are found in a deadenylated state (Eulalio et al. 2007; Zheng et al. 2008) and deadenylation is the first step in the mRNA decay pathway further. Some storage granules contain components for mRNA decay (Cougot 2004; Kedersha et al. 2005). The collection of these different protein aggregates with various cellular functions is often referred under the general terminology of processing bodies (p-bodies). Decay intermediates are typically stored in the p-bodies where decapping factors (DCP1 and DCP2) are concentrated. The mRNA can, however, resume translation by exiting the p-body, being re-adenylated, and interacting with polyribosomes (Brengues et al. 2005). This turnover is often observed to occur between periods of stress and cell growth.

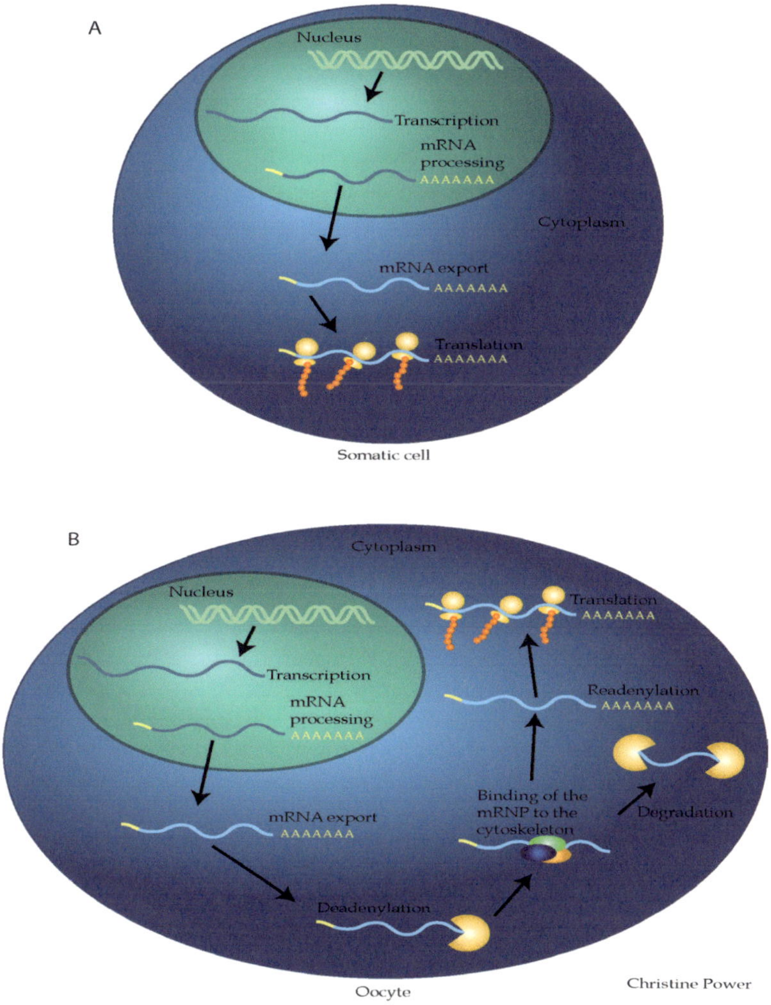

Fig. 1. The RNA pathway in a somatic cell (A) and in an oocyte (B)

The current state of knowledge regarding these processes is still fragmented as the detailed mechanisms of RNA storage in the oocyte and early embryos are still being determined. In the context of the oocyte, the mechanisms by which the transcripts must undergo to be stabilized are largely unknown, however, stored messengers are found to be deadenylated and this process does not result in RNA decay, but allows the RNA to be stored through protein interactions. Several key proteins and complexes have been identified to mitigate the poly(A) tail shortening. Such key players involve the poly(A) ribonuclease PARN in some species while in others, it can also be mediated by the Pumilio protein, which in turn interacts with the CCR4–Pop2–Not deadenylase complex (Radford et al. 2008). In drosophila the mRNA adenylation state is determined by a balance between the polyadenyl polymerase (PAP) involved in poly(A) tail lengthening and proteins with nuclease activity like the Caf1-Ccr4 complex (Eulalio et al. 2007). So far, the mammalian Ccr4 homolog has been localized in p-bodies and also acts to remove the poly(A) repeats (Zheng et al. 2008). Following this action, the length of the polyA tail of stored RNA has been estimated to be of less than 100 nucleotides reduced from over 200 nucleotides (Zheng et al. 2008). Other reports suggested that the extent of deadenylation is driven by sequence specific structures namely found in 3′ untranslated region (3′UTR) of mRNAs. For examples, it has been reported that the presence of a Cytoplasmic Polyadenylation Element (CPE) motif can influence the length of the remaining poly(A) tail where deadenylation of the poly A tail from 300-400 repeats down to 40 in absence of it or preserving a length of 40-100 when the CPE motif is present (Paynton and Bachvarova 1994). In all, poly(A) tail length of stored maternal mRNAs is still vaguely characterized as it is extremely difficult to clearly fractionate the mRNA pools to isolate the ones that are stored from the others that have been recruited. So far the extent of knowledge is restricted to general means in poly(A) tail fluctuations observed between developmental stages (Bachvarova et al. 1985; Paynton et al. 1988; Paynton and Bachvarova 1994; Brevini-Gandolfi et al. 1999).

Once bearing a shorter poly(A) tail, messenger storage requires stabilization to prevent destruction. This is conducted by the binding of proteins to form stable RNPs that aggregate in the oocyte's cytoplasm (Flemr et al. 2010). It has been suggested that as an oocyte approaches full size, there is a decrease in size of p-bodies and there is an increase in abundance of mRNA binding proteins in the cytoplasm. Transcript storage during oogenesis involves the binding of proteins, especially those of the Y-box family. These proteins called FRGY1 and FRGY2 were first studied in Xenopus (Bouvet and Wolffe 1994). These conserved factors are germ cell specific nucleic acid binding proteins and are homologous to the mouse MSY2 (Gu et al. 1998). In a fully grown murine oocyte, it has been estimated that MSY2 alone accounts for about 2% of the total protein content (Yu et al. 2001). These proteins are nuclease sensitive binding elements and have high sequence homology between mammalian species where identities match from 98% to 100% when using NCBI database Blast comparison. These proteins are conserved through evolution as nucleotide sequence identity between yps in D. Melanogaster and YBX1 in Human is still 79%. The full perspective on how these proteins are involved in maternal RNA storage is still under investigation. As mentioned, RNA storage is observed in other tissues than the oocyte and as such, a general perspective can be extrapolated from the other systems. These protein bound mRNA molecules form RNPs and can either aggregate in a granule like a P-body, or remain free in the cytoplasm. A variety of granules exists and are usually described based on the cell type they have been found in. Germ cells exhibit germ cell granules in oocytes, or chromatoid bodies in sperm (Nagamori et al. 2010), in neurons, neuronal granules exist, and in somatic cells there are typically p-bodies and stress granules reviews: (Anderson and Kedersha 2009; Voronina and Pshennikova 2010). Storage granule-like structures have been identified in single cell organisms, insects, plants, and mammals (Jansen 2001; Voronina and Pshennikova 2010). On a general perspective, storage granules share some basic RNA binding ability, often have exonuclease action, helicases, structural components, and are aggregations of RNPs (Anderson and Kedersha 2006). It is by studying the presence of these components that characterization of the granules is mainly being carried out. For instance, comparison of p-bodies and stress granules has been made as they were shown to remain functionally and spatially linked, but stress granule assembly requires eIF2α phosphorylation, but this is not necessary for p-bodies (Kedersha et al. 2005). Furthermore, eIF3, G3BP, eIF4G, and PABP-1 are found only in stress granules whereas decapping proteins are, however, found in p-bodies (Kedersha et al. 2005)

It is not known how many parallels can be drawn from the situation observed in somatic cells in comparison to the situation of long term maternal mRNAs storage. The knowledge of RNA storage in the mammalian context is still extremely fragmentary. In mouse, it was recently reported that there is a novel protein storing body that localizes in the subcortical region of the oocyte (Flemr et al. 2010). This storage form termed subcortical RNP domain (SCRD) is related to the components of a p-body as it shares similar protein components. Flemr and colleagues reported components that include "unidentified 18033 antibody-interacting protein", DDX6, YBX2 (previously termed MSY2 in the mouse and FRGY2 in xenopus), CPEB, and the exon junction complex or EJC, which is a variable complex based around 5 proteins (SRm160, DEK, RNPS1, Y14 and REF) that have a number of other interactions and are involved in enhancing nucleocytoplasmic shuttling of mRNAs (Le Hir et al. 2001). In a similar fashion to the storage mechanisms described in other cell types, two DCP1 containing bodies were proposed to be active in the mouse oocyte (Swetloff et al. 2009). Likewise, responsiveness to chemical treatments like cycloheximide and RNase A treatments (Lin et al. 2008) also helps to define the different granule types, with p-bodies being sensitive to the chemicals, unlike decapping bodies.

The makeup of storage sites is better described in other model organisms especially in drosophila; however, several distinctive features question the evolutionary conservation of these mechanisms. Perhaps these divergences may be due to the marked differences in the embryonic program duration and the number of cell cycles that must be conducted prior to the EGA. In drosophila, storage is known to be highly organized with protein sorting and delivering of the mRNA to a specific position. The sorting allows for polarity in the oocyte that helps set up the organization on the body and determines cell fate in the early embryo (Review (Bashirullah et al. 1998). For instance, in drosophila , Bicoid (bcd) polarity is mediated through several proteins such as exuperantia (exu), swallow (swa) and staufen (stau) (Schnorrer et al. 2000). Polarity is created in this case by the swa protein which interacts with a dynein light chain, and exu protein that is required for appropriate localization. Exu is also suspected to localize differently depending upon the mRNA it forms an RNP with (Jansen 2001). The polarity of stau containing complexes requires bcd polarity(Schnorrer et al. 2000). A staufen-like protein has been shown to have motor protein properties though association with cytoskeletal components (Hurst et al. 1999). In complement, transcript localization in this highly organized structure is encoded in the nucleotide sequence itself where zipcodes are part of the untranslated regions (UTR). RNA binding proteins called signal recognition proteins (SRP) can attach to this region and assist in the translocation. This interaction results in the formation of a RNP with specific cellular or cytoplasmic "address". Region specific signaling and coding is used to deliver proteins to their site of intended action. It has been proposed that this process of RNA movement is potentially less energetically demanding than protein translocation (Jansen 2001). The drosophila oocyte cytoplasm is compartmentalized by protein gradients determined by the

SRP-mRNA interaction creating a polarity that drives cell fate. These observations depict the cytoplasm has been highly structured for RNP storage where the cytoskeleton serves to anchor the RNPs awaiting to be used in the appropriate spatio-temporal manner. Unfortunately, Stau and other polarity related proteins have not been shown to function with the same effect in mammalian oocytes (Calder et al. 2008). In fact, Stau abundance has been shown to be homogeneously distributed thus raising doubts on its role in spatial organization in mammals. So far, the mammalian oocyte has not been shown to be highly and specifically compartmentalized as observed in non-mammalian models.

6. Using the stored resources

The complex series of events which orchestrate mRNA recruitment are still unclear and under continuous investigation. mRNAs can be recruited either for translation or degradation. It is still unknown if the mechanisms through which recruitment occurs are general or specific. Due to the presence of the highly organized structures in other model animals and the fact that mRNAs cannot be translated or degraded in a single wave of recruitment since development is a multi-stage process, it is believed that maternal RNA management must be under a yet unknown precise mechanism.

This need for a timely regulated management process is exemplified by the action of cyclins during the embryonic program. Cyclin degradation at the end of each cell-cycle check point is essential to allow the inactivation of cyclin-dependant kinases and in turn, this inactivation is needed to complete the essential steps that are spindle disassembly, cytokinesis and the transition into G1 phase (Irniger 2002). Obviously, new cyclin proteins have to be synthesized before each new cell division. Until EGA, this has to occur through the precise recruitment and translation of stored mRNAs to ensure the presence of the proper cyclin at the appropriate moments of early development. By similar reasoning, some stockpiled mRNAs have also to be destroyed at specific moments of early development. For example, some mRNAs involved in specific meiotic events are deleterious for further development if they are not rapidly degraded after fertilization. The dynamics of the proto-oncogene Mos which is part of the cytostatic factor necessary to halt meiosis in the second metaphase waiting for fertilization is a suitable example of this. It seems protein elimination is not sufficient as the Mos mRNA must be degraded rapidly after fertilization probably since this transcript is potentially harmful as the presence of the protein can cause a rapid embryonic arrest (Alizadeh et al. 2005). These examples illustrates that it is unlikely that maternal RNA management falls under the action of a single and global mechanism. It is expected that the different nature and roles of proteins encoded in the stored maternal transcripts require a vast array of processes directing the production of these proteins. So far, several different mechanisms have been shown to be involved to some extent in the management of at least a fraction of these stored maternal mRNAs.

7. Re-adenylation of stored mRNAs

The first step of mRNA recruitment from storage to translation is usually the lengthening of the poly(A) tail. As mentioned earlier, most mRNAs are stored in the cytoplasm with a short poly(A) tail containing less than 50 nucleotides. When the poly(A) tail of an mRNA is elongated to 200 nucleotides or more, it is recruited for translation (Kim and Richter 2006). For many stored transcripts, sequence encoded elements have been shown to be required for proper re-adenylation notably the presence of two 3'UTR cis-acting elements. The first one is the polyadenylation hexanucleotide (HEX), AAUAAA, which is always required for nuclear and cytoplasmic polyadenylation. The HEX sequence is bound by the cleavage and polyadenylation specificity factor (CPSF). The second one is the cytoplasmic polyadenylation element (CPE), whose consensus sequence is UUUUUAU (Stebbins-Boaz et al. 1999). It is bound by the CPE-Binding protein (CPEB) and is required for the cytoplasmic polyadenylation of many mRNAs following storage (Kim and Richter 2006). The presence of a specific sequence on all transcripts is insufficient to meet the requirements of gradual use throughout the embryonic program. The time dependant constraint of transcript utilization could be met if isoforms bearing different 3'UTR with different regulatory motifs are present in the maternal pools (Tremblay et al. 2005; Pique et al. 2008). It has been proposed that RNA accumulation during oogenesis may involve the production of a heterogenic RNA population. CPEB is also believed to be involved in other aspects of transcript storage from mediating mRNA deadenylation by interacting with the poly(A) ribonuclease PARN (Radford et al. 2008) to the control mRNA translation (presented below).

When mRNA is recruited for translation, mechanisms associated with the HEX and CPE sequences become active by promoting lengthening of the poly(A) tail. This probably occurs differently in each species. Most studies on this subject have been carried on oocytes and early embryos from species of Xenopus, since their large size and availability make them particularly well suited to such studies. Thus, in these non-mammalian animals, polyadenylation is induced by the poly(A) polymerase Gld2, which binds to both CPSF and CPEB proteins. Cytoplasmic readenylation seems to occur through opposing polymerase - deadenylase activities. Both the PARN ribonuclease and the Gld2 polymerase are components of the cytoplasmic polyadenylation apparatus and the length of the poly(A) tail is controlled by balancing the rates of both of these enzymes bearing antagonistic activities. Additionaly, CPEB can influence poly(A) tail length since its phosphorylation tends to expel PARN from the cytoplasmic polyadenylation complex, which seems to indicate that this phosphorylation event is involved in mRNA recruitment for translation. Once PARN is out of the way, Gld2 can finally extend the poly(A) tail (reviewed in (Kim and Richter 2006; Radford et al. 2008).

8. Involvement of the poly(A) binding proteins

The polyadenylation process stimulates translation. This stimulation is mediated by the association of poly(A) binding proteins (PABPs) that bind the poly(A) tail of mRNAs. Each PABP contains four RNA recognition motifs (RRMs) and a carboxyl-terminus domain that serves as an anchoring site for many interacting proteins. A physical association between PABP and the mRNA cap is involved in the circularization and translational stimulation of mRNAs (Imataka et al. 1998). This physical interaction is induced through the binding of one PABP with the eukaryotic initiation factor 4G (eIF4G). In turn, eIF4G binds to eIF4E, which binds the 5' cap of mRNAs. This interaction between a PABP and eIF4G could also stimulate binding of the 40S ribosomal subunit by stabilizing the eIF4F-cap interaction (Kahvejian et al. 2001).

Two Poly(A) binding protein interacting proteins i.e. Paip1 and Paip2, are known to interact with PABPs and regulate their function. Both have opposing effects on PABPs as Paip1 shows significant similarity with the central portion of eIF4G and, like it, interacts with the ATP-dependant RNA helicase eIF4A. In the same way, Paip1 interacts with eIF3, which acts as an adapter between the ribosome and the eIF4G protein (Craig et al. 1998; Martineau et al. 2008). Paip1 stimulates the action of PABP since the binding of eIF4A on the 5' UTR of the mRNA provokes the unwinding of mRNA secondary structures. This action enhances ribosome binding and translation initiation. Moreover, the possible interactions of Paip1 and eIF3 could link PABPs to the 40S ribosome subunit. This putative link is consistent with the idea that the 40S ribosome subunit could initiate a new translation cycle because of the proximity of the mRNA extremities. Conversely, Paip2 acts as a repressor of translation by decreasing the affinity of PABPs for polyadenylated mRNAs. As a matter of fact, Paip2 completely prevents PABP multimerization and thus prevents its poly(A)-organizing activity. The simplest model explaining Paip2 translation inhibition poses that Paip2 acts by disrupting the circularization of mRNAs. Evidence suggest that PABP cannot bind to eIF4G in the presence of Paip2 since the binding sites for Paip2 and eIF4G on PABP both overlap the second RRM (Khaleghpour et al. 2001). It was shown that Paip2 also inhibits the formation of the 80S ribosome initiation complex, demonstrating that Paip2 could affect a step that precedes the formation of this complex.

Nevertheless, the principal mode of action of Paip2 is to compete directly with Paip1 for binding PABP. Paip1 interacts with RRMs 1 and 2 of PABP whereas Paip2 interacts with RRMs 2 and 3. This overlap on RRM 2 explains the mutually exclusive binding of Paip1 and Paip2 on PABP. Thus, Paip1 and Paip2 regulation can be used to either stimulate or inhibit translation initiation. The mechanisms of Paip1/2 regulation do however, remain mostly unknown. Since Paip1 and Paip2 are both phosphoproteins, it is likely that their phosphorylation state could modulate their activities (Kahvejian et al. 2001).

9. Roles of RNA helicases

RNA molecules are highly prone to adopt secondary structures which play an important part in RNA processing. The classical example is the presence of hairpin structures in the 5′ UTR of the ferritin mRNA which prevents ribosome progression and thus control over translation. In this specific case, the proteins binding the stem-loop structure are responsive to environmental levels of iron, and appropriately, this region is referred to as the iron-response element (Kikinis et al. 1995; Cho et al. 2010). Another prime example is illustrated through the action of the stem-loop binding protein (SLBP) which binds to structures found in the 3′UTR region of histone mRNAs and regulates its translation (Allard et al. 2002; Whitfield et al. 2004). These examples clearly indicate that interactions between RNA and protein leads to important events of RNA processing involving the presence of secondary structures. These stable conformations can be destabilized by the action of RNA helicases that unwind the RNA molecules resulting in the displacement of bound proteins that can confer a new fate to the transcript.

Prokaryotic and eukaryotic genomes contain a large contingent of DNA and RNA helicases (Silverman et al. 2003). The latter are of interest to RNA processing and have been classified in five super-families that are distinguished by their respective domains and structure. Contrary to the last three super-families, members of the first two super-families form non-ring shaped complexes. From the RNA helicase database (http://www.rnahelicase.org/), the Human super-family 1 is composed of 11 members while the second super-family contains the DExD/H Proteins, a family of 62 members. RNA helicases are known to be involved in every aspect of RNA processing from transcription to mRNA splicing, including RNA transport, ribosome biogenesis and RNA decay (Cordin et al. 2006; Srivastava et al. 2010; Montpetit et al. 2011). They are generally thought as "RNA chaperones" or "maturases" that impact RNA-RNA, RNA-DNA and RNA-protein interactions (Tanner and Linder 2001).

This wide array of RNA helicases may be important for the complex regulation of the maternal RNA pools. Amongst these super-families the DEAD-box family contains the most proteins (36 in Human). The family is named after the D-E-A-D (asp-glu-ala-asp) conserved NTP binding motif and its most prestigious member is eIF4A (Rogers et al. 2002). As mentioned earlier, eIF4A (DDX2) is present in the eukaryotic translation initiation complex and unwinds secondary structures in the mRNA to allow the binding of the 40S ribosome subunit and facilitate its progression along the 5'UTR of the mRNA (Kahvejian et al. 2001). The DEAD-box proteins are known to have helicase, unwindase in addition to RNPase activities (Linder 2006; Naarmann et al. 2010). The later activity is related to the formation and destabilization of RNPs which is integral to the state in which maternal mRNAs are stored. Moreover, the analysis of the protein composition of germ cell granules in C. elegans highlighted the presence of several DEAD-box proteins including Vasa (DDX4) and Vasa-like proteins (Bezares-Calderon et al. 2010; Updike and Strome 2010). So far, the presence of DEAD-box proteins has been confirmed in mammalian oocytes and early embryos, though their association with maternal RNA processing still remains to be demonstrated.

10. Controlling translation through eIF4E binding proteins

Another mechanism by which translation of maternal RNA could be controlled involves eIF4E binding proteins (4E-BP). These small repressors interact with eIF4E to prevent eIF4G binding and thus inhibit the formation of the eukaryotic initiation complex. This complex is named eIF4F and is responsible for cap recognition and is composed of eIF4E, the aforementioned DEAD-box protein eIF4A (DDX2) and eIF4G. eIF4G is the scaffolding protein that binds many proteins involved in translation initiation. eIF4E sequestration by a 4E-BP complex is a reversible process and is modulated by the phosphorylation of 4E-BP (Kahvejian et al. 2001).

11. The closed-loop model

The interaction between proteins localized on the 3'end of the mRNAs (PABP, PAIBP, CPEB) and the translation initiation complex localized at the 5'end involves mRNA circularization by physical interactions between both of the extremities. The closed-loop model is important for translation initiation and efficacy of protein synthesis since in addition to protecting mRNA from degradation by limiting ribonuclease access, this interaction also allows for more efficient translation. Indeed, mRNA circularization could promote ribosome recycling on the same mRNA through the physical proximity of both extremities due to their interactions. This model also protects the cell against the potentially lethal production of truncated proteins, since circularization allows efficient translation only for intact mRNAs and thus prevents the translation of partially degraded mRNA (Kahvejian et al. 2001).

12. The CPEB-Maskin model

Along these lines, the 5' UTR and the 3' UTR of mRNAs are the key regions for translational regulation. Numerous models try to elucidate the pathways responsible for the temporal regulation of maternal stores. Most of them involve different 4E-BPs, different polyadenylation systems and various ways to promote the formation of the closed-loop.

One well known model (Stebbins-Boaz et al. 1999) involves the 4E-BP Maskin protein. This factor binds both CPEB and the cap-binding translation initiation factor eIF4E. Its presence on eIF4E prevents eIF4G binding and the formation of the eukaryotic initiation complex. It was shown that Maskin-eIF4E interactions are significantly reduced during oocyte maturation where many mRNAs are recruited for translation. The CPEB-Maskin regulation model functions so that, mRNA translation initiation is regulated by the release of Maskin from the CPEB-Maskin-eIF4E complex. The interaction between CPEB, Maskin and eIF4E forestalls the formation of the eukaryotic initiation complex by preventing eIF4G binding to eIF4E (Groisman et al. 2001). However, phosphorylation of CPEB by the protein kinase Aurora A enhances its affinity for CPSF, which binds the polyadenylation hexanucleotide HEX. CPSF binding to HEX promotes poly(A) polymerase recruitment, which elongates the poly(A) tail. PABPs can thereby bind the poly(A) tail which promotes the formation of the closed-loop through eIF4E-eIF4G interactions. eIF4G is a scaffold protein which allows the recruitment and binding of many proteins to form the eIF4F eukaryotic initiation complex. The RNA helicase eIF4A/DDX2 will join this complex to unwind the secondary structures of the 5'UTR of the mRNA. As for EIF3, it will act by promoting the recruitment of the 40S ribosomal subunit to initiate translation. Once the eIF4F complex is recruited, it journeys along the mRNA to reach the AUG initiation codon where the 60S subunit ribosome will join the complex and start mRNA translation.

The CPEB-Maskin model is probably one of the best known models of translation regulation applied to the context of maternal RNA management. Nevertheless, the portion of mRNAs regulated through this model is unknown. Furthermore, the model has been challenged as Maskin protein seems to be specific to non-mammalian species since no mammalian homologue has been identified yet despite sequence comparison (Cai et al. 2010). This discrepancy may again highlight some species specific means of regulating the early embryonic program through management of maternal RNAs.

13. A combinatorial code in the 3'UTR

The temporal control of protein production from stored maternal mRNAs through specific interactions of proteins requires the presence of a code imbedded in the UTR regions. Similarly to the HEX and CPE sequence known to drive mRNA polyadenylation, other sequences have been identified such as the embryo deadenylation element (EDEN) which is an AU-rich element found in the 3'UTR of certain mRNAs. It induces deadenylation in a subclass of mRNAs which undergoes deadenylation only after fertilization. An associated binding protein (EDEN-BP) is responsible for deadenylase recruitment such as the PARN or the CCR4–Pop2–Not complexes (Cosson et al. 2006). As an extent of these general processes, to regulate the complexe nature of maternal RNA management, it was proposed that the 3'UTR regions of stored mRNAs may contain a combinatorial code that could serve as a general molecular language to explain the temporal translation control. The proposed code involves the CPE and HEX sequences and explains how a specific mRNA is recruited for translation either early or late during oocyte maturation in mice (Pique et al. 2008). These observations were made from comparative analysis of the 3'UTR of mRNAs. The number and relative position of the two elements were shown to determine whether an mRNA is repressed or activated. An mRNA bearing a single CPE that does not overlap HEX is not repressed and translational activation will occur if the distance between the two sequences does not exceed 121 nucleotides. Furthermore, the distance between CPE and HEX will modulate the strength of activation. A maximal activation is induced by very close but non-overlapping sequences and increased distances induce a weaker polyadenylation (Pique et al. 2008). Additionally, an mRNA bearing a cluster of at least two CPEs is translationally repressed. The distance between the CPEs modulates the efficiency of the repression. An optimal separation between two CPEs is of 10 to 12 nucleotides. These results propose that Maskin binds a heterodimer of CPEB and cannot bind efficiently on only one CPEB. The HEX sequence is involved in allowing a differential translational activation depending on early or late polyadenylation. Early polyadenylation during oocyte maturation is triggered by Aurora A kinase, which phosphorylates CPEB. This phosphorylation increases CPEB affinity for CPSF, which can bind to the HEX sequence (Pique et al. 2008). Subsequently, the process presented earlier can get under way: i.e. PARN is expelled and the polyadenylation triggered by GLD2 initiates translation.

Late polyadenylation is specific to mRNAs where one of the CPE sequences overlaps the HEX sequence and prevents CPSF from binding. In this situation, mRNAs are silenced. During oocyte maturation this occurs until the synthesis of the cytostatic factor component Mos concomitantly with the phosphorylation of CPEB by CDK1 (formerly known as Cdc2). Once the cell cycle must resume, the conditions will lead to the degradation of most CPEBs which allows CPSF to bind on the HEX sequence triggering polyadenylation and stimulating translation (Pique et al. 2008).

In addition to managing the poly(A) tail length, sequences imbedded in the transcripts have also been shown to act downstream of messenger recruitment during initiation of translation. These sequences impact the rate of translation by destabilizing the binding of the initiation complex. Indeed, typical imitation of translation is conducted through the following sequence of events: after eIF4F complex association, the 40S ribosomal subunit can bind the mRNA and scan its 5'UTR region for the start codon. During this process, most of the eIF4F initiation factors are released letting the eIF5 initiation factors bind the mRNA. This promotes the association of the large 60S ribosomal subunit at the moment of the recognition of the initiation codon (Kahvejian et al. 2001). A sequence found in the 3'UTR of some mRNA called the Differentiation Control Element (DICE) is involved in a process that can interfere with the recruitment of the 60S ribosomal subunit and thus inhibit the formation of the monosome. In this manner, the DICE complex maintains translational silencing (Naarmann et al. 2010).

Embedding the fate of the transcript in the UTR regions of mRNAs is an appealing model. However, the proposed model is incomplete as it may fit the mouse embryonic program which only lasts the duration of a single cell cycle but in other species where the embryonic program must undergo several cell cycles, the coding of the transcripts would involve an extremely complex mixture of 3'UTR isoforms. With the recent development of NextGen sequencing, surveys of embryonic transcripts can be accomplished at a very complete depth and such messenger heterogeneity has not been demonstrated so far.

14. Potential involvement of non-coding RNAs

The properties of miRNAs are still being explored, however, the diversity of these short RNAs has been recognized (Williams 2008). As well as playing roles in cellular growth and differentiation, miRNAs function to alter transcript processing. Roles also exist for degradation of mRNAs, as well as sequestering mRNAs from translation (Ma et al. 2010). Along with small interfering (siRNAs), micro-RNAs (miRNAs) have been shown to play a role in the formation of storage granules (Eulalio et al. 2007). When miRNA attach to mRNA with the help of AGO2, transcriptional silencing can occur. The complex is referred to as a microRNP and mRISC (microRNA induced silencing complex) and can associate with p-bodies or related structures (Williams 2008). In the mouse oocyte, it was recently shown that miRNA function is considerably reduced in translational repression and mRNA degradation than previously thought (Ma et al. 2010). The authors discuss that in presence of high levels of miRNAs, the mRNAs are stabilized and this situation coincides with oocyte growth and RNA accumulation. It was also proposed that miRNA may be necessary for the maternal zygotic transition, suggesting that the miRNA activity inhibition may prepare the zygote's blastomeres for pluripotency, a program that assumes control over miRNA expression (Marson et al. 2008). The exact role the miRNAs may play in managing maternal RNAs in mammals still needs further investigation.

15. Concluding remarks

It is interesting to note that although focus has been directed at the understanding of how stored resources are managed to contribute to cell function and early embryogenesis, at least in mammals, it was shown that a large proportion of the maternal transcripts are never translated and are recruited to be sent for decay. In mouse, it has been shown that the content in maternal RNA decreases by about 19% during oocyte maturation (Bachvarova et al. 1985). Furthermore, it has also been proposed that complete degradation of maternal RNA is required for the mouse zygote to undergo the MZT (Schultz 2002). In the bovine, the EGA occurs when the embryonic RNA content are the lowest (Gilbert et al. 2009). The depletion of the maternal RNA content is massive and it is not paralleled by the amount of newly synthesized proteins during these developmental stages as determined by proteomic analysis (Massicotte et al. 2006). In addition, the abundance of ribosomal RNAs (rRNAs) during the pre-EGA stages show atypical profiles with low levels of 28S, the large rRNA component of the 60S ribosomal subunit, which may be indicative of lower translational potential in these early developmental stages (Gilbert et al. 2009). This would also support the observations of large reduction in RNA content that does not lead to massive protein synthesis thus supporting the fact that a large proportion of maternal RNAs are destroyed without ever being translated. So far, the physiological relevance of this apparent wastage is currently unknown.

Overall, it is clear that the processes that managed maternal RNAs have, for the main part, yet to be established. The knowledge so far is indicative of the complexity that underlies the regulation of the stored pools of RNAs during the embryonic program thus in absence of fully functional nuclear responsiveness. Species show marked divergence in the strategies employed to coordinate the use of the stored resources in a spatio-temporally manner. It is clear that regulation of protein synthesis from the stored pools of mRNA can be done at many different levels by interfering with the rates and efficacies during recruitment and/or initiation of translation. For every layer of potential regulation, several models are proposed and it is probable that a combination of many of these models exist to take into account the nature of the different classes of stored transcripts.

16. Reference

Akhtar, W. & G. J. Veenstra (2009). "TBP2 is a substitute for TBP in Xenopus oocyte transcription." *BMC Biol* 7: 45.

Alizadeh, Z., S. Kageyama & F. Aoki (2005). "Degradation of maternal mRNA in mouse embryos: selective degradation of specific mRNAs after fertilization." *Mol Reprod Dev* 72(3): 281-290.

Allard, P., M. J. Champigny, S. Skoggard, J. A. Erkmann, M. L. Whitfield, W. F. Marzluff & H. J. Clarke (2002). "Stem-loop binding protein accumulates during oocyte maturation and is not cell-cycle-regulated in the early mouse embryo." *J Cell Sci* 115(Pt 23): 4577-4586.

Anderson, J. E., R. L. Matteri, L. R. Abeydeera, B. N. Day & R. S. Prather (2001). "Degradation of maternal cdc25c during the maternal to zygotic transition is dependent upon embryonic transcription." *Mol Reprod Dev* 60(2): 181-188.

Anderson, P. & N. Kedersha (2006). RNA granules. *The Journal of Cell Biology*. 172: 803-808.

Anderson, P. & N. Kedersha (2009). RNA granules: post-transcriptional and epigenetic modulators of gene expression. *Nature Publishing Group*. 10: 430-436.

Bachvarova, R., V. De Leon, A. Johnson, G. Kaplan & B. V. Paynton (1985). "Changes in total RNA, polyadenylated RNA, and actin mRNA during meiotic maturation of mouse oocytes." *Dev Biol* 108(2): 325-331.

Bashirullah, A., R. L. Cooperstock & H. D. Lipshitz (1998). RNA localization in development. *Annual review of biochemistry*. 67: 335-394.

Bezares-Calderon, L. A., A. Becerra, L. S. Salinas, E. Maldonado & R. E. Navarro (2010). "Bioinformatic analysis of P granule-related proteins: insights into germ granule evolution in nematodes." *Dev Genes Evol* 220(1-2): 41-52.

Biggers, J., D. Whittingham & R. Donahue (1967). The pattern of energy metabolism in the mouse oöcyte and zygote. *Proceedings of the National Academy of Sciences of the United States of America*. 58: 560.

Bilodeau-Goeseels, S. & G. A. Schultz (1997). Changes in ribosomal ribonucleic acid content within in vitro-produced bovine embryos. *Biology of reproduction*. 56: 1323.

Bouniol-Baly, C., L. Hamraoui, J. Guibert, N. Beaujean, M. S. Szöllösi & P. Debey (1999). Differential transcriptional activity associated with chromatin configuration in fully grown mouse germinal vesicle oocytes. *Biology of Reproduction*. 60: 580.

Bouvet, P. & A. P. Wolffe (1994). A role for transcription and FRGY2 in masking maternal mRNA within Xenopus oocytes. *Cell*. 77: 931-941.

Braude, P., V. Bolton & S. Moore (1988). "Human gene expression first occurs between the four- and eight-cell stages of preimplantation development." *Nature* 332(6163): 459-461.

Brengues, M., D. Teixeira & R. Parker (2005). Movement of eukaryotic mRNAs between polysomes and cytoplasmic processing bodies. *Science*. 310: 486.

Brevini-Gandolfi, T. A., L. A. Favetta, L. Mauri, A. M. Luciano, F. Cillo & F. Gandolfi (1999). "Changes in poly(A) tail length of maternal transcripts during in vitro maturation of bovine oocytes and their relation with developmental competence." *Mol Reprod Dev* 52(4): 427-433.

Cai, C., K. Tamai & K. Molyneaux (2010). "KHDC1B is a novel CPEB binding partner specifically expressed in mouse oocytes and early embryos." *Mol Biol Cell* 21(18): 3137-3148.

Calder, M. D., P. Madan & A. J. Watson (2008). Bovine oocytes and early embryos express Staufen and ELAVL RNA-binding proteins. *Zygote*. 16: 1-8.

Chesnel, F. & J. J. Eppig (1995). "Synthesis and accumulation of p34cdc2 and cyclin B in mouse oocytes during acquisition of competence to resume meiosis." *Mol Reprod Dev* 40(4): 503-508.

Cho, H. H., C. M. Cahill, C. R. Vanderburg, C. R. Scherzer, B. Wang, X. Huang & J. T. Rogers (2010). "Selective translational control of the Alzheimer amyloid precursor protein transcript by iron regulatory protein-1." *J Biol Chem* 285(41): 31217-31232.

Combelles, C., N. Cekleniak, C. Racowsky & D. Albertini (2002). Assessment of nuclear and cytoplasmic maturation in in-vitro matured human oocytes. *Human Reproduction*. 17: 1006.

Conti, M., C. B. Andersen, F. Richard, C. Mehats, S. Y. Chun, K. Horner, C. Jin & A. Tsafriri (2002). Role of cyclic nucleotide signaling in oocyte maturation. *Molecular and cellular endocrinology*. 187: 153-159.

Cordin, O., J. Banroques, N. K. Tanner & P. Linder (2006). "The DEAD-box protein family of RNA helicases." *Gene* 367: 17-37.

Cosson, B., C. Gautier-Courteille, D. Maniey, O. Ait-Ahmed, M. Lesimple, H. B. Osborne & L. Paillard (2006). "Oligomerization of EDEN-BP is required for specific mRNA deadenylation and binding." *Biol Cell* 98(11): 653-665.

Cougot, N. (2004). Cytoplasmic foci are sites of mRNA decay in human cells. *The Journal of Cell Biology*. 165: 31-40.

Craig, A. W., A. Haghighat, A. T. Yu & N. Sonenberg (1998). "Interaction of polyadenylate-binding protein with the eIF4G homologue PAIP enhances translation." *Nature* 392(6675): 520-523.

Crosby, I. M., F. Gandolfi & R. M. Moor (1988). "Control of protein synthesis during early cleavage of sheep embryos." *J Reprod Fertil* 82(2): 769-775.

De La Fuente, R. & J. Eppig (2001). Transcriptional Activity of the Mouse Oocyte Genome: Companion Granulosa Cells Modulate Transcription and Chromatin Remodeling. *Developmental Biology*. 229: 224-236.

Deng, W. & H. Lin (1997). Spectrosomes and Fusomes Anchor Mitotic Spindles during Asymmetric Germ Cell Divisions and Facilitate the Formation of a Polarized Microtubule Array for Oocyte Specification inDrosophila* 1. *Developmental Biology*. 189: 79-94.

Elis, S., F. Batellier, I. Couty, S. Balzergue, M. L. Martin-Magniette, P. Monget, E. Blesbois & M. S. Govoroun (2008). "Search for the genes involved in oocyte maturation and early embryo development in the hen." *BMC Genomics* 9: 110.

Eulalio, A., I. Behm-Ansmant, D. Schweizer & E. Izaurralde (2007). P-Body Formation Is a Consequence, Not the Cause, of RNA-Mediated Gene Silencing. *Molecular and Cellular Biology*. 27: 3970-3981.

Fair, T., P. Hyttel & T. Greve (1995). Bovine oocyte diameter in relation to maturational competence and transcriptional activity. *Molecular reproduction and development*. 42: 437-442.

Flemr, M., J. Ma, R. M. Schultz & P. Svoboda (2010). P-Body Loss Is Concomitant with Formation of a Messenger RNA Storage Domain in Mouse Oocytes. *Biology of Reproduction*. 82: 1008-1017.

Gilbert, I., S. Scantland, E.-L. Sylvestre, C. Gravel, I. Laflamme, M.-A. Sirard & C. Robert (2009). The dynamics of gene products fluctuation during bovine pre-hatching development. *Mol. Reprod. Dev*. 76: 762-772.

Gougeon, A. (1986). Dynamics of follicular growth in the human: a model from preliminary results. *Human Reproduction*. 1: 81.

Groisman, I., Y. S. Huang, R. Mendez, Q. Cao & J. D. Richter (2001). "Translational control of embryonic cell division by CPEB and maskin." *Cold Spring Harb Symp Quant Biol* 66: 345-351.

Gu, W., S. Tekur, R. Reinbold, J. J. Eppig, Y. C. Choi, J. Z. Zheng, M. T. Murray & N. B. Hecht (1998). Mammalian male and female germ cells express a germ cell-specific Y-Box protein, MSY2. *Biology of Reproduction*. 59: 1266.

Henrion, G., A. Brunet, J. P. Renard & V. Duranthon (1997). "Identification of maternal transcripts that progressively disappear during the cleavage period of rabbit embryos." *Mol Reprod Dev* 47(4): 353-362.

Hulot, F. & J. C. Mariana (1985). "[Effect of genotype, age and season on preovulatory follicles in the rabbit 8 hours after mating]." *Reprod Nutr Dev* 25(1A): 17-32.

Hurst, S., N. J. Talbot & H. Stebbings (1999). A staufen-like RNA-binding protein in translocation channels linking nurse cells to oocytes in Notonecta shows nucleotide-dependent attachment to microtubules. *Journal of cell science.* 112: 2947.

Hussein, T., J. Thompson & R. Gilchrist (2006). Oocyte-secreted factors enhance oocyte developmental competence. *Developmental biology.* 296: 514-521.

Imataka, H., A. Gradi & N. Sonenberg (1998). "A newly identified N-terminal amino acid sequence of human eIF4G binds poly(A)-binding protein and functions in poly(A)-dependent translation." *EMBO J* 17(24): 7480-7489.

Irniger, S. (2002). "Cyclin destruction in mitosis: a crucial task of Cdc20." *FEBS Lett* 532(1-2): 7-11.

Jansen, R. P. (2001). mRNA localization: message on the move. *Nature Reviews Molecular Cell Biology.* 2: 247-256.

Kahvejian, A., G. Roy & N. Sonenberg (2001). "The mRNA closed-loop model: the function of PABP and PABP-interacting proteins in mRNA translation." *Cold Spring Harb Symp Quant Biol* 66: 293-300.

Kane, D. A. & C. B. Kimmel (1993). "The zebrafish midblastula transition." *Development* 119(2): 447-456.

Kedersha, N., G. Stoecklin, M. Ayodele, P. Yacono, J. Lykke-Andersen, M. J. Fritzler, D. Scheuner, R. J. Kaufman, D. E. Golan & P. Anderson (2005). Stress granules and processing bodies are dynamically linked sites of mRNP remodeling. *The Journal of cell biology.* 169: 871.

Khaleghpour, K., Y. V. Svitkin, A. W. Craig, C. T. DeMaria, R. C. Deo, S. K. Burley & N. Sonenberg (2001). "Translational repression by a novel partner of human poly(A) binding protein, Paip2." *Mol Cell* 7(1): 205-216.

Kikinis, Z., R. S. Eisenstein, A. J. Bettany & H. N. Munro (1995). "Role of RNA secondary structure of the iron-responsive element in translational regulation of ferritin synthesis." *Nucleic Acids Res* 23(20): 4190-4195.

Kim, J. H. & J. D. Richter (2006). "Opposing polymerase-deadenylase activities regulate cytoplasmic polyadenylation." *Mol Cell* 24(2): 173-183.

Knox, R. (2005). Recruitment and selection of ovarian follicles for determination of ovulation rate in the pig. *Domestic Animal Endocrinology.* 29: 385-397.

Kocabas, A. M., J. Crosby, P. J. Ross, H. H. Otu, Z. Beyhan, H. Can, W. L. Tam, G. J. M. Rosa, R. G. Halgren & B. Lim (2006). The transcriptome of human oocytes. *Proceedings of the National Academy of Sciences.* 103: 14027.

Krawetz, S. A. (2005). Paternal contribution: new insights and future challenges. *Nat Rev Genet.* 6: 633-642.

Lalancette, C., D. Miller, Y. Li & S. A. Krawetz (2008). Paternal contributions: New functional insights for spermatozoal RNA. *J. Cell. Biochem.* 104: 1570-1579.

Le Hir, H., D. Gatfield, E. Izaurralde & M. J. Moore (2001). The exon–exon junction complex provides a binding platform for factors involved in mRNA export and nonsense-mediated mRNA decay. *The EMBO journal.* 20: 4987-4997.

Lequarre, A. S. (2004). Poly(A) RNA Is Reduced by Half During Bovine Oocyte Maturation but Increases when Meiotic Arrest Is Maintained with CDK Inhibitors. *Biology of Reproduction.* 71: 425-431.

Lin, M.-D., X. Jiao, D. Grima, S. F. Newbury, M. Kiledjian & T.-B. Chou (2008). Drosophila processing bodies in oogenesis. *Developmental Biology.* 322: 276-288.

Linder, P. (2006). "Dead-box proteins: a family affair--active and passive players in RNP-remodeling." *Nucleic Acids Res* 34(15): 4168-4180.

Lodde, V., S. Modina, P. Maddox-Hyttel, F. Franciosi, A. Lauria & A. M. Luciano (2008). Oocyte morphology and transcriptional silencing in relation to chromatin remodeling during the final phases of bovine oocyte growth. *Mol. Reprod. Dev.* 75: 915-924.

Ma, J., M. Flemr, P. Stein, P. Berninger, R. Malik, M. Zavolan, P. Svoboda & R. M. Schultz (2010). MicroRNA Activity Is Suppressed in Mouse Oocytes. *Current Biology*. 20: 265-270.

Marson, A., S. S. Levine, M. F. Cole, G. M. Frampton, T. Brambrink, S. Johnstone, M. G. Guenther, W. K. Johnston, M. Wernig & J. Newman (2008). Connecting microRNA genes to the core transcriptional regulatory circuitry of embryonic stem cells. *Cell*. 134: 521-533.

Martineau, Y., M. C. Derry, X. Wang, A. Yanagiya, J. J. Berlanga, A. B. Shyu, H. Imataka, K. Gehring & N. Sonenberg (2008). "Poly(A)-binding protein-interacting protein 1 binds to eukaryotic translation initiation factor 3 to stimulate translation." *Mol Cell Biol* 28(21): 6658-6667.

Massicotte, L., K. Coenen, M. Mourot & M. A. Sirard (2006). "Maternal housekeeping proteins translated during bovine oocyte maturation and early embryo development." *Proteomics* 6(13): 3811-3820.

Masui, Y. (2001). "From oocyte maturation to the in vitro cell cycle: the history of discoveries of Maturation-Promoting Factor (MPF) and Cytostatic Factor (CSF)." *Differentiation* 69(1): 1-17.

McCleland, M. L., A. W. Shermoen & P. H. O'Farrell (2009). "DNA replication times the cell cycle and contributes to the mid-blastula transition in Drosophila embryos." *J Cell Biol* 187(1): 7-14.

Memili, E., T. Dominko & N. L. First (1998). "Onset of transcription in bovine oocytes and preimplantation embryos." *Mol Reprod Dev* 51(1): 36-41.

Miyara, F. A., C. Migne, M. Dumont-Hassan, A. L. Meur, P. Cohen-Bacrie, F. O.-X. Aubriot, A. L. Glissant, C. Nathan, S. P. Douard, A. Stanovici & P. Debey (2003). Chromatin configuration and transcriptional control in human and mouse oocytes. *Mol. Reprod. Dev.* 64: 458-470.

Montpetit, B., N. D. Thomsen, K. J. Helmke, M. A. Seeliger, J. M. Berger & K. Weis (2011). "A conserved mechanism of DEAD-box ATPase activation by nucleoporins and InsP6 in mRNA export." *Nature* 472(7342): 238-242.

Moore, G. & S. Lintern-Moore (1978). Transcription of the mouse oocyte genome. *Biology of Reproduction*. 18: 865.

Motlik J, K. V., Travnik P, Pivko J (1984). "RNA synthesis in pig follicular oocytes. Autoradiographic and cytochemical study." *Biol. Cell* 50(3): 7.

Naarmann, I. S., C. Harnisch, G. Muller-Newen, H. Urlaub, A. Ostareck-Lederer & D. H. Ostareck (2010). "DDX6 recruits translational silenced human reticulocyte 15-lipoxygenase mRNA to RNP granules." *RNA* 16(11): 2189-2204.

Nagamori, I., A. Cruickshank & P. Sassone-Corsi (2010). Epigenetics and Human Reproduction: 311-328.

Newport, J. & M. Kirschner (1982). "A major developmental transition in early Xenopus embryos: II. Control of the onset of transcription." *Cell* 30(3): 687-696.

Olszańska, B. & A. Borgul (1993). Maternal RNA content in oocytes of several mammalian and avian species. *Journal of Experimental Zoology*. 265: 317-320.

Osteen, K. G. & T. M. Mills (1980). Changes in the size, distribution and steroid content of rabbit ovarian follicles during early pseudopregnancy. *Biology of Reproduction*. 22: 1040.

Paynton, B. V. & R. Bachvarova (1994). "Polyadenylation and deadenylation of maternal mRNAs during oocyte growth and maturation in the mouse." *Mol Reprod Dev* 37(2): 172-180.

Paynton, B. V. & R. Bachvarova (1994). Polyadenylation and deadenylation of maternal mRNAs during oocyte growth and maturation in the mouse. *Molecular reproduction and development*. 37: 172-180.

Paynton, B. V., R. Rempel & R. Bachvarova (1988). "Changes in state of adenylation and time course of degradation of maternal mRNAs during oocyte maturation and early embryonic development in the mouse." *Dev Biol* 129(2): 304-314.

Pedersen, T. & H. Peters (1968). Proposal for a classification of oocytes and follicles in the mouse ovary. *Reproduction*. 17: 555.

Piko, L. & K. B. Clegg (1982). Quantitative changes in total RNA, total poly (A), and ribosomes in early mouse embryos* 1. *Developmental Biology*. 89: 362-378.

Pique, M., J. M. Lopez, S. Foissac, R. Guigo & R. Mendez (2008). "A combinatorial code for CPE-mediated translational control." *Cell* 132(3): 434-448.

Radford, H. E., H. A. Meijer & C. H. de Moor (2008). "Translational control by cytoplasmic polyadenylation in Xenopus oocytes." *Biochim Biophys Acta* 1779(4): 217-229.

Robert, C., I. Hue, S. McGraw, D. Gagne & M. A. Sirard (2002). "Quantification of cyclin B1 and p34(cdc2) in bovine cumulus-oocyte complexes and expression mapping of genes involved in the cell cycle by complementary DNA macroarrays." *Biol Reprod* 67(5): 1456-1464.

Rodman, T. C. & R. Bachvarova (1976). "RNA synthesis in preovulatory mouse oocytes." *J Cell Biol* 70(1): 251-257.

Rogers, G. W., Jr., A. A. Komar & W. C. Merrick (2002). "eIF4A: the godfather of the DEAD box helicases." *Prog Nucleic Acid Res Mol Biol* 72: 307-331.

Rose, U., R. Hanssen & H. Kloosterboer (1999). Development and characterization of an in vitro ovulation model using mouse ovarian follicles. *Biology of Reproduction*. 61: 503.

Russo, V., A. Martelli, P. Berardinelli, O. Di Giacinto, N. Bernabò, D. Fantasia, M. Mattioli & B. Barboni (2007). Modifications in chromatin morphology and organization during sheep oogenesis. *Microsc. Res. Tech.* 70: 733-744.

Schnorrer, F., K. Bohmann & C. Nüsslein-Volhard (2000). The molecular motor dynein is involved in targeting swallow and bicoid RNA to the anterior pole of Drosophila oocytes. *Nat Cell Biol*. 2: 185-190.

Schultz, R. M. (1993). "Regulation of zygotic gene activation in the mouse." *Bioessays* 15(8): 531-538.

Schultz, R. M. (2002). "The molecular foundations of the maternal to zygotic transition in the preimplantation embryo." *Hum Reprod Update* 8(4): 323-331.

Schultz, R. M. & P. M. Wassarman (1977). Specific changes in the pattern of protein synthesis during meiotic maturation of mammalian oocytes in vitro. *Proceedings of the National Academy of Sciences of the United States of America*. 74: 538.

Shalgi, R., A. Magnus, R. Jones & D. M. Phillips (1994). Fate of sperm organelles during early embryogenesis in the rat. *Molecular reproduction and development*. 37: 264-271.

Silverman, E., G. Edwalds-Gilbert & R. J. Lin (2003). "DExD/H-box proteins and their partners: helping RNA helicases unwind." *Gene* 312: 1-16.

Srivastava, L., Y. R. Lapik, M. Wang & D. G. Pestov (2010). "Mammalian DEAD box protein Ddx51 acts in 3' end maturation of 28S rRNA by promoting the release of U8 snoRNA." *Mol Cell Biol* 30(12): 2947-2956.

Stebbins-Boaz, B., Q. Cao, C. H. de Moor, R. Mendez & J. D. Richter (1999). "Maskin is a CPEB-associated factor that transiently interacts with elF-4E." *Mol Cell* 4(6): 1017-1027.

Sternlicht, A. L. & R. M. Schultz (1981). Biochemical studies of mammalian oogenesis: Kinetics of accumulation of total and poly (A)-containing RNA during growth of the mouse oocyte. *Journal of Experimental Zoology*. 215: 191-200.

Sun, X.-S., Y. Liu, K.-Z. Yue, S.-F. Ma & J.-H. Tan (2004). Changes in germinal vesicle (GV) chromatin configurations during growth and maturation of porcine oocytes. *Mol. Reprod. Dev.* 69: 228-234.

Sutovsky, P., C. S. Navara & G. Schatten (1996). Fate of the sperm mitochondria, and the incorporation, conversion, and disassembly of the sperm tail structures during bovine fertilization. *Biology of reproduction*. 55: 1195.

Swann, K. (2004). The cytosolic sperm factor that triggers Ca2+ oscillations and egg activation in mammals is a novel phospholipase C: PLC *Reproduction*. 127: 431-439.

Swetloff, A., B. Conne, J. Huarte, J. L. Pitetti, S. Nef & J. D. Vassalli (2009). Dcp1-bodies in mouse oocytes. *Molecular Biology of the Cell*. 20: 4951.

Tan, J.-H., H.-L. Wang, X.-S. Sun, Y. Liu, H.-S. Sui & J. Zhang (2009). Chromatin configurations in the germinal vesicle of mammalian oocytes. *Molecular Human Reproduction*. 15: 1-9.

Tanner, N. K. & P. Linder (2001). "DExD/H box RNA helicases: from generic motors to specific dissociation functions." *Mol Cell* 8(2): 251-262.

Tomek, W., H. Torner & W. Kanitz (2002). Comparative analysis of protein synthesis, transcription and cytoplasmic polyadenylation of mRNA during maturation of bovine oocytes in vitro. *Reproduction in Domestic Animals*. 37: 86-91.

Tremblay, K., C. Vigneault, S. McGraw & M. A. Sirard (2005). "Expression of cyclin B1 messenger RNA isoforms and initiation of cytoplasmic polyadenylation in the bovine oocyte." *Biol Reprod* 72(4): 1037-1044.

Turnbull, K., A. Braden & P. Mattner (1977). The pattern of follicular growth and atresia in the ovine ovary. *Australian Journal of Biological Sciences*. 30: 229-242.

Updike, D. & S. Strome (2010). "P granule assembly and function in Caenorhabditis elegans germ cells." *J Androl* 31(1): 53-60.

Voronina, A. S. & E. S. Pshennikova (2010). mRNPs: From informosomes to stress granules. *Mol Biol*. 44: 520-528.

Wang, H., N. Isobe, K. Kumamoto, H. Yamashiro, Y. Yamashita & T. Terada (2006). Studies of the role of steroid hormone in the regulation of oocyte maturation in cattle. *Reproductive Biology and Endocrinology*. 4: 4.

Wassarman, P. M. & G. E. Letourneau (1976). RNA synthesis in fully-grown mouse oocytes.

Whitfield, M. L., H. Kaygun, J. A. Erkmann, W. H. Townley-Tilson, Z. Dominski & W. F. Marzluff (2004). "SLBP is associated with histone mRNA on polyribosomes as a component of the histone mRNP." *Nucleic Acids Res* 32(16): 4833-4842.

Williams, A. E. (2008). Functional aspects of animal microRNAs. *Cell. Mol. Life Sci*. 65: 545-562.

Yu, J., N. B. Hecht & R. M. Schultz (2001). Expression of MSY2 in mouse oocytes and preimplantation embryos. *Biology of reproduction*. 65: 1260.

Zheng, D., N. Ezzeddine, C.-Y. A. Chen, W. Zhu, X. He & A.-B. Shyu (2008). Deadenylation is prerequisite for P-body formation and mRNA decay in mammalian cells. *The Journal of Cell Biology*. 182: 89-101.

Žitný, J., P. Massányi, A. Trakovická, J. Rafaj & R. Toman (2004). Quantification of the ovarian follicular growth in rabbits. *Bull. Vet. Inst. Pulawy*. 48: 37-40.

Part 4

RNA Processing Factors

10

Recent Advances in Understanding of Alternative Splicing in Neuronal Pathogenesis

Hung-Hsi Chen, Jung-Chun Lin and Woan-Yuh Tarn
Institute of Biomedical Sciences
Academia Sinica
Taiwan

1. Introduction

The nervous system is an intricate and highly specialized network of neurons. Neuronal differentiation involves complex reprogramming of gene expression. Alternative splicing of precursor mRNAs increases the complexity of transcriptomes and diversifies protein functions at the post-transcriptional level. Indeed, alternative splicing plays an important role in neuronal differentiation, axon guidance, synaptogenesis, synaptic transmission, and plasticity. Because the delicate structure and function of neurons make them particularly susceptible to dysregulation of splicing, aberrant expression or function of splicing factors may cause neuronal disorders. Therefore, it is important to improve our understanding of the mechanisms and physiological functions of alternative splicing regulation in neurons. Regulation of alternative splicing primarily involves the binding of regulatory factors to specific *cis*-elements of precursor mRNAs, and interplay between splicing factors may lead to fine tuning of splicing regulation, thereby diversifying the cadre of mature products. In addition, transcription rate and the availability of the basal splicing machinery may also influence alternative splicing. Recently, our understanding of the mechanisms underlying alternative splicing have been advanced from studies of several neuronal splicing factors; these studies have utilized genetic knockout or disease models as well as genome-wide analysis of mRNA isoforms. In this chapter, we review current understanding of alternative splicing in neurons.

2. Introduction to alternative splicing

Recent estimates have indicated that as many as 95% of human genes generate alternatively spliced mRNAs (Pan, et al., 2008; E. T. Wang, et al., 2008). Alternative splicing of precursor mRNAs (pre-mRNAs) may alter the coding sequence and hence change the function or stability of the encoded proteins. Moreover, alternative splicing may create pre-mature termination codons within the coding region due to frame shift, thereby inducing mRNA destruction via the nonsense-mediated decay pathway (Isken & Maquat, 2007; McGlincy & Smith, 2008; Moore & Proudfoot, 2009). Alterative splicing may also occur in the 3' untranslated region of a pre-mRNA and thus create or eliminate *cis*-regulatory elements that may change the kinetics of mRNA decay or translation (Khabar, 2010; Thiele, et al., 2006). Therefore, alternative splicing is a mechanism that not only increases protein diversity but also may post-transcriptionally modulate the level of gene expression. Moreover, a growing body of evidence suggests that coordinated control of alternative splicing of functionally related transcripts allows for proper orchestration of cellular processes and thus the maintenance of homoeostasis (Allen, et al., 2010; Calarco, et al., 2011; Licatalosi & Darnell, 2010).

Alternative splicing plays a critical role in many fundamental biological processes, such as cell differentiation and specification during development and specificity of function in diverse cell types (Keren, et al., 2010; Nilsen & Graveley, 2010). The nervous system also adopts alternative splicing for cell differentiation, morphogenesis, and even for formation of complex neuronal networks and delicate synapse formation/plasticity (Calarco, et al., 2009; Grabowski, 2011; Li, et al., 2007). An extreme case of alternative splicing is the gene encoding *Drosophila* Down syndrome cell adhesion molecule (Dscam), which potentially could generate >38000 mRNA isoforms by mutually exclusive selection of cassette exons (Hattori, et al., 2008). Dscam encodes neuronal recognition proteins that act as axon guidance receptors. Homotypic interaction between identical Dscam isoforms on opposing membranes causes repulsion between sister neurites (J. W. Park & Graveley, 2007). Therefore, accurate alternative splicing control is critical for establishment of neural circuits in *Drosophila*. In the mammalian brain, alternative splicing is also an important regulatory mechanism for creating the remarkable capacity for plasticity and adaptation. For example, the splicing-mediated splicing of exon 21 in the ionotropic glutamate receptor *N*-methyl *D*-aspartate (NMDA) receptor subunit 1 mRNA affects the membrane trafficking of the NMDA receptor (Ares, 2007). Interestingly, inclusion of exon 21 can be suppressed, likely by the calmodulin-dependent protein kinase IV pathway, which is activated upon cell depolarization (Ares, 2007). Therefore, splicing control provides an intricate and rapid means for regulating mRNA isoform expression.

Alternative splicing is primarily controlled by splicing regulatory factors that bind to *cis*-elements within exons and/or introns of pre-mRNAs. Their binding may modulate the loading of the spliceosomal components to the splice sites and thereby influence alternative splice site utilization (Chen & Manley, 2009; Witten & Ule, 2011). Several neuron-specific splicing regulatory factors have been discovered; some of them, such as the neuro-oncological ventral antigen (Nova), have been studied intensively (Licatalosi & Darnell, 2010; C. Zhang, et al., 2010). In particular, identification of mRNA targets and potential binding sites of Nova have benefited greatly from recent genome-wide splicing arrays and sequencing technology. Therefore, the study of Nova has provided a detailed picture of a splicing regulatory network as well as the combinatorial action of multiple splicing factors (Nilsen & Graveley, 2010; Z. Wang & Burge, 2008).

The repertoire of splicing factors is adjusted during neuronal differentiation and perhaps for functional specification of different neuronal cell types. For example, the switch in the expression of the polypyrimidine tract-binding protein (PTB) to its neuronal homolog, nPTB, may tune neuronal transcriptomes during differentiation (Coutinho-Mansfield, et al., 2007; Tang, et al., 2011). In addition to RNA-binding factors, altered abundance of basic splicing machinery components may also modulate splice site selection (Calarco, et al., 2011; Saltzman, et al., 2011). The survival of motor neuron (SMN) protein is a key factor for the assembly of spliceosomal small nuclear ribonucleoproteins (snRNPs). SMN deficiency may reduce snRNP abundance and thus influence splicing. Defective Nova and/or SMN proteins are associated with disease (Robert B. Darnell, 2011; Lorson, et al., 2010; Lukong, et al., 2008; G. H. Park, et al., 2010). Therefore, to understand how defects of Nova and SMN induce pathological effects on neurons via misregulated splicing control is an interesting and important question. Therefore, a complete understanding of such diseases will require knowledge of how misregulated splicing control in Nova or SMN causes neuronal pathology.

We hereby discuss our current knowledge of Nova, PTB/nPTB, and SMN with respect to their splicing regulation mechanisms, physiological roles, and functions.

3. Nova

3.1 Nova proteins and expression

Nova was discovered as a target of the autoantibodies in cancer patients with paraneoplastic opsoclonus myoclonus ataxia, a type of rare paraneoplastic neurologic disease that causes motor disorders (Buckanovich, et al., 1993; R. B. Darnell & Posner, 2003; Yang, et al., 1998). The amino acid sequences of the two mammalian Nova proteins (1 and 2) are highly similar throughout their lengths, and both contain three heterogeneous nuclear RNP (hnRNP) K-homology (KH) RNA-binding domains (Buckanovich, et al., 1996; Yang, et al., 1998). In mice, Nova-1 expression is restricted in subcortical regions of developing and mature neurons, whereas Nova-2 is more broadly expressed in the central nervous system (Buckanovich, et al., 1993; Buckanovich, et al., 1996; Yang, et al., 1998). Moreover, Nova-1 and Nova-2 appear to be reciprocally expressed in the nervous system, i.e., the level of Nova-2 is generally low in regions where Nova-1 is abundant, which may reflect their distinct biological functions (Yang, et al., 1998). Nevertheless, Nova-1 and -2 primarily act as splicing regulatory factors and also play a role in alternative polyadenylation and mRNA trafficking in neuronal dendrites (Licatalosi, et al., 2008; Racca, et al., 2010).

3.2 RNA-binding specificity of Nova

The RNA-binding specificity of the Nova proteins has been examined by various methods. Initially, the results of *in vitro* systematic selection of ligands and RNP immunoprecipitation indicated that Nova-1 binds to long stem-loop RNAs containing UCAU repeats (Buckanovich & Darnell, 1997). Nova-2-selected RNA ligands also appear to form a stem-loop structure encompassing the UCAU motif (Yang, et al., 1998). Structural studies have shown that both Nova-1 and -2 bind to UCAU-containing sequences via their KH3 domains, of which the residues involved in UCAU interaction are conserved (Lewis, et al., 2000). Nevertheless, the KH1 and KH2 domains of both Nova proteins can also bind to the UCAU motif (Musunuru & Darnell, 2004). Perhaps cooperativity between several KH domains promotes protein binding to RNAs (Chmiel, et al., 2006; Valverde, et al., 2008). The similar RNA-binding properties of Nova-1 and Nova-2 suggest that they may regulate common RNA targets.

Next, ultraviolet cross-linking in conjunction with ribonucleoprotein immunoprecipitation (CLIP) was developed to identify *in vivo* targets of RNA-binding proteins. CLIP analysis has been applied to identify Nova-associated RNA fragments in mouse brain; approximately 340 Nova-1/-2 CLIP tags (~70 nucleotides each) contained, on average, four YCAY repeats (Y, pyrimidine) (Ule, et al., 2003). Detailed analysis of these tag sequences revealed an overrepresentation of YCAU tetramers flanked by pyrimidines. It is currently believed that YCAY repeats are the principal elements in the mRNAs to which Nova proteins bind. More recently, an unbiased method using CLIP combined with high-throughput sequencing (HITS) of RNA was used to identify genome-wide functional protein-RNA interactions (R.

B. Darnell, 2010; Ule, et al., 2005a). A HITS-CLIP analysis showed that Nova-2 tags in mouse cortex, as expected, also harbor ~3.6 YCAY repeats per tag (Ule, et al., 2005a). The results of all these CLIP analyses of Nova coincide with previous observations from RNA selection experiments (Licatalosi, et al., 2008).

Moreover, the aforementioned CLIP analyses also revealed that the largest set of Nova tags is located within introns and even flanking alternative exons (Licatalosi, et al., 2008), which is consistent with the primary role of Nova proteins in regulating pre-mRNA splicing (see below). In addition, Nova tags are also found in protein-coding regions and 3' untranslated region of mRNAs. The results of HITS-CLIP experiments have confirmed the high frequency of potential Nova-binding elements in 3' untranslated regions, thus disclosing a role for Nova in alternative polyadenylation and mRNA transport regulation in brain (Licatalosi, et al., 2008; Racca, et al., 2010).

3.3 Alternative splicing regulated by Nova

Earlier studies have shown that two neuronal transcripts, encoding the inhibitory glycine receptor α2 (GlyRα2) and Nova-1 itself, contain the Nova-1-binding elements adjacent to the alternatively spliced exons and indeed bound to the Nova-1 protein (Buckanovich & Darnell, 1997). The role of Nova-1 in splicing regulation was first analyzed by genetic knockout of Nova-1 in mice (Jensen, et al., 2000); in those mice, selection of GlyRα2 exon 3A is diminished. Further experiments demonstrated that Nova-1 binds to three consecutive YCAY repeats in the intron upstream of exon 3A and thereby increases exon 3A inclusion. Alternative exon selection in another neuronal ionotropic receptor, $GABA_A$ Rγ2, is also impaired in Nova-1 null mice (Dredge & Darnell, 2003; Jensen, et al., 2000). Nova-1 was subsequently shown to promote $GABA_A$ Rγ2 exon 9 inclusion via a distal downstream intronic YCAY-rich splicing enhancer. Notably, the Nova-1 gene itself harbors five YCAY repeats in its exon 4 that are indeed essential for Nova-1 autoregulation (Dredge, et al., 2005). Inclusion of exon 4 in Nova-1 transcripts was increased in haploinsufficient $Nova^{+/-}$ mice. Accordingly, exon 4 inclusion in a Nova-1 splicing reporter was suppressed upon Nova-1 overexpression. In this case, Nova-1 acts via binding to the YCAY repeats in the alternative exon. Therefore, Nova can function either as a positive or negative splicing regulator via binding to intronic or exonic YCAY elements. Further study by swapping of Nova-1-binding sites between various splicing substrates of Nova-1 indicated that the action of Nova-1 is determined by the position of the Nova-binding elements (Dredge, et al., 2005). This positional effect has also been found in other splicing regulators (see below).

Through CLIP and exon junction arrays, a large number of the potential targets of Nova, including some previously defined targets, have been identified (Ule, et al., 2003). Alternative splicing of several candidates was indeed altered in Nova knockout mice, confirming that those transcripts undergo Nova-mediated splicing control. This systematic and genome-wide identification also indicted that Nova may coregulate a set of synaptic and axonal transcripts by controlling alternative splicing. Such coordinated control of alternative exon usage may perhaps provide a powerful means to rapidly modulate synaptic function in response to stimuli.

More recently, HITS-CLIP analysis established functional RNA binding maps of Nova (Licatalosi, et al., 2008). That analysis predicted ~600 differentially spliced exons in brain that are potentially targeted by Nova-2. The transcripts harboring some of the identified exons showed a severe splicing defect in the neocortex of Nova-2 null mice, where Nova-2 is exclusively expressed. However, minor effects were seen in the spinal cord, cerebellum, and midbrain perhaps owing to redundancy of Nova-1 and Nova-2 in these tissues (Licatalosi, et al., 2008). Other work has indicated that Nova proteins regulate alternative splicing across all members of the spectrin-ankyrin-protein 4.1-CASK scaffold complex and the Cav2.2 voltage-gated calcium channels and thereby may finely modulate synaptic function in a coordinated way (Licatalosi, et al., 2008; Ule, et al., 2005b). A genome-wide search in combination with gene ontology analysis revealed that Nova-2-regulated transcripts encode a group of synaptic proteins located at the cell membrane, most often at cell-cell junctions, and are implicated in synapse biogenesis and synaptic transmission. Therefore, Nova-1 and -2 may function analogously in regulating alternative splicing of pre-mRNAs encoded by functionally related genes in neurons.

Drosophila pasilla is the homolog of mammalian Nova proteins (Seshaiah, et al., 2001). Pasilla localizes primarily to nuclear puncta in *Drosophila* cells, indicating its role in splicing. Interestingly, identification of the mRNA targets of pasilla also revealed an enrichment of YCAY repeats near pasilla-regulated cassette exons (Brooks, et al., 2011). Like Nova, pasilla suppresses alternative exon inclusion when it binds predominantly upstream of the exon, whereas it activates splicing when it binds downstream of the exon. Therefore, the RNA-binding specificity and regulatory activity of Nova orthologs apparently have been preserved throughout evolution (Irimia, et al., 2011; Jelen, et al., 2007).

3.4 Mechanisms of Nova-mediated splicing regulation

The interplay between Nova proteins and *cis*-elements was revealed by CLIP-based analyses. CLIP followed by genome-wide detection has identified a considerable number of Nova-binding sites and Nova-regulated transcripts. Bioinformatics analysis revealed the mechanism of Nova-mediated alternative splicing regulation (Ule, et al., 2006). Consistent with previous reports using minigene splicing assays, the position of Nova-binding sites in pre-mRNAs determines the effect of Nova proteins on splicing (Dredge, et al., 2005). For a cassette exon, Nova binding to its downstream intronic YCAY clusters enhances exon inclusion, whereas exon skipping occurs when Nova binds either immediately upstream of or within the exon. Therefore, Nova binding to its target *cis*-elements may result in an asymmetric action on splicing regulation. Indeed, such a positional effect has also been observed for some other splicing regulatory factors (see below, (Konig, et al., 2010; Xue, et al., 2009; Yeo, et al., 2009)).

Bioinformatic analysis of the Nova HITS-CLIP data using Bayesian networks has further provided a comprehensive view of alternative splicing coordinately regulated by Nova and cofactors (C. Zhang, et al., 2010). This analysis initially predicted more than 600 Nova-regulated alternative splicing events. Gene ontology classification supported the hypothesis that Nova may regulate a subgroup of functionally coherent genes involved in synaptic plasticity. This analysis also revealed that the avidity with which Nova binds YCAY clusters may modulate how Nova affects splicing. Moreover, Nova binding to multiple regions may result in a different effect on alternative exon selection from binding to a single region (Figure 1). For example, Nova binding to both the regulated exon and its upstream intron increases the probability of exon exclusion. Moreover, it is estimated that ~15% of Nova targets harbor binding sites for the splicing factors Fox-1 and Fox-2, implying combinatory splicing regulation by Nova and Fox (C. Zhang, et al., 2010). Therefore, an intriguing issue is how the relative location of Nova and Fox binding sites dictates splicing regulation (Chen & Manley, 2009; Licatalosi & Darnell, 2010).

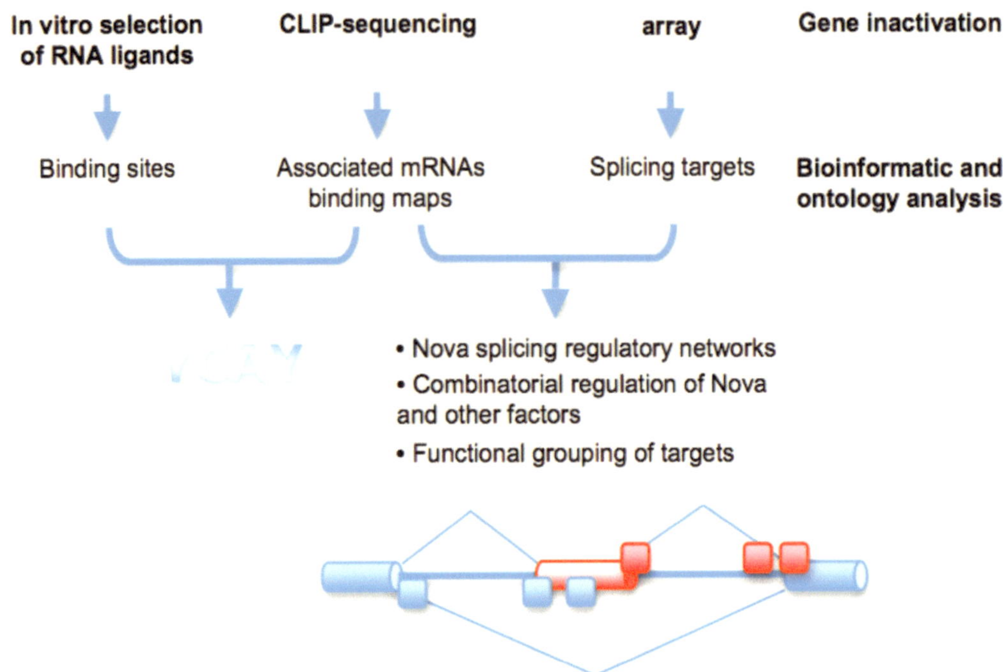

Fig. 1. **Establishment of a Nova regulatory network.** The binding sites and target mRNAs of Nova proteins are identified through *in vitro* RNA selection and *in vivo* crosslinking followed by sequencing or array analysis. In addition, comparative genome-wide transcriptome profiling of Nova knockout mutants also facilitates identification of the transcripts regulated by Nova. Bioinformatic and ontology analysis helps to establish binding and functional maps for Nova. Methods used are denoted by bold type. The bottom diagram shows a model of Nova-mediated splicing control. Positive and negative *cis*-elements that appear with high frequency in CLIP datasets are depicted by red and blue rectangles, respectively. Red and blue cylinders are alternative and constitutive exons, respectively.

Previous studies have also revealed how Nova proteins may modulate the activity of the spliceosome. For example, Nova binding to exons may interfere with U1 snRNP binding to the 5' splice site, thereby inhibiting splicing (Dredge, et al., 2005). When Nova binds to the downstream intron of a regulated exon, it may facilitate spliceosome assembly and promote exon inclusion (Dredge, et al., 2005). As described above, Nova and Fox proteins may coregulate alternative splicing of a considerable number of transcripts in a cooperative or antagonistic manner (C. Zhang, et al., 2010). Notably, neuronal depolarization can induce exon 19 exclusion of Fox-1, producing a Fox-1 isoform with higher splicing activity (Lee, et al., 2009). Therefore, under certain circumstances this Fox-1 isoform may function coordinately with Nova to modulate splicing of Fox-1/Nova-coregulated mRNAs. Moreover, the neuron-enriched nPTB can antagonize Nova action to increase inclusion of GlyRα2 exon 3A (Polydorides, et al., 2000). The physical and functional interactions between Nova and other splicing regulatory factors certainly complicate Nova splicing networks, but the detailed mechanisms remain to be investigated.

3.5 Cellular signaling pathways affect Nova expression level and activity

In contrast to the abundant information about Nova-target interactions, we have only rudimentary knowledge of whether Nova's function can be modulated by cellular signaling pathways. However, several reports have indicated that Nova expression may be regulated at different gene expression levels. It has been shown that the neuronal protein embryonic lethal abnormal visual (nELAV) can increase the stability of the Nova-1 mRNA via binding to its AU-rich elements in the highly conserved 3'-untranslated region (Ratti, et al., 2008; Rossi, et al., 2009). In addition, protein kinase C–induced phosphorylation of nELAV can promote Nova-1 translation (Ratti, et al., 2008). Therefore, nELAV can increase Nova-1 abundance. Moreover, nELAV can modulate the splicing activity of Nova-1 on its target pre-mRNAs (Ratti, et al., 2008). Glucocorticoids can also regulate Nova-1-mediated alternative splicing by downregulating Nova-1 (E. Park, et al., 2009). Moreover, cholinergic stimulation may decrease Nova-2 transcripts but increase Nova-1 transcripts in striatum (Jelen, et al., 2010). Therefore, the expression switch between these two Nova proteins may modify Nova activity in neurons. Finally, it is noteworthy that Nova-1 can autoregulate its exon 4 inclusion by acting as a splicing repressor (Dredge, et al., 2005). Because exon 4 contains multiple phosphorylation sites for serine/threonine kinases, it would be interesting to know whether Nova-1 may modulate its own activity via autoregulation of alternative splicing in response to activation of specific cellular signaling pathways.

3.6 Physiological function and pathological implications of Nova

Early studies of Nova-1 and -2 showed that these proteins have a reciprocal expression pattern in the neocortex and hippocampus in postnatal mouse brain and may have slightly different RNA-binding specificity and/or affinity (Buckanovich & Darnell, 1997; Yang, et al., 1998). Genetic knockout studies then provided further hints to their different physiological roles. Nova-1 knockout mice died 7-10 days after birth owing to a motor deficit caused by apoptotic death of spinal and brainstem neurons, indicating that Nova-1 is an essential gene in mice (Jensen, et al., 2000; Yang, et al., 1998). Nova-2 null mice died in the second postnatal week, whereas double Nova knockout caused perinatal death (Ruggiu, et al., 2009; Ule, et al., 2006). Microarray analysis revealed distinct splicing defects for Nova-1 vs. Nova-2 knockout mice (Ule, et al., 2005b; C. Zhang, et al., 2010). These results indicate that these two Nova genes have non-redundant physiological functions.

Identified targets of Nova have implicated a role for Nova in synaptic plasticity. As predicted, long-term potentiation induced by $GABA_B$ receptor-mediated slow inhibitory postsynaptic current in hippocampal neurons is abolished in Nova-2 knockout mice (Huang, et al., 2005). Moreover, a recent report showed a migration deficiency in cortical and Purkinje neurons in Nova-2 null mice (Yano, et al., 2010). These observations are consistent with the role of Nova-2 in alternative splicing regulation of GABA receptor subunits and of disabled-1, a regulatory factor of the reelin signaling pathway essential for cell positioning during neurogenesis. Therefore, Nova-2 can regulate neuronal migration and synaptic plasticity via its control of alternative splicing.

Certain Nova targets have been implicated in genetic disorders. For example, reelin-disabled-1 signaling may be associated with epilepsy, schizophrenia, and autism (Frotscher, 2010; Pardo & Eberhart, 2007). Interestingly, Fox-1, a functional partner of the Nova proteins, has been implicated in autism (Martin, et al., 2007; Smith & Sadee, 2011). Indeed, the genes coregulated by Nova and Fox appear to be more frequently associated with autism (C. Zhang, et al., 2010). Therefore, aberrant regulation of Nova proteins may contribute to autism.

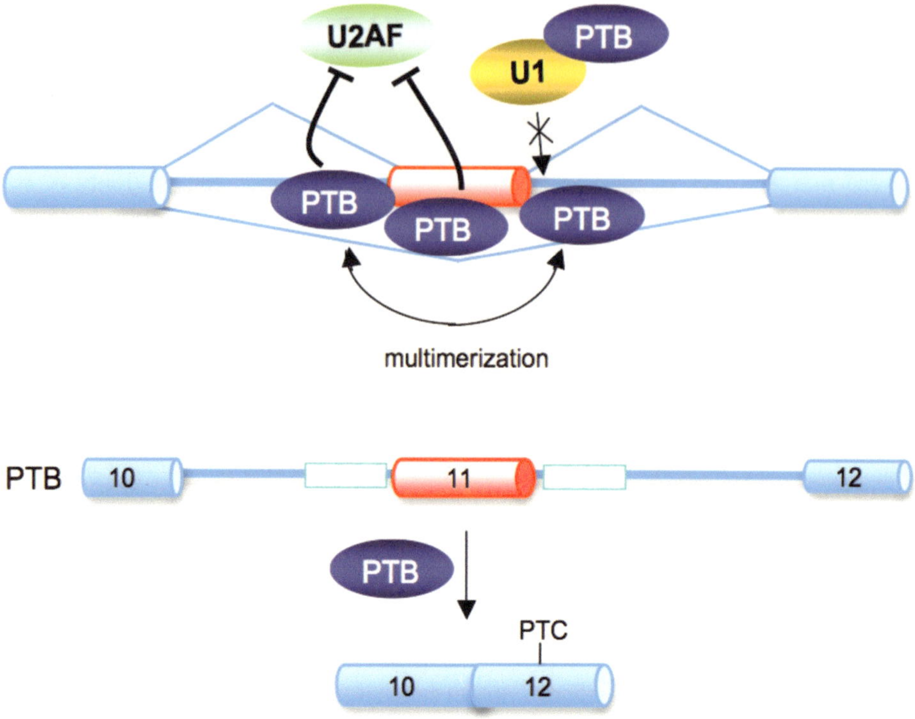

Fig. 2. **PTB-mediated splicing regulation and autoregulation.** Top diagram: PTB suppresses exon inclusion when bound to silencing elements located upstream or downstream of an alternative exon (red cylinder) or even within the exon. Blue cylinders represent constitutive exons. PTB may compete with U2AF for binding to the intron 3' end, prevent U1 snRNP recognition of the 5' splice site, or loop-out the regulated exon. However, PTB can promote exon inclusion when it binds downstream of an alternative exon or close to a strong constitutive splice site (not depicted). This model suggests a positional effect of PTB binding on splicing. (B) PTB activates exon 11 skipping in its own transcript via binding to phylogenetically conserved CU-rich sequences (green hatched boxes) surrounding exon 11, which fits well with the model shown in panel A. The resulting mRNA contains a premature termination codon (PTC) and is degraded by nonsense-mediated decay. Therefore, PTB downregulates the level of its own mRNA.

4. PTB and nPTB

4.1 PTB/nPTB proteins

PTB is a ubiquitously expressed RNA-binding protein containing four RNA recognition motifs with high affinity for CU-rich sequences (Xue, et al., 2009). nPTB is predominant in neurons although also present in other tissues and is remarkably similar to PTB in domain structure and RNA-binding specificity (Spellman, et al., 2007). Both PTB and nPTB primarily function as splicing regulators, and PTB can also regulate translation of specific mRNAs and internal ribosome entry site-mediated translation (Mitchell, et al., 2001; Sawicka, et al., 2008). PTB localizes primarily to the nucleus but can shuttle between the nucleus and cytoplasm

(Michael, et al., 1995). Protein kinase A-mediated phosphorylation of PTB can cause its accumulation in the cytoplasm, thereby promoting its cytoplasmic functions such as translation control and RNA transport (Ma, et al., 2007; Xie, et al., 2003).

4.2 Mechanisms of PTB/nPTB-controlled alternative spicing

Multiple mechanisms underlie PTB/nPTB-induced splicing regulation. In general, PTB and nPTB function as splicing inhibitors. Because CU-rich sequences frequently appear in the 3' end of most constitutive introns, binding of PTB to this region interferes with recognition of the 3' splice site by the essential splicing factor, U2AF, thus preventing spliceosome assembly (Sharma, et al., 2005). Moreover, CU-rich elements are also located in other discrete intronic regions surrounding alternative exons. PTB can loop out a regulated exon via binding to both its upstream and downstream intronic CU-rich sequences and forming homomultimers, which thus drives exon exclusion (Lamichhane, et al., 2010). Consistently, a recent genome-wide mapping of PTB-binding sites revealed a position effect for PTB-mediated splicing regulation (Sawicka, et al., 2008) (Figure 2). When PTB binds near an alternative exon, it generally induces exon skipping. However, PTB can also promote exon inclusion when it binds close to a strong constitutive splice site. Besides self-interaction, PTB can also interact with other splicing factors to form complexes that often compete with the splicing machinery, thereby interfering with splicing (Sharma, et al., 2011). A recent report showed that PTB can interact with a pyrimidine-rich loop of U1 snRNA and alter its recognition of the 5' splice site (Coutinho-Mansfield, et al., 2007). nPTB may use similar mechanisms as PTB to suppress exon inclusion. However, nPTB appears to be a weaker splicing suppressor compared with PTB, and nPTB may interact with additional transcripts that are implicated in neuronal activity (Spellman, et al., 2007). Thus, PTB and nPTB have distinct properties in regulating alternative splicing.

4.3 The PTB/nPTB switch during neuronal differentiation

Immunocytochemistry has shown that PTB is detected in neuronal precursor cells as well as non-neuronal lineages of the brain whereas nPTB is specifically expressed in post-mitotic neurons (Boutz, et al., 2007). Therefore, a switch in expression from PTB to nPTB likely occurs during neuronal differentiation. To date, two post-transcriptional mechanisms have been implicated in mutually exclusive expression of PTB and nPTB (Boutz, et al., 2007; Makeyev, et al., 2007). One mechanism involves alternative splicing-coupled nonsense-mediated decay, and the other involves microRNA-mediated translation control. Skipping of exon 11 of PTB and exon 10 of nPTB generates transcripts containing a premature termination codon that subsequently undergo nonsense-mediated decay. PTB is responsible for such exon suppression by binding to highly conserved CU-rich elements flanking the alternative PTB/nPTB exons (Figure 2). Through this activity, PTB may negatively autoregulate its own expression, perhaps to maintain appropriate levels of the protein and restrict the expression of nPTB in non-neuronal cells. In addition, the neuron-specific microRNA miR-124 can directly target to the PTB mRNA and suppresses its translation (Makeyev, et al., 2007). Therefore, PTB expression is down-regulated in neurons, which thus relieves nPTB suppression.

4.4 The PTB/nPTB switch reprograms specific splicing events

Although nPTB and PTB have overlapping function, their different spatial and timely expression patterns in neurons suggest that they have diverse physiological functions in splicing regulation. Indeed, a recent report showed that ~25% of neuron-specific alternative splicing events may result from a decrease of PTB and increase of nPTB during neuronal differentiation (Boutz, et al., 2007). The possible distinct target specificity of PTB and nPTB may be important for establishing unique and neuron-specific splicing programs during neuronal differentiation. Therefore, the PTB/nPTB switch may have evolved as a post-transcriptional mechanism to fine tune the existing program and alter the transcriptome to promote cell differentiation.

As described above, Nova-1 and Nova-2, although having highly similar sequences, contribute to neuron-specific splicing in different types of neurons (C. Zhang, et al., 2010). Given that Nova-1 can drive its own exon 4 skipping, the Nova-1/Nova-2 reciprocal expression may in part proceed through a negative feedback control mechanism similar to that used by PTB/nPTB (Coutinho-Mansfield, et al., 2007; Dredge, et al., 2005). Therefore, the switch between two highly similar but still distinct splicing factors may provide a potent and rapid means to adjust cellular function in a specific environment.

5. SMN

5.1 SMN genes and expression

Spinal muscular atrophy (SMA) is an autosomal recessive disorder characterized by degeneration of lower motor neurons in the spinal cord with subsequent muscle atrophy (Pearn, 1978). SMA is caused by deletions or mutations of the survival of motor neuron 1 (SMN1) gene (Lefebvre, et al., 1995). In human, the SMN2 gene is almost identical to SMN1 but contains a C to T transition at position 6 in exon 7. This nucleotide change induces SMN2 exon 7 skipping during splicing and results in an unstable truncated SMN protein (Cho & Dreyfuss, 2010). Therefore, SMN2 fails to produce a sufficient amount of functional SMN protein to compensate for the loss of SMN1 (Lorson, et al., 1999; Monani, et al., 1999). Multiple factors have been proposed to regulate exon 7 inclusion/exclusion of the SMN transcripts. In principle, SMN1 exon 7 harbors a splicing enhancer for the splicing activator SF2/ASF, which promotes exon 7 inclusion in the SMN1 transcript, whereas the C to U change in SMN2 pre-mRNA disrupts the binding of SF2/ASF but creates a recognition site for the suppressor hnRNP A1 that excludes exon 7 (Cartegni, et al., 2006; Cartegni & Krainer, 2002; Kashima & Manley, 2003; Kashima, et al., 2007). Besides, other SMN regulators may function via direct binding to exon 7 or even to intronic elements or through a protein complex to modulate exon 7 selection (Doktor, et al., 2011; Nlend Nlend, et al., 2010; Pedrotti & Sette, 2010). SMN splicing regulation has been reviewed elsewhere; this section thus focuses on SMN function in pre-mRNA splicing and regulation.

5.2 SMN and its cellular localization

SMN expression is not restricted to neurons, and in fact it is expressed in all cell types Unlike Nova and PTB, SMN lacks a typical RNA-binding domain but contains a Tudor domain that mediates its interaction with the Sm proteins of spliceosomal snRNPs. Indeed, SMN participates in snRNP biogenesis, which is an important housekeeping function, and also in splicing, transcription, and neuronal mRNA trafficking (Burghes & Beattie, 2009; Coady & Lorson, 2011) (Figure 3). In the nucleus, SMN is particularly concentrated in discrete nuclear bodies that are very close to Cajal bodies (Carvalho, et al., 1999; Young, et al., 2000). This nuclear localization pattern suggests a role for SMN in nuclear snRNP maturation and regeneration. In neurons, SMN forms cytoplasmic granules in neurites and growth cones and participates in active bidirectional transport of mRNAs (Fallini, et al., 2011; Todd, et al., 2010; H. Zhang, et al., 2006). SMN deficiency disrupts Cajal bodies and impairs mRNA trafficking in motor neuron axons (Girard, et al., 2006; Rossoll, et al., 2003; Shpargel & Matera, 2005), indicating that the diverse subcellular distribution of SMN is functionally important. Moreover, a recent observation that SMN associates and colocalizes with the α subunit of "coatomer", a protein coat for vesicles that mediate intracellular transport, indicates a role for Golgi-associated COPI vesicles in SMN transport (Peter, et al., 2011).

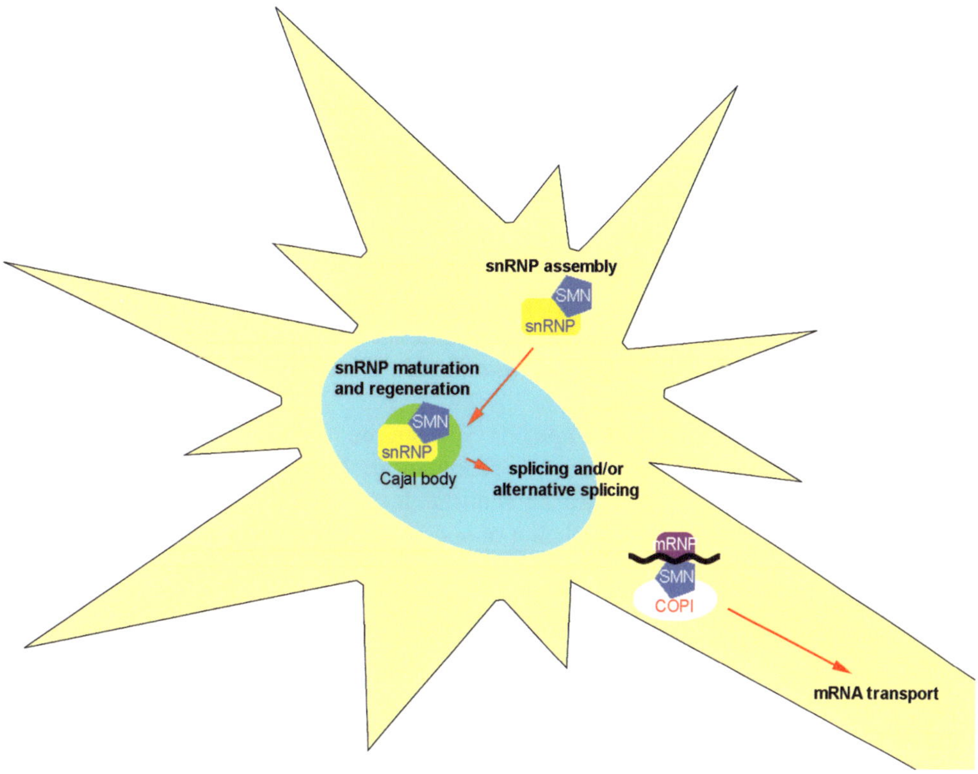

Fig. 3. **Functions of SMN in neurons.** In the cytoplasm, SMN forms a protein complex to facilitate snRNP biogenesis. Moreover, SMN along with other RNA-binding proteins participates in mRNA transport; the role of COPI-containing vesicles in SMN transport is unclear. In the nucleus, SMN is highly concentrated in Cajal bodies and possibly plays a role in snRNP maturation and multi-snRNP assembly. SMN deficiency may indirectly induce aberrant splicing.

5.3 SMN in snRNP biogenesis

The role of SMN in snRNP biogenesis has been well characterized. Assembly of the heptameric Sm cores with each spliceosomal snRNA occurs in a highly ordered manner (Burghes & Beattie, 2009; Cauchi, 2010; Coady & Lorson, 2011). Initially, the chaperon factor pICln brings methylated Sm protein subcomplexes to the SMN complex, which is composed of SMN, Gemin2-8, and unr-interacting proteins. The SMN complex facilitates the arrangement of the Sm proteins on a single-stranded region of snRNA to form a ring-shaped structure of the snRNP. An initial report showed that ~80% depletion of SMN by RNA interference in cultured mammalian cells had no significant loss-of-function effect on snRNP assembly (Girard, et al., 2006). Perhaps excess SMN complex exists in cells to maintain normal levels of the basal splicing machinery. However, further reduction of SMN differentially impaired snRNP assembly (Gabanella, et al., 2007; Workman, et al., 2009; Z. Zhang, et al., 2008). In particular, the levels of several U12-type spliceosomal snRNAs decreased more significantly in SMA mice, and formation of the U12-type tri-snRNPs was also impeded in lymphoblasts derived from SMA patients (Gabanella, et al., 2007; Workman, et al., 2009; Z. Zhang, et al., 2008). The latter observation is also in accordance with the assumption that SMN is possibly involved in tri-snRNP assembly in Cajal bodies (Carvalho, et al., 1999; Novotny, et al., 2011; Young, et al., 2000). Although direct evidence for defective snRNP assembly or reduced snRNP levels in SMA pathogenesis is lacking, one hint has been provided by the observation that knockdown of SMN or other snRNP assembly factors in zebrafish causes motor axon defects (Winkler, et al., 2005).

5.4 SMN in pre-mRNA splicing

It is clear that SMN has an essential function for snRNP biogenesis, and possibly that insufficient SMN causes various degrees of snRNP assembly defects. However, whether loss of SMN affects splicing of a wide range or a specific set of transcripts and whether the effect of SMN in splicing, if any, indeed results from impaired snRNP assembly have just begun to be investigated.

Exon array analysis has shown that splicing of numerous transcripts is affected in various tissues of late-symptomatic SMA mice (Z. Zhang, et al., 2008). It is unclear whether such a widespread splicing defect is caused by reduced levels of SMN. It is suspected that the decrease in SMN level may affect splicing of specific transcripts in motor neurons that are most vulnerable to degeneration in SMA (Briese, et al., 2005; Liu, et al., 2010; Monani, 2005). A recent report showed that the tri-snRNP of the U12-type splicing machinery is most affected in SMA patients and, consistently, the splicing of a subgroup of U12-type introns is affected (Boulisfane, et al., 2011). Because U12-type introns are present in a number of genes involved in cytoskeletal organization, defects in their excision may impair motor neuron function. Finally, the error rate of exon inclusion/skipping is higher in fibroblasts of SMA patients, perhaps owing to poor recognition of the splice sites by a low abundance of functional snRNPs (Fox-Walsh & Hertel, 2009).

5.5 How does SMN deficiency cause SMA pathogenesis

To date, two plausible possibilities have been raised to explain how SMN deficiency causes specific neurological defects of motor neurons. First, as discussed above, inefficient snRNP assembly may affect the splicing of a specific set of transcripts that are critical to motor neuron functions. However, issues such as which transcripts are most sensitive to SMN deficiency and whether their splicing defects lead to SMA pathogenesis remain to be investigated. In addition, it has been shown that SMN forms RNA granules with other RNA-binding proteins such as hnRNP R to deliver β-actin mRNA in motor axons (Glinka, et al., 2010; Rossoll, et al., 2003). A recent report showed that clustering of Cav2.2 calcium channels is impaired in axonal growth cones of SMA animals, and such a defect can be restored by rescue of SMN expression (Jablonka, et al., 2007). It is possible that SMN plays a role in actin filament formation via β-actin mRNA trafficking, and such an activity of SMN is critical for motor neuron functions.

SMA patients and animal models show a variable extent of defects in neuromuscular junction functions, axonal arborization, synaptic transport, and neurodevelopment. Such complexity may result from different residual levels of SMN in different systems as well as multiple cellular functions and interacting partners of SMN (Boyer, et al., 2010; Burghes & Beattie, 2009; Cauchi, 2010; Wu, et al., 2011). Nevertheless, restoration of SMN levels or function is certainly a primary therapeutic strategy for SMA treatment (Kolb & Kissel, 2011). For example, activation of SMN2 transcription and restoration of SMN2 splicing ameliorate symptoms of SMA mice and thus provide promise for future SMA treatment.

6. Conclusions

Our understanding of splicing regulation mechanisms and splicing regulatory networks has been advanced substantially by recent studies using gene inactivation techniques and genome-wide experimental and computational examination of alternative splicing events. In the past decade, CLIP in conjunction with various types of mRNA identification systems has been used extensively for *in vitro* study of splicing factors and their regulation mechanisms. Ablation of splicing factors in cultured cells by RNA interference has also been widely used for mechanistic studies of alternative splicing of endogenous or reporter minigene transcripts. Nevertheless, we are still at the beginning of our understanding of the mechanistic and, in particular, physiological aspects of alternative splicing regulation.

Our understanding of the physiological consequences of alternative splicing still largely relies on genetic approaches. For example, knockout of splicing factors in animals in combination of mRNA isoform comparison can facilitate the identification of their *in vivo* targets and biological functions. Study of disease-related splicing factors can in particular provide insights into pathogenesis of aberrant splicing. Moreover, knock-in or knockout of specific mRNA isoforms can help to unveil their functional consequence(s), which is poorly understood, and may even allow delineation of causal effects (Moroy & Heyd, 2007). However, progress has been relatively slow owing to limitations of genetic techniques in mammalian systems. At present, efficient recombination technologies are being developed to facilitate high-throughput gene knockout in embryonic stem cells (Valenzuela, et al., 2003), which may allow large-scale analysis of biological functions of splicing factors as well as mRNA isoforms. Besides more efficient/convenient genetic tools, high-throughput whole-transcriptome sequencing and extensive bioinformatics tools have proved their advantage. With these techniques, we will begin to establish a more accurate paradigm for mRNA splicing regulatory networks with physiological significance.

7. Acknowledgements

We acknowledge support from intramural funds of the Institute of Biomedical Sciences, Academia Sinica, and the Academia Sinica Investigator Award to W.-Y. Tarn.

8. References

Allen, S. E.; Darnell, R. B. & Lipscombe, D. (2010). The neuronal splicing factor Nova controls alternative splicing in N-type and P-type CaV2 calcium channels. *Channels (Austin)*, Vol.4, No.6, (Nov-Dec, 2010), pp. 483-489

Ares, M., Jr. (2007). Sing the genome electric: excited cells adjust their splicing. *PLoS Biol*, Vol.5, No.2, (Feb, 2007), pp. e55

Boulisfane, N.; Choleza, M.; Rage, F.; Neel, H.; Soret, J. & Bordonne, R. (2011). Impaired minor tri-snRNP assembly generates differential splicing defects of U12-type introns in lymphoblasts derived from a type I SMA patient. *Hum Mol Genet*, Vol.20, No.4, (Feb 15, 2011), pp. 641-648

Boutz, P. L.; Stoilov, P.; Li, Q.; Lin, C. H.; Chawla, G.; Ostrow, K.; Shiue, L.; Ares, M., Jr. & Black, D. L. (2007). A post-transcriptional regulatory switch in polypyrimidine tract-binding proteins reprograms alternative splicing in developing neurons. *Genes Dev*, Vol.21, No.13, (Jul 1, 2007), pp. 1636-1652

Boyer, J. G.; Bowerman, M. & Kothary, R. (2010). The many faces of SMN: deciphering the function critical to spinal muscular atrophy pathogesis. *Future Neurol*, Vol.5, No.6, 2010), pp. 873-890

Briese, M.; Esmaeili, B. & Sattelle, D. B. (2005). Is spinal muscular atrophy the result of defects in motor neuron processes? *Bioessays*, Vol.27, No.9, (Sep, 2005), pp. 946-957

Brooks, A. N.; Yang, L.; Duff, M. O.; Hansen, K. D.; Park, J. W.; Dudoit, S.; Brenner, S. E. & Graveley, B. R. (2011). Conservation of an RNA regulatory map between Drosophila and mammals. *Genome Res*, Vol.21, No.2, (Feb, 2011), pp. 193-202

Buckanovich, R. J. & Darnell, R. B. (1997). The neuronal RNA binding protein Nova-1 recognizes specific RNA targets in vitro and in vivo. *Mol Cell Biol*, Vol.17, No.6, (Jun, 1997), pp. 3194-3201

Buckanovich, R. J.; Posner, J. B. & Darnell, R. B. (1993). Nova, the paraneoplastic Ri antigen, is homologous to an RNA-binding protein and is specifically expressed in the developing motor system. *Neuron*, Vol.11, No.4, (Oct, 1993), pp. 657-672

Buckanovich, R. J.; Yang, Y. Y. & Darnell, R. B. (1996). The onconeural antigen Nova-1 is a neuron-specific RNA-binding protein, the activity of which is inhibited by paraneoplastic antibodies. *J Neurosci*, Vol.16, No.3, (Feb 1, 1996), pp. 1114-1122

Burghes, A. H. & Beattie, C. E. (2009). Spinal muscular atrophy: why do low levels of survival motor neuron protein make motor neurons sick? *Nat Rev Neurosci*, Vol.10, No.8, (Aug, 2009), pp. 597-609

Calarco, J. A.; Superina, S.; O'Hanlon, D.; Gabut, M.; Raj, B.; Pan, Q.; Skalska, U.; Clarke, L.; Gelinas, D.; van der Kooy, D.; Zhen, M.; Ciruna, B. & Blencowe, B. J. (2009). Regulation of vertebrate nervous system alternative splicing and development by an SR-related protein. *Cell*, Vol.138, No.5, (Sep 4, 2009), pp. 898-910

Calarco, J. A.; Zhen, M. & Blencowe, B. J. (2011). Networking in a global world: Establishing functional connections between neural splicing regulators and their target transcripts. *RNA*, Vol.17, No.5, (May, 2011), pp. 775-791

Cartegni, L.; Hastings, M. L.; Calarco, J. A.; de Stanchina, E. & Krainer, A. R. (2006). Determinants of exon 7 splicing in the spinal muscular atrophy genes, SMN1 and SMN2. *Am J Hum Genet*, Vol.78, No.1, (Jan, 2006), pp. 63-77

Cartegni, L. & Krainer, A. R. (2002). Disruption of an SF2/ASF-dependent exonic splicing enhancer in SMN2 causes spinal muscular atrophy in the absence of SMN1. *Nat Genet*, Vol.30, No.4, (Apr, 2002), pp. 377-384

Carvalho, T.; Almeida, F.; Calapez, A.; Lafarga, M.; Berciano, M. T. & Carmo-Fonseca, M. (1999). The spinal muscular atrophy disease gene product, SMN: A link between snRNP biogenesis and the Cajal (coiled) body. *J Cell Biol*, Vol.147, No.4, (Nov 15, 1999), pp. 715-728

Cauchi, R. J. (2010). SMN and Gemins: 'we are family' ... or are we?: insights into the partnership between Gemins and the spinal muscular atrophy disease protein SMN. *Bioessays*, Vol.32, No.12, (Dec, 2010), pp. 1077-1089

Chen, M. & Manley, J. L. (2009). Mechanisms of alternative splicing regulation: insights from molecular and genomics approaches. *Nat Rev Mol Cell Biol*, Vol.10, No.11, (Nov, 2009), pp. 741-754

Chmiel, N. H.; Rio, D. C. & Doudna, J. A. (2006). Distinct contributions of KH domains to substrate binding affinity of Drosophila P-element somatic inhibitor protein. *RNA*, Vol.12, No.2, (Feb, 2006), pp. 283-291

Cho, S. & Dreyfuss, G. (2010). A degron created by SMN2 exon 7 skipping is a principal contributor to spinal muscular atrophy severity. *Genes Dev*, Vol.24, No.5, (Mar 1, 2010), pp. 438-442

Coady, T. H. & Lorson, C. L. (2011). SMN in spinal muscular atrophy and snRNP biogenesis. *Wiley Interdisciplinary Reviews: RNA*, 2011), pp. n/a-n/a

Coutinho-Mansfield, G. C.; Xue, Y.; Zhang, Y. & Fu, X. D. (2007). PTB/nPTB switch: a post-transcriptional mechanism for programming neuronal differentiation. *Genes Dev*, Vol.21, No.13, (Jul 1, 2007), pp. 1573-1577

Darnell, R. B. (2010). HITS-CLIP: panoramic views of protein-RNA regulation in living cells. *WIREs RNA*, Vol.1, 2010), pp. 266-286

Darnell, R. B. (2011). RNA regulation in Neurodegeneration and Cancer, In: *Two Faces of Evil: Cancer and Neurodegeneration*, Curran, T. & Christen, Y., pp. 103-111, Springer Berlin Heidelberg, 978-3-642-16602-0,

Darnell, R. B. & Posner, J. B. (2003). Paraneoplastic syndromes involving the nervous system. *N Engl J Med*, Vol.349, No.16, (Oct 16, 2003), pp. 1543-1554

Doktor, T. K.; Schroeder, L. D.; Vested, A.; Palmfeldt, J.; Andersen, H. S.; Gregersen, N. & Andresen, B. S. (2011). SMN2 exon 7 splicing is inhibited by binding of hnRNP A1 to a common ESS motif that spans the 3' splice site. *Hum Mutat*, Vol.32, No.2, (Feb, 2011), pp. 220-230

Dredge, B. K. & Darnell, R. B. (2003). Nova regulates GABA(A) receptor gamma2 alternative splicing via a distal downstream UCAU-rich intronic splicing enhancer. *Mol Cell Biol*, Vol.23, No.13, (Jul, 2003), pp. 4687-4700

Dredge, B. K.; Stefani, G.; Engelhard, C. C. & Darnell, R. B. (2005). Nova autoregulation reveals dual functions in neuronal splicing. *EMBO J*, Vol.24, No.8, (Apr 20, 2005), pp. 1608-1620

Fallini, C.; Zhang, H.; Su, Y.; Silani, V.; Singer, R. H.; Rossoll, W. & Bassell, G. J. (2011). The Survival of Motor Neuron (SMN) Protein Interacts with the mRNA-Binding Protein HuD and Regulates Localization of Poly(A) mRNA in Primary Motor Neuron Axons. *J Neurosci*, Vol.31, No.10, (Mar 9, 2011), pp. 3914-3925

Fox-Walsh, K. L. & Hertel, K. J. (2009). Splice-site pairing is an intrinsically high fidelity process. *Proc Natl Acad Sci U S A*, Vol.106, No.6, (Feb 10, 2009), pp. 1766-1771

Frotscher, M. (2010). Role for Reelin in stabilizing cortical architecture. *Trends Neurosci*, Vol.33, No.9, (Sep, 2010), pp. 407-414

Gabanella, F.; Butchbach, M. E.; Saieva, L.; Carissimi, C.; Burghes, A. H. & Pellizzoni, L. (2007). Ribonucleoprotein assembly defects correlate with spinal muscular atrophy severity and preferentially affect a subset of spliceosomal snRNPs. *PLoS One*, Vol.2, No.9, 2007), pp. e921

Girard, C.; Neel, H.; Bertrand, E. & Bordonne, R. (2006). Depletion of SMN by RNA interference in HeLa cells induces defects in Cajal body formation. *Nucleic Acids Res*, Vol.34, No.10, 2006), pp. 2925-2932

Glinka, M.; Herrmann, T.; Funk, N.; Havlicek, S.; Rossoll, W.; Winkler, C. & Sendtner, M. (2010). The heterogeneous nuclear ribonucleoprotein-R is necessary for axonal beta-actin mRNA translocation in spinal motor neurons. *Hum Mol Genet*, Vol.19, No.10, (May 15, 2010), pp. 1951-1966

Grabowski, P. (2011). Alternative splicing takes shape during neuronal development. *Curr Opin Genet Dev*, (Apr 19, 2011), pp.

Hattori, D.; Millard, S. S.; Wojtowicz, W. M. & Zipursky, S. L. (2008). Dscam-mediated cell recognition regulates neural circuit formation. *Annu Rev Cell Dev Biol*, Vol.24, 2008), pp. 597-620

Huang, C. S.; Shi, S. H.; Ule, J.; Ruggiu, M.; Barker, L. A.; Darnell, R. B.; Jan, Y. N. & Jan, L. Y. (2005). Common molecular pathways mediate long-term potentiation of synaptic excitation and slow synaptic inhibition. *Cell*, Vol.123, No.1, (Oct 7, 2005), pp. 105-118

Irimia, M.; Denuc, A.; Burguera, D.; Somorjai, I.; Martin-Duran, J. M.; Genikhovich, G.; Jimenez-Delgado, S.; Technau, U.; Roy, S. W.; Marfany, G. & Garcia-Fernandez, J. (2011). Stepwise assembly of the Nova-regulated alternative splicing network in the vertebrate brain. *Proc Natl Acad Sci U S A*, Vol.108, No.13, (Mar 29, 2011), pp. 5319-5324

Isken, O. & Maquat, L. E. (2007). Quality control of eukaryotic mRNA: safeguarding cells from abnormal mRNA function. *Genes Dev*, Vol.21, No.15, (Aug 1, 2007), pp. 1833-1856

Jablonka, S.; Beck, M.; Lechner, B. D.; Mayer, C. & Sendtner, M. (2007). Defective Ca2+ channel clustering in axon terminals disturbs excitability in motoneurons in spinal muscular atrophy. *J Cell Biol*, Vol.179, No.1, (Oct 8, 2007), pp. 139-149

Jelen, N.; Ule, J. & Zivin, M. (2010). Cholinergic regulation of striatal Nova mRNAs. *Neuroscience*, Vol.169, No.2, (Aug 25, 2010), pp. 619-627

Jelen, N.; Ule, J.; Zivin, M. & Darnell, R. B. (2007). Evolution of Nova-dependent splicing regulation in the brain. *PLoS Genet*, Vol.3, No.10, (Oct, 2007), pp. 1838-1847

Jensen, K. B.; Dredge, B. K.; Stefani, G.; Zhong, R.; Buckanovich, R. J.; Okano, H. J.; Yang, Y. Y. & Darnell, R. B. (2000). Nova-1 regulates neuron-specific alternative splicing and is essential for neuronal viability. *Neuron*, Vol.25, No.2, (Feb, 2000), pp. 359-371

Kashima, T. & Manley, J. L. (2003). A negative element in SMN2 exon 7 inhibits splicing in spinal muscular atrophy. *Nat Genet*, Vol.34, No.4, (Aug, 2003), pp. 460-463

Kashima, T.; Rao, N.; David, C. J. & Manley, J. L. (2007). hnRNP A1 functions with specificity in repression of SMN2 exon 7 splicing. *Hum Mol Genet*, Vol.16, No.24, (Dec 15, 2007), pp. 3149-3159

Keren, H.; Lev-Maor, G. & Ast, G. (2010). Alternative splicing and evolution: diversification, exon definition and function. *Nat Rev Genet*, Vol.11, No.5, (May, 2010), pp. 345-355

Khabar, K. S. (2010). Post-transcriptional control during chronic inflammation and cancer: a focus on AU-rich elements. *Cell Mol Life Sci*, Vol.67, No.17, (Sep, 2010), pp. 2937-2955

Kolb, S. J. & Kissel, J. T. (2011). Spinal Muscular Atrophy: A Timely Review. *Arch Neurol*, (Apr 11, 2011), pp.

Konig, J.; Zarnack, K.; Rot, G.; Curk, T.; Kayikci, M.; Zupan, B.; Turner, D. J.; Luscombe, N. M. & Ule, J. (2010). iCLIP reveals the function of hnRNP particles in splicing at individual nucleotide resolution. *Nat Struct Mol Biol*, Vol.17, No.7, (Jul, 2010), pp. 909-915

Lamichhane, R.; Daubner, G. M.; Thomas-Crusells, J.; Auweter, S. D.; Manatschal, C.; Austin, K. S.; Valniuk, O.; Allain, F. H. & Rueda, D. (2010). RNA looping by PTB: Evidence using FRET and NMR spectroscopy for a role in splicing repression. *Proc Natl Acad Sci U S A*, Vol.107, No.9, (Mar 2, 2010), pp. 4105-4110

Lee, J. A.; Tang, Z. Z. & Black, D. L. (2009). An inducible change in Fox-1/A2BP1 splicing modulates the alternative splicing of downstream neuronal target exons. *Genes Dev*, Vol.23, No.19, (Oct 1, 2009), pp. 2284-2293

Lefebvre, S.; Burglen, L.; Reboullet, S.; Clermont, O.; Burlet, P.; Viollet, L.; Benichou, B.; Cruaud, C.; Millasseau, P.; Zeviani, M. & et al. (1995). Identification and characterization of a spinal muscular atrophy-determining gene. *Cell*, Vol.80, No.1, (Jan 13, 1995), pp. 155-165

Lewis, H. A.; Musunuru, K.; Jensen, K. B.; Edo, C.; Chen, H.; Darnell, R. B. & Burley, S. K. (2000). Sequence-specific RNA binding by a Nova KH domain: implications for paraneoplastic disease and the fragile X syndrome. *Cell*, Vol.100, No.3, (Feb 4, 2000), pp. 323-332

Li, Q.; Lee, J. A. & Black, D. L. (2007). Neuronal regulation of alternative pre-mRNA splicing. *Nat Rev Neurosci*, Vol.8, No.11, (Nov, 2007), pp. 819-831

Licatalosi, D. D. & Darnell, R. B. (2010). RNA processing and its regulation: global insights into biological networks. *Nat Rev Genet*, Vol.11, No.1, (Jan, 2010), pp. 75-87

Licatalosi, D. D.; Mele, A.; Fak, J. J.; Ule, J.; Kayikci, M.; Chi, S. W.; Clark, T. A.; Schweitzer, A. C.; Blume, J. E.; Wang, X.; Darnell, J. C. & Darnell, R. B. (2008). HITS-CLIP yields genome-wide insights into brain alternative RNA processing. *Nature*, Vol.456, No.7221, (Nov 27, 2008), pp. 464-469

Liu, H.; Shafey, D.; Moores, J. N. & Kothary, R. (2010). Neurodevelopmental consequences of Smn depletion in a mouse model of spinal muscular atrophy. *J Neurosci Res*, Vol.88, No.1, (Jan, 2010), pp. 111-122

Lorson, C. L.; Hahnen, E.; Androphy, E. J. & Wirth, B. (1999). A single nucleotide in the SMN gene regulates splicing and is responsible for spinal muscular atrophy. *Proc Natl Acad Sci U S A*, Vol.96, No.11, (May 25, 1999), pp. 6307-6311

Lorson, C. L.; Rindt, H. & Shababi, M. (2010). Spinal muscular atrophy: mechanisms and therapeutic strategies. *Hum Mol Genet*, Vol.19, No.R1, (Apr 15, 2010), pp. R111-118

Lukong, K. E.; Chang, K. W.; Khandjian, E. W. & Richard, S. (2008). RNA-binding proteins in human genetic disease. *Trends Genet*, Vol.24, No.8, (Aug, 2008), pp. 416-425

Ma, S.; Liu, G.; Sun, Y. & Xie, J. (2007). Relocalization of the polypyrimidine tract-binding protein during PKA-induced neurite growth. *Biochim Biophys Acta*, Vol.1773, No.6, (Jun, 2007), pp. 912-923

Makeyev, E. V.; Zhang, J.; Carrasco, M. A. & Maniatis, T. (2007). The MicroRNA miR-124 promotes neuronal differentiation by triggering brain-specific alternative pre-mRNA splicing. *Mol Cell*, Vol.27, No.3, (Aug 3, 2007), pp. 435-448

Martin, C. L.; Duvall, J. A.; Ilkin, Y.; Simon, J. S.; Arreaza, M. G.; Wilkes, K.; Alvarez-Retuerto, A.; Whichello, A.; Powell, C. M.; Rao, K.; Cook, E. & Geschwind, D. H. (2007). Cytogenetic and molecular characterization of A2BP1/FOX1 as a candidate gene for autism. *Am J Med Genet B Neuropsychiatr Genet*, Vol.144B, No.7, (Oct 5, 2007), pp. 869-876

McGlincy, N. J. & Smith, C. W. (2008). Alternative splicing resulting in nonsense-mediated mRNA decay: what is the meaning of nonsense? *Trends Biochem Sci*, Vol.33, No.8, (Aug, 2008), pp. 385-393

Michael, W. M.; Siomi, H.; Choi, M.; Pinol-Roma, S.; Nakielny, S.; Liu, Q. & Dreyfuss, G. (1995). Signal sequences that target nuclear import and nuclear export of pre-mRNA-binding proteins. *Cold Spring Harb Symp Quant Biol*, Vol.60, 1995), pp. 663-668

Mitchell, S. A.; Brown, E. C.; Coldwell, M. J.; Jackson, R. J. & Willis, A. E. (2001). Protein factor requirements of the Apaf-1 internal ribosome entry segment: roles of polypyrimidine tract binding protein and upstream of N-ras. *Mol Cell Biol*, Vol.21, No.10, (May, 2001), pp. 3364-3374

Monani, U. R. (2005). Spinal muscular atrophy: a deficiency in a ubiquitous protein; a motor neuron-specific disease. *Neuron*, Vol.48, No.6, (Dec 22, 2005), pp. 885-896

Monani, U. R.; Lorson, C. L.; Parsons, D. W.; Prior, T. W.; Androphy, E. J.; Burghes, A. H. & McPherson, J. D. (1999). A single nucleotide difference that alters splicing patterns distinguishes the SMA gene SMN1 from the copy gene SMN2. *Hum Mol Genet*, Vol.8, No.7, (Jul, 1999), pp. 1177-1183

Moore, M. J. & Proudfoot, N. J. (2009). Pre-mRNA processing reaches back to transcription and ahead to translation. *Cell*, Vol.136, No.4, (Feb 20, 2009), pp. 688-700

Moroy, T. & Heyd, F. (2007). The impact of alternative splicing in vivo: mouse models show the way. *RNA*, Vol.13, No.8, (Aug, 2007), pp. 1155-1171

Musunuru, K. & Darnell, R. B. (2004). Determination and augmentation of RNA sequence specificity of the Nova K-homology domains. *Nucleic Acids Res*, Vol.32, No.16, 2004), pp. 4852-4861

Nilsen, T. W. & Graveley, B. R. (2010). Expansion of the eukaryotic proteome by alternative splicing. *Nature*, Vol.463, No.7280, (Jan 28, 2010), pp. 457-463

Nlend Nlend, R.; Meyer, K. & Schumperli, D. (2010). Repair of pre-mRNA splicing: prospects for a therapy for spinal muscular atrophy. *RNA Biol*, Vol.7, No.4, (Nov 19, 2010), pp. 430-440

Novotny, I.; Blazikova, M.; Stanek, D.; Herman, P. & Malinsky, J. (2011). In vivo kinetics of U4/U6.U5 tri-snRNP formation in Cajal bodies. *Mol Biol Cell*, Vol.22, No.4, (Feb 15, 2011), pp. 513-523

Pan, Q.; Shai, O.; Lee, L. J.; Frey, B. J. & Blencowe, B. J. (2008). Deep surveying of alternative splicing complexity in the human transcriptome by high-throughput sequencing. *Nat Genet*, Vol.40, No.12, (Dec, 2008), pp. 1413-1415

Pardo, C. A. & Eberhart, C. G. (2007). The neurobiology of autism. *Brain Pathol*, Vol.17, No.4, (Oct, 2007), pp. 434-447

Park, E.; Lee, M. S.; Baik, S. M.; Cho, E. B.; Son, G. H.; Seong, J. Y.; Lee, K. H. & Kim, K. (2009). Nova-1 mediates glucocorticoid-induced inhibition of pre-mRNA splicing of gonadotropin-releasing hormone transcripts. *J Biol Chem*, Vol.284, No.19, (May 8, 2009), pp. 12792-12800

Park, G. H.; Kariya, S. & Monani, U. R. (2010). Spinal muscular atrophy: new and emerging insights from model mice. *Curr Neurol Neurosci Rep*, Vol.10, No.2, (Mar, 2010), pp. 108-117

Park, J. W. & Graveley, B. R. (2007). Complex alternative splicing. *Adv Exp Med Biol*, Vol.623, 2007), pp. 50-63

Pearn, J. (1978). Incidence, prevalence, and gene frequency studies of chronic childhood spinal muscular atrophy. *J Med Genet*, Vol.15, No.6, (Dec, 1978), pp. 409-413

Pedrotti, S. & Sette, C. (2010). Spinal muscular atrophy: a new player joins the battle for SMN2 exon 7 splicing. *Cell Cycle*, Vol.9, No.19, (Oct 1, 2010), pp. 3874-3879

Peter, C. J.; Evans, M.; Thayanithy, V.; Taniguchi-Ishigaki, N.; Bach, I.; Kolpak, A.; Bassell, G. J.; Rossoll, W.; Lorson, C. L.; Bao, Z. Z. & Androphy, E. J. (2011). The COPI vesicle complex binds and moves with survival motor neuron within axons. *Hum Mol Genet*, Vol.20, No.9, (May 1, 2011), pp. 1701-1711

Polydorides, A. D.; Okano, H. J.; Yang, Y. Y.; Stefani, G. & Darnell, R. B. (2000). A brain-enriched polypyrimidine tract-binding protein antagonizes the ability of Nova to regulate neuron-specific alternative splicing. *Proc Natl Acad Sci U S A*, Vol.97, No.12, (Jun 6, 2000), pp. 6350-6355

Racca, C.; Gardiol, A.; Eom, T.; Ule, J.; Triller, A. & Darnell, R. B. (2010). The Neuronal Splicing Factor Nova Co-Localizes with Target RNAs in the Dendrite. *Front Neural Circuits*, Vol.4, 2010), pp. 5

Ratti, A.; Fallini, C.; Colombrita, C.; Pascale, A.; Laforenza, U.; Quattrone, A. & Silani, V. (2008). Post-transcriptional regulation of neuro-oncological ventral antigen 1 by the neuronal RNA-binding proteins ELAV. *J Biol Chem*, Vol.283, No.12, (Mar 21, 2008), pp. 7531-7541

Rossi, D.; Amadio, M.; Carnevale Baraglia, A.; Azzolina, O.; Ratti, A.; Govoni, S.; Pascale, A. & Collina, S. (2009). Discovery of small peptides derived from embryonic lethal abnormal vision proteins structure showing RNA-stabilizing properties. *J Med Chem*, Vol.52, No.16, (Aug 27, 2009), pp. 5017-5019

Rossoll, W.; Jablonka, S.; Andreassi, C.; Kroning, A. K.; Karle, K.; Monani, U. R. & Sendtner, M. (2003). Smn, the spinal muscular atrophy-determining gene product, modulates axon growth and localization of beta-actin mRNA in growth cones of motoneurons. *J Cell Biol*, Vol.163, No.4, (Nov 24, 2003), pp. 801-812

Ruggiu, M.; Herbst, R.; Kim, N.; Jevsek, M.; Fak, J. J.; Mann, M. A.; Fischbach, G.; Burden, S. J. & Darnell, R. B. (2009). Rescuing Z+ agrin splicing in Nova null mice restores synapse formation and unmasks a physiologic defect in motor neuron firing. *Proc Natl Acad Sci U S A*, Vol.106, No.9, (Mar 3, 2009), pp. 3513-3518

Saltzman, A. L.; Pan, Q. & Blencowe, B. J. (2011). Regulation of alternative splicing by the core spliceosomal machinery. *Genes Dev*, Vol.25, No.4, (Feb 15, 2011), pp. 373-384

Sawicka, K.; Bushell, M.; Spriggs, K. A. & Willis, A. E. (2008). Polypyrimidine-tract-binding protein: a multifunctional RNA-binding protein. *Biochem Soc Trans*, Vol.36, No.Pt 4, (Aug, 2008), pp. 641-647

Seshaiah, P.; Miller, B.; Myat, M. M. & Andrew, D. J. (2001). pasilla, the Drosophila homologue of the human Nova-1 and Nova-2 proteins, is required for normal secretion in the salivary gland. *Dev Biol*, Vol.239, No.2, (Nov 15, 2001), pp. 309-322

Sharma, S.; Falick, A. M. & Black, D. L. (2005). Polypyrimidine tract binding protein blocks the 5' splice site-dependent assembly of U2AF and the prespliceosomal E complex. *Mol Cell*, Vol.19, No.4, (Aug 19, 2005), pp. 485-496

Sharma, S.; Maris, C.; Allain, F. H. & Black, D. L. (2011). U1 snRNA directly interacts with polypyrimidine tract-binding protein during splicing repression. *Mol Cell*, Vol.41, No.5, (Mar 4, 2011), pp. 579-588

Shpargel, K. B. & Matera, A. G. (2005). Gemin proteins are required for efficient assembly of Sm-class ribonucleoproteins. *Proc Natl Acad Sci U S A*, Vol.102, No.48, (Nov 29, 2005), pp. 17372-17377

Smith, R. M. & Sadee, W. (2011). Synaptic signaling and aberrant RNA splicing in autism spectrum disorders. *Front Synaptic Neurosci*, Vol.3, 2011), pp. 1

Spellman, R.; Llorian, M. & Smith, C. W. (2007). Crossregulation and functional redundancy between the splicing regulator PTB and its paralogs nPTB and ROD1. *Mol Cell*, Vol.27, No.3, (Aug 3, 2007), pp. 420-434

Tang, Z. Z.; Sharma, S.; Zheng, S.; Chawla, G.; Nikolic, J. & Black, D. L. (2011). Regulation of the Mutually Exclusive Exons 8a and 8 in the CaV1.2 Calcium Channel Transcript by Polypyrimidine Tract-binding Protein. *J Biol Chem*, Vol.286, No.12, (Mar 25, 2011), pp. 10007-10016

Thiele, A.; Nagamine, Y.; Hauschildt, S. & Clevers, H. (2006). AU-rich elements and alternative splicing in the beta-catenin 3'UTR can influence the human beta-catenin mRNA stability. *Exp Cell Res*, Vol.312, No.12, (Jul 15, 2006), pp. 2367-2378

Todd, A. G.; Morse, R.; Shaw, D. J.; McGinley, S.; Stebbings, H. & Young, P. J. (2010). SMN, Gemin2 and Gemin3 associate with beta-actin mRNA in the cytoplasm of neuronal cells in vitro. *J Mol Biol*, Vol.401, No.5, (Sep 3, 2010), pp. 681-689

Ule, J.; Jensen, K.; Mele, A. & Darnell, R. B. (2005a). CLIP: a method for identifying protein-RNA interaction sites in living cells. *Methods*, Vol.37, No.4, (Dec, 2005a), pp. 376-386

Ule, J.; Jensen, K. B.; Ruggiu, M.; Mele, A.; Ule, A. & Darnell, R. B. (2003). CLIP identifies Nova-regulated RNA networks in the brain. *Science*, Vol.302, No.5648, (Nov 14, 2003), pp. 1212-1215

Ule, J.; Stefani, G.; Mele, A.; Ruggiu, M.; Wang, X.; Taneri, B.; Gaasterland, T.; Blencowe, B. J. & Darnell, R. B. (2006). An RNA map predicting Nova-dependent splicing regulation. *Nature*, Vol.444, No.7119, (Nov 30, 2006), pp. 580-586

Ule, J.; Ule, A.; Spencer, J.; Williams, A.; Hu, J. S.; Cline, M.; Wang, H.; Clark, T.; Fraser, C.; Ruggiu, M.; Zeeberg, B. R.; Kane, D.; Weinstein, J. N.; Blume, J. & Darnell, R. B. (2005b). Nova regulates brain-specific splicing to shape the synapse. *Nat Genet*, Vol.37, No.8, (Aug, 2005b), pp. 844-852

Valenzuela, D. M.; Murphy, A. J.; Frendewey, D.; Gale, N. W.; Economides, A. N.; Auerbach, W.; Poueymirou, W. T.; Adams, N. C.; Rojas, J.; Yasenchak, J.; Chernomorsky, R.; Boucher, M.; Elsasser, A. L.; Esau, L.; Zheng, J.; Griffiths, J. A.; Wang, X.; Su, H.; Xue, Y.; Dominguez, M. G.; Noguera, I.; Torres, R.; Macdonald, L. E.; Stewart, A. F.; DeChiara, T. M. & Yancopoulos, G. D. (2003). High-throughput engineering of the mouse genome coupled with high-resolution expression analysis. *Nat Biotechnol*, Vol.21, No.6, (Jun, 2003), pp. 652-659

Valverde, R.; Edwards, L. & Regan, L. (2008). Structure and function of KH domains. *FEBS J*, Vol.275, No.11, (Jun, 2008), pp. 2712-2726

Wang, E. T.; Sandberg, R.; Luo, S.; Khrebtukova, I.; Zhang, L.; Mayr, C.; Kingsmore, S. F.; Schroth, G. P. & Burge, C. B. (2008). Alternative isoform regulation in human tissue transcriptomes. *Nature*, Vol.456, No.7221, (Nov 27, 2008), pp. 470-476

Wang, Z. & Burge, C. B. (2008). Splicing regulation: from a parts list of regulatory elements to an integrated splicing code. *RNA*, Vol.14, No.5, (May, 2008), pp. 802-813

Winkler, C.; Eggert, C.; Gradl, D.; Meister, G.; Giegerich, M.; Wedlich, D.; Laggerbauer, B. & Fischer, U. (2005). Reduced U snRNP assembly causes motor axon degeneration in an animal model for spinal muscular atrophy. *Genes Dev*, Vol.19, No.19, (Oct 1, 2005), pp. 2320-2330

Witten, J. T. & Ule, J. (2011). Understanding splicing regulation through RNA splicing maps. *Trends Genet*, Vol.27, No.3, (Mar, 2011), pp. 89-97

Workman, E.; Saieva, L.; Carrel, T. L.; Crawford, T. O.; Liu, D.; Lutz, C.; Beattie, C. E.; Pellizzoni, L. & Burghes, A. H. (2009). A SMN missense mutation complements SMN2 restoring snRNPs and rescuing SMA mice. *Hum Mol Genet*, Vol.18, No.12, (Jun 15, 2009), pp. 2215-2229

Wu, C. Y.; Whye, D.; Glazewski, L.; Choe, L.; Kerr, D.; Lee, K. H.; Mason, R. W. & Wang, W. (2011). Proteomic assessment of a cell model of spinal muscular atrophy. *BMC Neurosci*, Vol.12, 2011), pp. 25

Xie, J.; Lee, J. A.; Kress, T. L.; Mowry, K. L. & Black, D. L. (2003). Protein kinase A phosphorylation modulates transport of the polypyrimidine tract-binding protein. *Proc Natl Acad Sci U S A*, Vol.100, No.15, (Jul 22, 2003), pp. 8776-8781

Xue, Y.; Zhou, Y.; Wu, T.; Zhu, T.; Ji, X.; Kwon, Y. S.; Zhang, C.; Yeo, G.; Black, D. L.; Sun, H.; Fu, X. D. & Zhang, Y. (2009). Genome-wide analysis of PTB-RNA interactions reveals a strategy used by the general splicing repressor to modulate exon inclusion or skipping. *Mol Cell*, Vol.36, No.6, (Dec 25, 2009), pp. 996-1006

Yang, Y. Y.; Yin, G. L. & Darnell, R. B. (1998). The neuronal RNA-binding protein Nova-2 is implicated as the autoantigen targeted in POMA patients with dementia. *Proc Natl Acad Sci U S A*, Vol.95, No.22, (Oct 27, 1998), pp. 13254-13259

Yano, M.; Hayakawa-Yano, Y.; Mele, A. & Darnell, R. B. (2010). Nova2 regulates neuronal migration through an RNA switch in disabled-1 signaling. *Neuron*, Vol.66, No.6, (Jun 24, 2010), pp. 848-858

Yeo, G. W.; Coufal, N. G.; Liang, T. Y.; Peng, G. E.; Fu, X. D. & Gage, F. H. (2009). An RNA code for the FOX2 splicing regulator revealed by mapping RNA-protein interactions in stem cells. *Nat Struct Mol Biol*, Vol.16, No.2, (Feb, 2009), pp. 130-137

Young, P. J.; Le, T. T.; thi Man, N.; Burghes, A. H. & Morris, G. E. (2000). The relationship between SMN, the spinal muscular atrophy protein, and nuclear coiled bodies in differentiated tissues and cultured cells. *Exp Cell Res*, Vol.256, No.2, (May 1, 2000), pp. 365-374

Zhang, C.; Frias, M. A.; Mele, A.; Ruggiu, M.; Eom, T.; Marney, C. B.; Wang, H.; Licatalosi, D. D.; Fak, J. J. & Darnell, R. B. (2010). Integrative modeling defines the Nova splicing-regulatory network and its combinatorial controls. *Science*, Vol.329, No.5990, (Jul 23, 2010), pp. 439-443

Zhang, H.; Xing, L.; Rossoll, W.; Wichterle, H.; Singer, R. H. & Bassell, G. J. (2006). Multiprotein complexes of the survival of motor neuron protein SMN with Gemins traffic to neuronal processes and growth cones of motor neurons. *J Neurosci*, Vol.26, No.33, (Aug 16, 2006), pp. 8622-8632

Zhang, Z.; Lotti, F.; Dittmar, K.; Younis, I.; Wan, L.; Kasim, M. & Dreyfuss, G. (2008). SMN deficiency causes tissue-specific perturbations in the repertoire of snRNAs and widespread defects in splicing. *Cell*, Vol.133, No.4, (May 16, 2008), pp. 585-600

11

The Lsm Proteins: Ring Architectures for RNA Capture

Jens M. Moll, Meghna Sobti[1] and Bridget C. Mabbutt
Department of Chemistry and Biomolecular Sciences, Macquarie University, Australia

1. Introduction

It is today recognized that the vast majority of the cellular pool of RNA (nearly 98% in humans) comprises non-coding RNA (ncRNA) species (Mattick, 2001), with only a small proportion serving as direct template for protein synthesis. The diverse ncRNA forms are themselves capable of function, involved in a plethora of tasks such as protein scaffolding, *cis* and *trans* regulatory roles and catalysis (Lilley, 2005; Mattick & Makunin, 2006). Many of these functions are carried out in tight partnership with specific ancillary proteins within large ribonucleo-protein complexes (RNPs) (Eddy, 2001).

Various types of ncRNA, as well as RNPs containing tRNA, rRNA or snRNA, directly interact with mRNA at different stages of its life. Figure 1 presents an overview of the maturation of pre-mRNA and the fate of the mRNA generated. Pre-mRNA initially undergoes modification to enhance its stability: a 5′ methyl guanosine (m_7G) cap added during transcription (Wen & Shatkin, 1999) and a poly(A)-tail placed in the 3′ region by the polyadenylation machinery (Proudfoot et al., 2002; Balbo & Bohm, 2007). Following initiation of spliceosomal assembly by recruitment of core particles in the cytoplasm, non-coding introns are spliced from the pre-mRNA sequence by the mature spliceosome in the nucleus (Crick, 1979; Pozzoli et al., 2002). This multi-megadalton complex itself contains 170 protein components and various types of snRNA, rivaling the ribosome in molecular complexity (Wahl et al., 2009).

Within the spliceosome, several distinct small nuclear RNP (snRNP) core complexes each contain snRNA organized around specific ring-structured protein assemblies. For those known as U1-, U2-, U4- and U5-snRNPs, these ring scaffolds are provided by members of the Sm protein family (Luhrmann et al., 1990), recruited to their specific snRNA partners in the cytoplasm at a distinct Sm-site of bases (Urlaub et al., 2001; Peng & Gallwitz 2004). The core snRNPs are reimported into the nucleus for further processing and spliceosome assembly (Will & Luhrmann, 2001; Patel & Bellini 2008). In contrast, U6 snRNA is first modified within the nucleoli and then engages with a related protein ring, in this case containing Lsm ("Sm-like") proteins Lsm2-Lsm8. Together with the U1-U5 particles, the U6 snRNP is translocated to Cajal bodies for formation of the U4/U6*U5 tri-snRNP (Patel & Bellini, 2008). The mature snRNPs eventually assemble on pre-mRNA for intron removal steps (Will & Luhrmann, 2001; Patel & Bellini 2008).

[1] Present address: Structural and Computational Biology Division, Victor Chang Cardiac Research Institute, Australia

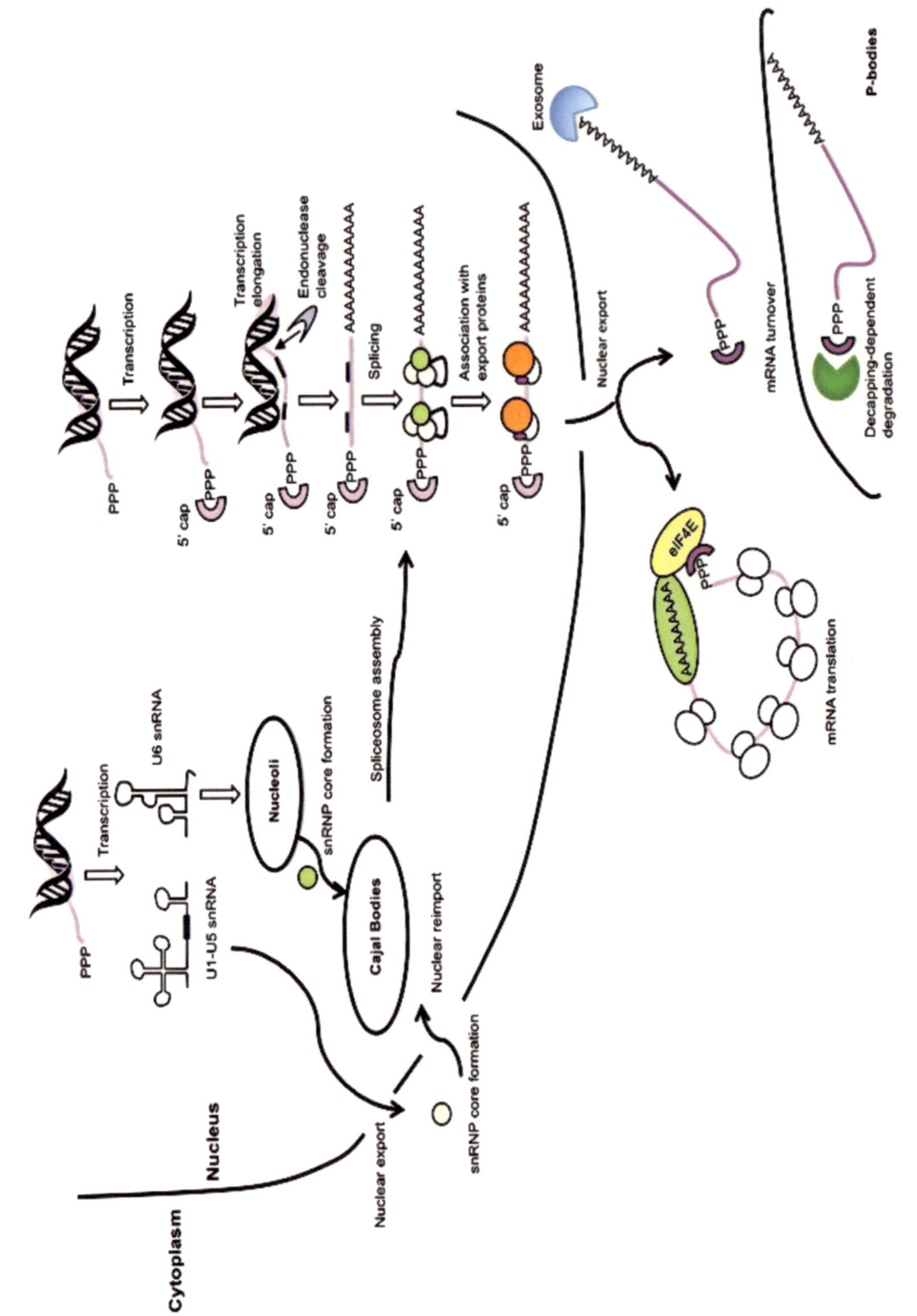

Fig. 1. Lifecycle of mRNA from transcription to decay.

Following excision of introns, mRNA enters the cytoplasm via the nuclear pore complex to be either translated or degraded. In eukaryotes, two pathways are utilized for mRNA decay: i) 3′-to-5′ degradation by the exosome or ii) 5′-decapping, followed by 5′-to-3′ exonuclease degradation (Garneau et al., 2007). In either event, decay is initiated by shortening of the poly(A)-tail by deadenylases (Tucker et al., 2001; Garneau et al., 2007; Nissan et al., 2010). Protein machinery required for the 5′-decapping pathway is found enriched in cytoplasmic foci known as processing or P-bodies (Sheth & Parker 2003), which appear to control the sorting and storage of mRNA. Within P-bodies, a specific assembly of Lsm proteins (Lsm1-Lsm7) and ancilliary protein factors expedites mRNA decapping and subsequent breakdown by ribonuclease (Nissan et al., 2010). While the extent to which mRNA decay is restricted to P-bodies is unclear, sequestered mRNA species are observed to leave P-bodies and may re-enter translation (Brengues et al., 2005).

2. Phylogeny of Lsm protein sequences

The Lsm proteins recur as molecular chaperones for RNA during the many steps of its processing, sorting and regulation (Beggs, 2005). While Sm proteins were first found enriched in a patient with systemic lupus erythematosis (Lerner & Steitz 1979), the wider protein family has since been described across all domains of life (Beggs, 2005; Ma et al., 2005). Members include eukaryotic Lsm (Salgado-Garrido et al., 1999), Sm (Kambach et al., 1999) and SMN/Gemin proteins (Selenko et al., 2001; Ma et al., 2005), archaeal Lsm proteins (Collins et al., 2001), the bacterial protein Hfq (Schumacher et al., 2002) and a recently identified Lsm homolog of cyanophage origin (Das et al., 2009). Eukaryotic genomes can contain up to 16 Lsm and 7 Sm proteins (Albrecht & Lengauer 2004), yet 2-3 Lsm proteins are generally encoded in archaea (Collins et al., 2001; Toro et al., 2002; Mura et al., 2003) and only a single form is evident in bacteria and cyanophage (Schumacher et al., 2002; Das et al., 2009).

A characteristic feature of the Lsm proteins is their natural tendency to form ring-shaped quaternary complexes, each of a precise composition related to cellular location and RNA target (Beggs, 2005; Spiller et al., 2007). In prokaryotes and archaea, homomeric complexes of six or seven Lsm protomers appear to be functional, whilst discrete heteromeric assemblies of seven distinct Lsm proteins are found in eukaryotes. The individual Lsm proteins vary in size from 8-25 kDa (78-240 amino acids); representative sequences are depicted in Figure 2. Within each, a bipartite consensus sequence (designated Sm1 and Sm2 motifs) can be identified. These motifs arise from strands β1-β3 and β4-β5 of the core β-sheet structure, respectively. A variable stretch of residues between these conserved segments is created by a surface-exposed interconnecting loop (Kambach et al., 1999; Collins et al., 2001). The N- and C-terminal tail regions of each Lsm sequence are often highly charged and differ markedly between members; these are considered to provide contact points for additional protein or RNA interactions (Reijns et al., 2008; Reijns et al., 2009; Weber et al., 2010). In the case of the eukaryotic Lsm1 and Lsm4 proteins, these tail segments are notably elongated.

The most highly conserved sequence segments across the Lsm family include specific amino acid sidechains implicated in RNA-binding. These are localized to two specific loop features, as outlined in Figure 2. For archaeal and eukaryotic Lsm proteins, sequence motifs Asp-x-ϕ-ϕ-Asn (ϕ = hydrophobic) and Arg-Gly-(Asp) (Kambach et al., 1999; Collins et al., 2001; Toro et al., 2001) are characteristic of loops L3 and L5, respectively. In bacterial Hfq, these RNA-binding segments occur as Asp-x-ϕ-ϕ-ϕ (L3) and Tyr-Lys-His (L5) (Schumacher

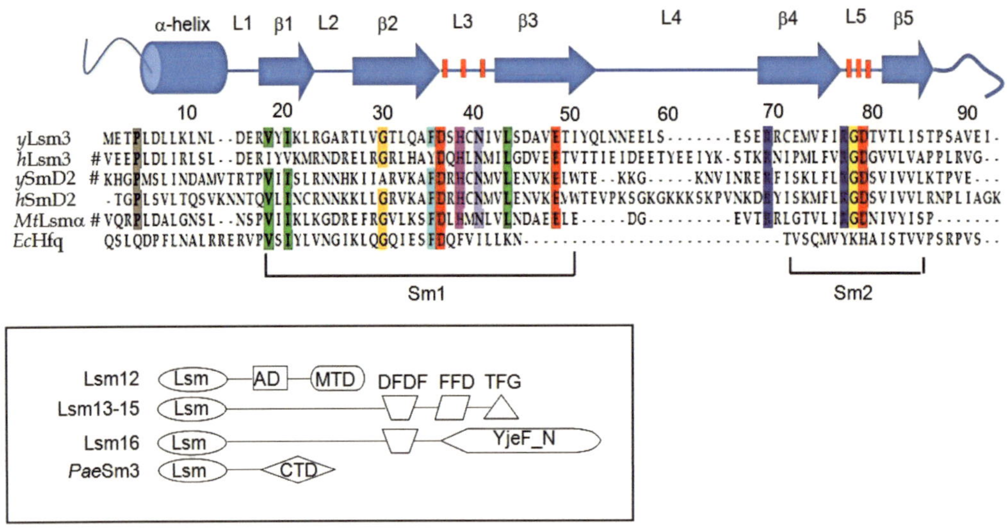

Fig. 2. Structure-based Lsm protein sequence alignment. Sequences displayed are for *S. cerevisiae* Lsm3 (*y*Lsm3), *H. sapiens* Lsm3 (*h*Lsm3), *S. cerevisiae* SmD2 (*y*SmD2), human SmD2 (*h*SmD2), *M. thermoautotrophicum* Lsmα (*Mt*Lsmα) and *E. coli* Hfq (*Ec*Hfq). Shaded residues represent areas with ≥ 80% sequence homology. Secondary structure assignment is based on the crystal structure of *y*Lsm3 (Naidoo et al., 2008). Red bars indicate conserved residues implicated in RNA binding. # indicates additional truncated residues not displayed. Boxed insert shows organization of other Lsm multidomain proteins: AD, anticodon binding domain; MTD, methyl transferase domain; DFDF, DFDF-x(7)-F containing domain; FFD, Y-x-K-x(3)-FFD-x-(IL)-S containing motif; TFG: [RKH]-x(2-5)-E-x(0-2)-[RK]-x(3-4)-[DE]-TFG containing domain. CTD, C-terminal domain2.

et al., 2002). For this bacterial ortholog, a highly conserved Gln residue on the N-terminal α-helix is also implicated in RNA-binding (Schumacher et al., 2002).

Overall, the bacterial protein Hfq shows little sequence conservation with its archaeal and eukaryotic orthologs, yet the archaeal and eukaryotic Lsm proteins share some limited sequence similarity (>20 %). The following Lsm-Sm protein paralogs are identifiable: Lsm1-SmB, Lsm2-SmD1, Lsm3-SmD2, Lsm4-SmD3, Lsm5-SmE, Lsm6-SmF, Lsm7-SmG, Lsm8-SmB (Fromont-Racine et al., 2000). These specific sequence relationships suggest the eukaryotic Lsm proteins to have evolved from a common archaeal ancestor in two waves (Khusial et al., 2005; Veretnik et al., 2009). A first gene duplication event likely created eight distinct Lsm proteins, from which later evolved the Sm protein group. The diversity of biological activities of Lsm proteins compared to their more specialized Sm counterparts supports this two-step evolution model (Beggs, 2005; Khusial et al., 2005). The presence of up to three Lsm proteins in archaea, as well as an Hfq-like protein in archaeal *M. jannaschii*, further supports a common ancestor of eukaryotic and archaeal Lsm proteins (Fischer et al., 2011).

A few multidomain proteins incorporating Lsm components have been observed (summarized, Figure 2). Lsm12 includes t-RNA and methyltransferase domains (Albrecht & Lengauer, 2004), and Lsm13, Lsm14 and Lsm15 all contain a central DFDF-x(7)-F domain (Albrecht & Lengauer, 2004; Anantharaman & Aravind, 2004). Lsm16 features a remarkably disrupted Lsm variant (lacking both the N-terminal α-helix and a complete β4 strand) in addition to FDF and YjeF-N domains (Albrecht & Lengauer, 2004; Tritschler et al., 2007). This protein is suggested to be dimeric in solution (Ling et al., 2008). The archaeal protein Pa-Sm3 contains an Lsm-like domain in addition to a C-terminal domain of unknown function adopting an α/β-fold (Mura et al., 2003).

3. Structures of Lsm protein ring complexes

Crystal structures of Lsm and Sm proteins from diverse sources today provide many high-resolution views of the ring morphology of their assemblies. As shown in Figure 3, Lsm rings have been observed to range 58-75 Å in diameter and to contain a central pore of 6-15 Å. Some crystal structures solved to date (Table 1) have been obtained in the presence of specific RNA partners. The recent solving of the human U1-snRNP structures containing the Sm assembly bound together with U1 snRNA and proteins U1-70K and U1-A have been significant and exciting advances (Pomeranz Krummel et al., 2009; Weber et al., 2010). These provide the first molecular detail of L/Sm rings bound to the highly intertwined protein-RNA network within RNP complexes.

Within the various Lsm ring assemblies, each protomer occurs as a highly bent five-stranded antiparallel β-sheet overlaid in most cases by an N-terminal α-helix (Figure 4A). The pronounced twist of the β-sheet aligns strand β5 against β1, so forming an SH3-type barrel loosely related to the OB-fold (Kambach et al., 1999; Collins et al. 2001). Strands β4 and β5 each present on opposite ends of the module, so providing interaction sites for adjacent Lsm subunits via β4-β5′ pairing (Figure 4). Stacking of five to eight protomers in such a manner ultimately results in the formation of the toroid assembly characteristic of all Lsm assemblies (Figure 4).

Within this ring organisation, the N-terminal amphipathic α-helices of each Lsm component are gathered across one face of the toroid, from which also project the unstructured N- and

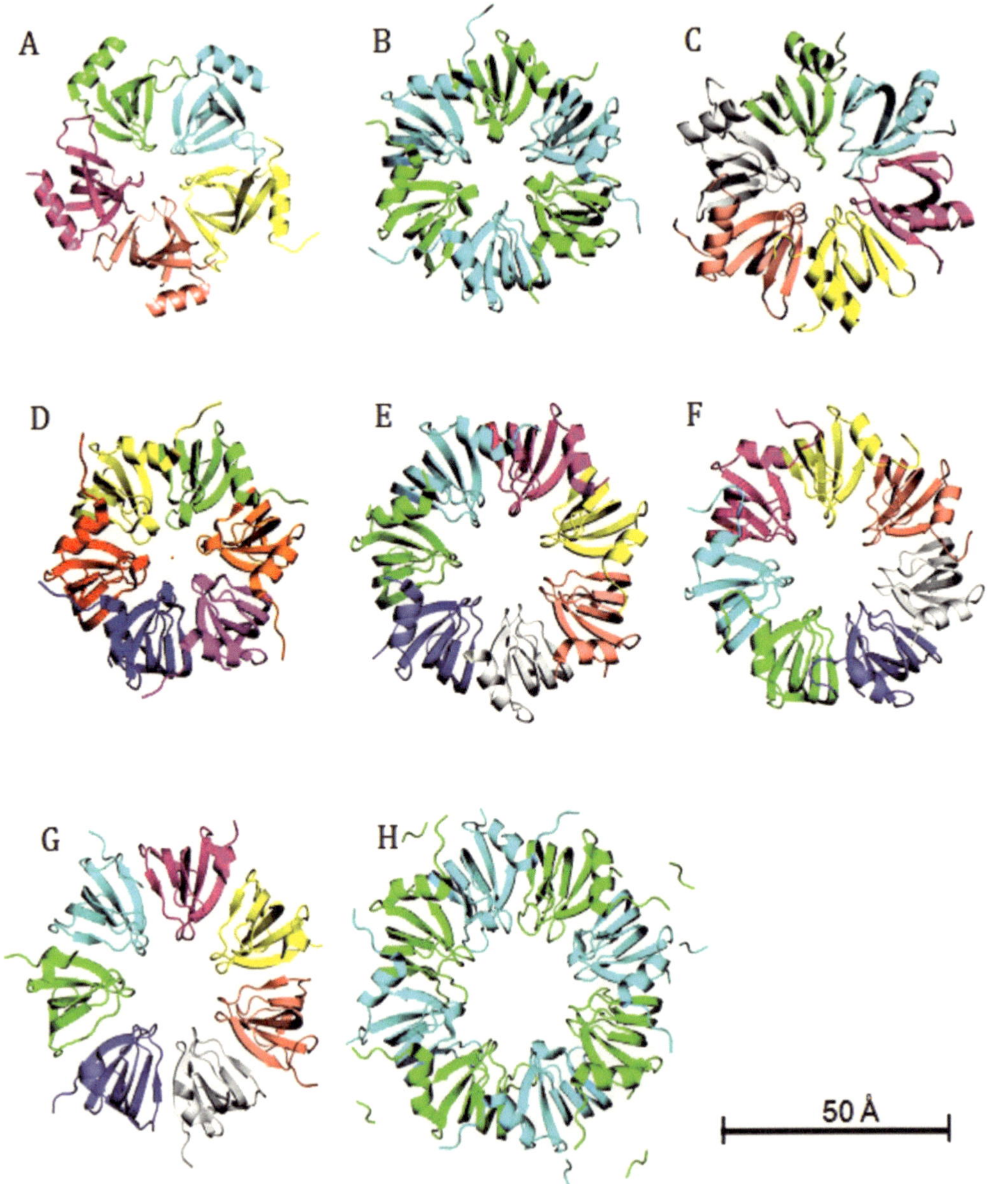

Fig. 3. Selected crystal structures solved for Lsm assemblies. A) Pentamer, cyanophage ECX21941 (PDB 3BY7) 60 Å ring, 9 Å pore. B) Hexamer, of *C. parvum* Lsm5 (PDB 3PGG) 60 Å ring, 10 Å pore. C) Hexamer, *S. aureus* Hfq (PDB 1KQ1) 65 Å ring, 11 Å pore. D) Hexamer, *A. fulgidus* Sm2 (PDB 1LJO) 58 Å ring, 6 Å pore. E) Hexamer, *A. fulgidus* Sm2 (PDB 1LJO) 58 Å ring, 6 Å pore. F) Heptamer, *A. fulgidus* Sm1 (PDB 1I4K) 65 Å ring, 13 Å pore. G) Heptamer, *M. thermoautotrophicum* Lsmα (PDB 1I81) 65 Å ring, 10-15 Å pore. F) Heptamer, *S. cerevisiae* Sm-F (PDB 1N9R) 65 Å ring, 10-15 Å pore. H) Octamer, *S. cerevisiae* Lsm3 (PDB 3BW1) 75 Å ring, 15 Å pore.

	Protein[1]	PDB ID	Resolution (Å)	Organism	Reference
Hexameric	*Hs*SmD3B	1D3B	2.00	*H. sapiens*	Kambach et al., 1999
	*Sa*Hfq	1KQ1	1.55	*S. aureus*	Schumacher et al., 2002
	*Sa*Hfq*	1KQ2	2.71	*S. aureus*	Schumacher et al., 2002
	*Af*Sm2	1LJO	1.95	*A. fulgidus*	Toro et al., 2002
	*Ec*Hfq	1HK9	2.15	*E. coli*	Sauter et al., 2003
	*Pa*Hfq	1U1S	1.60	*P. aeruginosa*	Nikulin et al., 2003
	*Pa*Hfq	1U1T	1.90	*P. aeruginosa*	Nikulin et al., 2003
	*Mj*Sm	2QTX	2.50	*M. jannaschii*	Nielsen et al., 2007
	*Cp*Lsm5	3PGG	2.14	*C. parvum*	Vedadi et al., 2007
	*A*Hfq	3HFN	2.31	*Anabena sp.*	Boggild et al., 2009
	*Ec*Hfq*	3GIB	2.40	*E. coli*	Link et al., 2009
	*S*Hfq	3HFO	1.30	*Synchocystis sp.*	Boggild et al., 2009
	*Pa*H57THfq	3INZ	1.70	*P. aeruginosa*	Moskaleva et al., 2010
	*Pa*H57AHfq	3M4G	2.05	*P. aeruginosa*	Moskaleva et al., 2010
	*Bs*Hfq	3HSB	2.20	*B. subtilis*	Someya et al., 2010[3]
Heptameric	*Mt*Lsmα	1I81, 1MGQ	2.00, 1.70	*M. thermoautotrophicum*	Collins et al., 2001
	*Pae*Sm1	1I8F	1.75	*P. aerophilum*	Mura et al., 2001
	*Af*Sm1	1I4K	2.50	*A. fulgidus*	Toro et al., 2001
	*Af*Sm1*	1I5L	2.75	*A. fulgidus*	Toro et al., 2001
	*Mt*Lsmα	1JBM	1.85	*M. thermoautotrophicum*	Mura et al., 2003b
	*Pae*Sm1	1JRI	1.75	*P. aerophilum*	Mura et al., 2003b
	*Pae*Sm1	1LNX	2.05	*P. aerophilum*	Mura et al., 2003b
	*Pab*Sm1	1H64	1.90	*P. abysii*	Thore et al., 2003
	*Pab*Sm1*	1M8V	2.60	*P. abysii*	Thore et al., 2003
	*Pae*Sm3	1M5Q	2.00	*P. aerophilum*	Mura et al., 2003a
	*Pae*Sm1	1LOJ	1.90	*M. thermoautotrophicum*	Mura et al., 2003b
	*Sc*SmF	1N9R	2.80	*S. cerevisiae*	Collins et al., 2003
	*Sc*SmF	1N9S	3.50	*S. cerevisiae*	Collins et al., 2003
	*Ss*Sm1	1TH7	1.68	*S. solfataricus*	Kilic et al., 2005
	U1-snRNP*	3CW1	5.49	*H. sapiens*	Pomeranz Krummel et al., 2009
	U1-snRNP*	3PGW	4.40	*H. sapiens*	Weber et al., 2010
Other	*Cph*Lsm	3BY7	2.60	*Cyanophage*	Das et al., 2009
	*Sc*Lsm3	3BW1	2.50	*S. cerevisiae*	Naidoo et al., 2008
	*Pfu*Q8TZN2[2]	1YCY	2.80	*P. furiosus*	Huang et al., 2004[3]

[1]Proteins are named by the first letters of the species, followed by the type of protein. Asterisked entries indicate structures solved in the presence of RNA.
[2]Hypothetical protein adopting an Lsm fold.
[3]Structure deposited without supporting publication.

Table 1. Crystal structures solved for Lsm assemblies (to 2010)

C-terminal extensions. The opposite face of the ring, named the distal face, is predominantly composed of residues of the variable loop L4 segments. All the Lsm ring structures (across eukarya, archaea and bacteria) reveal clusters of positive residues lining the internal pore, as well as pronounced positive elements on the distal face (Toro et al., 2001; Brennan & Link, 2007; Naidoo et al., 2008).

The body of structural data adds to biochemical understanding concerning L/Sm-RNA interactions, and distinct RNA sites within the protein oligomer. These include i) a binding site within the lumen of the ring, ii) an external contact site on the helix face and iii) residues located on the distal face of the complex (Figure 4). The first of these sites engages residues from loops L3 and L5, contributed from all Lsm components to create a nucleotide-binding pocket running around the inner rim (Weber et al., 2010). The specific architecture and repeated circular location of these specific, highly conserved, sidechains enables one nucleotide base to be bound per L/Sm protomer. Crystal structures of archaeal and bacterial Lsm complexed with RNA clearly show the oligonucleotides to be threaded around this rim of the toroid (Toro et al., 2001; Schumacher et al., 2002). Each binding "slot" allows specific base stacking to a hydrophobic sidechain of loop L3, as well as contact with the signature Arg residues of loop L5 and H-bonding with Asn residues (strand β4). Further electrostatic contacts (involving conserved Asp (strand β2), Arg (loop L5) and Gly (loop L5) residues) enhance the stability of the Lsm-RNA complex (Toro et al., 2001). Figure 5 displays these relevant binding interactions for U_5 within the lumen site of archaeal *Af*Sm1.

An external contact site for RNA at the helix face of the Lsm toroid (site ii) is suggested by the crystal structure of *Pa*Sm1 bound with U_7 oligonucleotide (Thore et al. 2003). In this case, each of two sandwiched Lsm rings engage two nucleotides at the N-terminal α-helix (Arg, His) and strands β2 (Tyr) via base stacking and H-bonding.

A third distinct RNA-binding site (iii) is likely to be unique to the bacterial Hfq assembly, and its tripartite form has been detailed in the crystal structure of Hfq bound to poly(A) RNA (Link *et al.* 2009). The protein Hfq engages poly(A) sequences on its distal face via specific residues exposed from strands β2 and β4. There is, however, no evidence for poly(A) binding by eukaryotic Lsm proteins. In the structure of the Hfq/RNA complex, RNA contacts include electrostatic interactions from Lys (strand β2) and Gln (strand β4) sidechains, as well as stacking of bases between Tyr, Leu (strand β2) and Leu and Ile (strand β2') of adjacent subunits. It is in this region of the toroid that sequence variability of the loop L4 across the Lsm family results in non-conservation of distal face chemistry, so explaining the unique binding properties of Hfq.

Within the crystal structures of the human U1-snRNP complex, multiple RNA interactions made by the ring of Sm proteins include binding sites i) and ii) outlined above (Weber et al., 2010). However, the U1-snRNP structure also clearly demonstrates the role of the Sm sequence extensions and loop regions as additional interaction sites, particularly the C-terminal extensions of SmD3 and SmB. In the lumen of the toroid (i.e. site i), snRNA threads to stack single nucleotides of the Sm site against the key loop L3 and L5 residues, noteably the aromatic sidechains. From the helix face of the ring are projected residues of the N-terminal α-helix and loop L3 of SmD2, forming an external contact site (reminiscent of site ii) that guides the snRNA into the ring pore. Residues from the loop L2 regions of SmD1 and SmD2 appear to guide RNA out from the Sm ring. Protruding beyond the distal face, residues of the elongated L4 loops of SmD2 and SmB provide another important interaction point to clamp and secure a stem-loop of the snRNA.

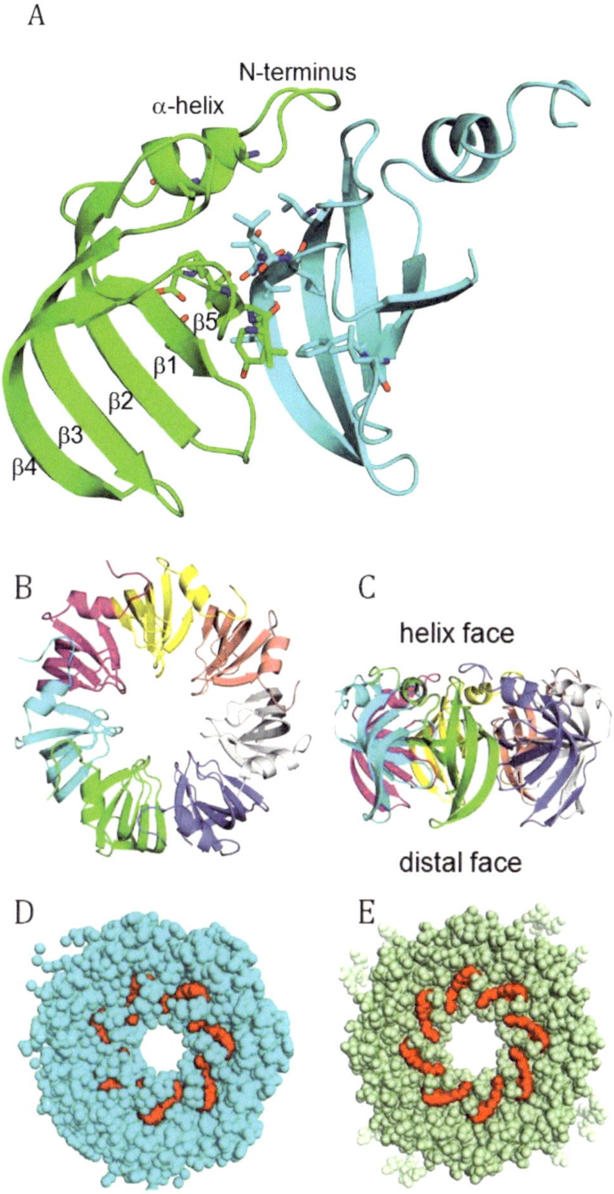

Fig. 4. Lsm fold and quaternary structure. Ribbon diagrams of *Mt*Lsmα (A, B; PDB 1I81) are displayed. A) Dimer interface of *Mt*Lsmα. Chain A is represented in green, chain B in blue. Residues involved in hydrophobic packing at the dimer interface (Chain A: Ile27, Val77, Tyr78 of chain A; Chain B: Leu 30, Phe36, Leu66, Val69, Ile71) are shown in stick representation. B-C) Top and side view of heptameric *Mt*Lsmα. D) Homo-heptameric *Mt*Lsmα (PDB 1I81). E) Homo-octameric yeast Lsm3 (PDB 3BW1). Space-filled models highlight in red conserved residues implicated in RNA binding: Asp in β2, Asn in L3, Arg and Gly in L5.

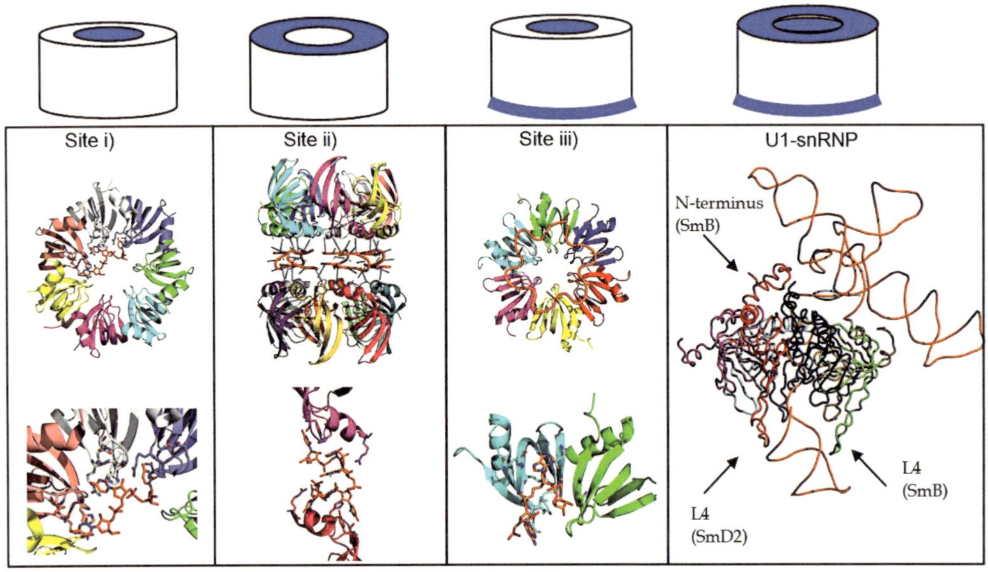

Fig. 5. Three general sites for RNA binding within specific examples of Lsm complexes. Site i) *Af*Sm1 (PDB 1I5L) bound to U_5 RNA viewed from helix face. Site ii) Two *Pa*Sm1 (PDB 1M8V) heptamers are bridged by uridine heptamer. Site iii) *Ec*Hfq (PDB 3GIB) bound to poly(A) viewed from distal face. U1-snRNP) Figure includes side view of the Sm-core of the human U1 snRNP structure (PDB 3PGW).

The majority of crystal structures of Lsm obtained to date portray the hexa- and heptameric protein assemblies that correspond to fully functional homomeric or heteromeric protein groupings. It is, for instance, assumed that complexes of SmD1-SmD2, SmD3-SmB and SmE-SmF-SmG can exist independently in the cytoplasm, yet rearrange into mixed heptamers in the presence of RNA during snRNP formation (Peng & Gallwitz, 2004). However, a few crystal structures suggest that other compositions, e.g. pentamers and octamers, may be stable for eukaryotic Lsm (Naidoo et al., 2008; Das et al., 2009). While it is currently not clear if these organizations are peculiar to recombinant preparations of the Lsm family, they suggest possibilities for a variety of multimeric assemblies *in vivo*. Our own interaction studies indicate that Lsm assemblies may be relatively dynamic in solution, providing capacity to engage in alternative protein partnerships and stable groupings (Sobti et al., 2010).

4. Functional roles for Lsm proteins

Sm and Lsm proteins are known to interact with a diversity of RNA partner species. Specific RNA sequences recognized by various Lsm complexes include the Sm-site (A_2U_5GA) (Raker et al., 1999) and U-rich stretches at the 3′ end of oligoadenylated mRNA (Chowdhury et al., 2007) and RNA polymerase III transcripts, including snRNA (Achsel et al., 1999). Other binding partners include snoRNA (Kufel et al., 2003a), P RNA (Kufel et al., 2002), tRNA (Kufel et al., 2002) and rRNA (Kufel et al., 2003b). Depletion of Lsm proteins 2-5 and 8 in yeast results in defects in post-transcriptional processing of tRNA, P RNA, rRNA, snoRNA and snRNA precursors (Kufel et al., 2002; Kufel et al., 2003b; Kufel et al., 2003a). Yet only minor (or no) effects are observed on depletion of Lsm6 and Lsm7. A summary of some specific Lsm-ncRNA interactions is presented in Table 2.

The Lsm2-Lsm8 complex plays a key role in U6 snRNA maturation, so impacting on the formation of spliceosomal snRNPs (Karaduman et al., 2006). U6 snRNA is the most conserved of all snRNA species and key to the catalytic activity of the spliceosome (Brow, 2002). Newly transcribed U6 pre-snRNA is targeted to the nucleoli following binding of the La protein (Lhp1 in yeast) at its U-rich 3′ region (Wolin & Cedervall, 2002). Following cyclic phosphorylation, La (or Lhp1) is displaced from the U6 snRNA by the Lsm2-Lsm8 assembly (Achsel et al., 1999; Licht et al., 2008), which induces conformational changes that stimulate binding of a recycling factor (p110 or Prp24) (Rader & Guthrie, 2002; Ryan et al., 2002; Karaduman et al., 2006). These conformational changes have been suggested to assist in the formation and recycling of the U4/U6 di-snRNP by exposing single stranded nucleotides for base pairing (Beggs, 2005; Karaduman et al., 2006; Karaduman et al., 2008). The Lsm2-Lsm8 complex is also implicated in decapping steps of mRNA in the nucleus. This was suggested by the finding that Lsm6 and Lsm8 were required for nuclear mRNA decay (Kufel et al., 2004).

A specific role for Lsm1-Lsm7 concerns activation of mRNA decay in P-bodies; depletion of individual yeast Lsm proteins results in the accumulation of capped, oligoadenylated mRNA transcripts (Boeck et al., 1998; Bonnerot et al., 2000; Bouveret et al., 2000; Tharun et al., 2000). This specific Lsm complex is recruited alongside other decay factors to U-rich tracts by the protein Pat1, after its displacement of cap-binding translation factors (Parker & Sheth, 2007). It is likely that Pat1 and Lsm1-Lsm7 are then involved in subsequent activation of the Dcp1-Dcp2 enzyme (Nissan et al., 2010). A variety of studies have demonstrated the interaction of Lsm1-Lsm7 with decapping factors and exoribonuclease Xrn1 (Bonnerot et al., 2000; Bouveret et al., 2000; Tharun et al., 2000; Coller et al., 2001).

RNA species	Lsm function	Selected experimental evidence	References
snRNA	assembly, processing	Lsm2-8 binds 3′ end of U6 snRNA	Achsel et al., 1999
		Lsm2-8 initiates structural rearrangements of U6 snRNA	Karaduman et al., 2006; 2008
		Depletion of Lsm2-Lsm8 results in splicing defects	Mayes et al., 1999
		Splicing activity recovered through recombinant Lsm proteins	Verdone et al., 2004
	and nuclear localization	Lsm2-8 localizes U6 snRNA to the nucleus	Spiller et al., 2007
tRNA	splicing, 3′ and 5′ end-processing	Accumulation of unprocessed pre-tRNA and reduced La/Lhp1 binding upon Lsm2-Lsm5 and Lsm8 depletion	Kufel et al., 2002
		Direct interaction of Lsm3 with tRNA and its splicing factors	Fromont-Racine et al., 1997
P RNA	chaperone	Depletion of Lsm2-Lsm5 and Lsm8 reduces pre-PRNA levels	Mayes et al., 1999
		Reduced La/Lhp1 binding upon Lsm2-Lsm5 and Lsm8 depletion	Kufel et al., 2002
		Lsm2-Lsm7 proteins coprecipitate with pre-PRNA	Salgado-Garrido et al., 1999
rRNA	3′ and 5′ end-processing	Depletion of Lsm2-Lsm5 and Lsm8 delays pre-rRNA processing and increases rRNA decay rate	Kufel et al., 2003b
		Pre-rRNA coprecipitates with Lsm3 but not Lsm1	Kufel et al., 2003b
		Deletion of Lsm6 and Lsm7 genes impairs 20S pre-rRNA processing	Li et al., 2009
snoRNA	3′ end-processing	Lsm2-Lsm5 and Lsm8 depletion results in U3-snoRNA degradation and loss of its 3′ extended precursor	Kufel et al., 2003a
		Reduced La/Lhp1 binding upon Lsm3 or Lsm5 depletion	Kufel et al., 2003a
		Lsm2-Lsm7 but not Lsm1 or Lsm8 coprecipitate with snR5 snoRNA	Fernandez et al., 2004
		Lsm2-4 and 6-8 but not Lsm5 coprecipitate with U8 snoRNA	Tomasevic & Peculis, 2002

Table 2. Lsm binding interactions with ncRNA

In contrast to its enhancement of mRNA decay, however, the Lsm1-Lsm7 complex can also protect mRNA against 3′ end trimming (He & Parker, 2001). This may involve steric hindrance of nuclease attack at mRNA locations on which Lsm1-Lsm7 and Pat1 proteins are bound.

5. Specific functions of bacterial Hfq

Bacterial Hfq is observed to interact with bacterial sRNA and so promote the formation of sRNA-mRNA complexes (Wassarman et al., 2001; Gottesman & Storz, 2010). Bacterial sRNAs are small non-coding RNA species (50-500 nucleotides), which regulate gene expression via base pairing with mRNA transcripts in a similar mechanism to eukaryotic siRNA or miRNA (Storz et al., 2004; Majdalani et al., 2005; Livny & Waldor, 2007; Gottesman & Storz, 2010). Hfq controls gene expression either by rearranging the RNA secondary structure, or by increasing the concentration of RNA locally to promote RNA-RNA interactions (Moll et al., 2003; Lease & Woodson, 2004; Afonyushkin et al., 2005). A similar mode of binding to sRNA was recently observed for the archaeal Lsm from *Haloferax volcanii* (Fischer et al., 2011).

As for the eukaryotic Lsm proteins, Hfq is required for deadenylation-dependent mRNA decay. An RNase E-Hfq-sRNA complex is thought to function in translational repression and subsequent mRNA destabilization and degradation (Morita et al., 2005; Morita et al., 2006). Additional functions of Hfq include ATPase activity (Sukhodolets & Garges, 2003), cellular stress response and modulation of virulence in some bacterial strains (Tsui et al., 1994; Fantappie et al., 2009; Liu et al., 2010). Interestingly, the virulence of the multi-drug resistant human pathogen *S. aureus* was decreased in Hfq-deletion strains. (Liu et al., 2010).

6. Lsm proteins in human disease and viral replication

Aberrations in functions of Lsm proteins have been associated with a number of human diseases. Sm proteins are known to be targeted by auto-antibodies in systemic lupus erythematosis (Lerner & Steitz, 1979). In fact, the proteins were first identified in nuclear extracts of a patient suffering from this disease. A mutation of the SMN gene resulting in diminished assembly of snRNPs is the cause of spinal muscular atrophy (Lefebvre et al., 1995; Wan et al., 2005). Three Lsm proteins (Lsm1, Lsm3 and Lsm7) have now been directly connected to different cancer types. Lsm1 (also named cancer associated Sm-like protein, CaSm) was upregulated in pancreatic, prostate and breast cancer, as well as in several cancer-derived cell lines (Schweinfest et al., 1997; Fraser et al., 2005; Streicher et al., 2007). Remarkably, overexpression of antisense Lsm1 has been demonstrated to promote tumor reduction (Kelley et al., 2000; Kelley et al., 2001; Yan et al., 2006). Elevated levels of Lsm7 have been identified in malignant thyroid tumors, and a reduction in Lsm7 expression was observed in breast cancers (Conte et al., 2002; Rosen et al., 2005). The copy number and expression for the Lsm3 gene was found to be elevated in cervical cancer (Lyng et al., 2006).

Observations concerning Lsm proteins in viral replication underlines some interesting functional diversity. Bacterial Hfq was initially described as a host factor required for phage Qß replication (Franze de Fernandez et al., 1968). A role for Lsm1 as an effector of HIV replication has been reported (Chable-Bessia et al., 2009). It has also been suggested more recently that positive-strand RNA viruses may directly bind to the host Lsm1-7 protein complex via tRNA-like structures and A-rich stretches, so diverting normal mRNA regulation (Galao et al., 2010). The requirement of host Lsm proteins for the replication of this class of virus has additionally been demonstrated in plant brome mosaic virus (Diez et al., 2000; Noueiry et al., 2003; Mas et al., 2006) and human hepatitis C virus (Scheller et al., 2009).

7. References

Achsel, T., Brahms, H., Kastner, B., Bachi, A., Wilm, M., and Luerhmann, R. (1999), 'A doughnut-shaped heteromer of human Sm-like proteins binds to the 3' end of U6 snRNA, thereby facilitating U4/U6 duplex formation in vitro', *EMBO J*, 18 (20), 5789-802.

Afonyushkin, T., Vecerek, B., Moll, I., Blasi, U., and Kaberdin, V. R. (2005), 'Both RNase E and RNase III control the stability of sodB mRNA upon translational inhibition by the small regulatory RNA RyhB', *Nucleic Acids Res*, 33 (5), 1678-89.

Albrecht, M. and Lengauer, T. (2004), 'Novel Sm-like proteins with long C-terminal tails and associated methyltransferases', *FEBS Lett*, 569 (1-3), 18-26.

Anantharaman, V. and Aravind, L. (2004), 'Novel conserved domains in proteins with predicted roles in eukaryotic cell-cycle regulation, decapping and RNA stability', *BMC Genomics*, 5 (1), 45.

Balbo, P. B. and Bohm, A. (2007), 'Mechanism of poly(A) polymerase: structure of the enzyme-MgATP-RNA ternary complex and kinetic analysis', *Structure*, 15 (9), 1117-31.

Beggs, J. D. (2005), 'Lsm proteins and RNA processing', *Biochem Soc Trans* 33, 439-501.

Boeck, R., Lapeyre, B., Brown, C. E., and Sachs, A. B. (1998), 'Capped mRNA degradation intermediates accumulate in the yeast spb8-2 mutant', *Mol Cell Biol*, 18 (9), 5062-72.

Bonnerot, C., Boeck, R., and Lapeyre, B. (2000), 'The two proteins Pat1p (Mrt1p) and Spb8p interact in vivo, are required for mRNA decay, and are functionally linked to Pab1p.', *Mol Cell Biol*, 20.

Bouveret, E., Rigaut, G., Shevchenko, A., Wilm, M., and Seraphin, B. (2000), 'A Sm-like protein complex that participates in mRNA degradation', *EMBO J*, 19 (7), 1661-71.

Brengues, M., Teixeira, D., and Parker, R. (2005), 'Movement of eukaryotic mRNAs between polysomes and cytoplasmic processing bodies', *Science*, 310 (5747), 486-9.

Brennan, R. G. and Link, T. M. (2007), 'Hfq structure, function and ligand binding', *Curr Opin Microbiol*, 10 (2), 125-33.

Brow, D. A. (2002), 'Allosteric cascade of spliceosome activation', *Annu Rev Genet*, 36, 333-60.

Chable-Bessia, C., Meziane, O., Latreille, D., Triboulet, R., Zamborlini, A., Wagschal, A., Jacquet, J. M., Reynes, J., Levy, Y., Saib, A., Bennasser, Y., and Benkirane, M. (2009), 'Suppression of HIV-1 replication by microRNA effectors', *Retrovirology*, 6, 26.

Chowdhury, A., Mukhopadhyay, J. , and Tharun, S. (2007), 'The decapping activator Lsm1p-7p–Pat1p complex has the intrinsic ability to distinguish between oligoadenylated and polyadenylated RNAs', *RNA*, 13.

Coller, JM., Tucker, M., Sheth, U., Valencia-Sanchez, MA., and Parker, R. (2001), 'The DEAD box helicase, Dhh1p, functions in mRNA decapping and interacts with both the decapping and deadenylase complexes.', *RNA*, 7.

Collins, BM., Harrop, SJ., Kornfeld, GD., Ian, DW, Curmi, PMG., and Mabbutt, BC. (2001), 'Crystal Structure of a Heptameric Sm-like Protein Complex from Archea: Implications for the Structure and Evolution of snRNPs', *J Mol Biol*, 309, 915-23.

Conte, N., Charafe-Jauffret, E., Delaval, B., Adelaide, J., Ginestier, C., Geneix, J., Isnardon, D., Jacquemier, J., and Birnbaum, D. (2002), 'Carcinogenesis and translational controls: TACC1 is down-regulated in human cancers and associates with mRNA regulators', *Oncogene,* 21 (36), 5619-30.

Crick, F. (1979), 'Split genes and RNA splicing', *Science,* 204 (4390), 264-71.

Das, D., Kozbial, P., Axelrod, H. L., Miller, M. D., McMullan, D., Krishna, S. S., Abdubek, P., Acosta, C., Astakhova, T., Burra, P., Carlton, D., Chen, C., Chiu, H. J., Clayton, T., Deller, M. C., Duan, L., Elias, Y., Elsliger, M. A., Ernst, D., Farr, C., Feuerhelm, J., Grzechnik, A., Grzechnik, S. K., Hale, J., Han, G. W., Jaroszewski, L., Jin, K. K., Johnson, H. A., Klock, H. E., Knuth, M. W., Kumar, A., Marciano, D., Morse, A. T., Murphy, K. D., Nigoghossian, E., Nopakun, A., Okach, L., Oommachen, S., Paulsen, J., Puckett, C., Reyes, R., Rife, C. L., Sefcovic, N., Sudek, S., Tien, H., Trame, C., Trout, C. V., van den Bedem, H., Weekes, D., White, A., Xu, Q., Hodgson, K. O., Wooley, J., Deacon, A. M., Godzik, A., Lesley, S. A., and Wilson, I. A. (2009), 'Crystal structure of a novel Sm-like protein of putative cyanophage origin at 2.60 A resolution', *Proteins,* 75 (2), 296-307.

Diez, J., Ishikawa, M., Kaido, M., and Ahlquist, P. (2000), 'Identification and characterization of a host protein required for efficient template selection in viral RNA replication', *Proc Natl Acad Sci U S A,* 97 (8), 3913-8.

Eddy, S. R. (2001), 'Non-coding RNA genes and the modern RNA world', *Nat Rev Genet,* 2 (12), 919-29.

Fantappie, L., Metruccio, M. M., Seib, K. L., Oriente, F., Cartocci, E., Ferlicca, F., Giuliani, M. M., Scarlato, V., and Delany, I. (2009), 'The RNA chaperone Hfq is involved in stress response and virulence in Neisseria meningitidis and is a pleiotropic regulator of protein expression', *Infect Immun,* 77 (5), 1842-53.

Fernandez, C. F., Pannone, B. K., Chen, X., Fuchs, G., and Wolin, S. L. (2004), 'An Lsm2-Lsm7 complex in Saccharomyces cerevisiae associates with the small nucleolar RNA snR5', *Mol Biol Cell,* 15 (6), 2842-52.

Fischer, S., Benz, J., Spath, B., Maier, L. K., Straub, J., Granzow, M., Raabe, M., Urlaub, H., Hoffmann, J., Brutschy, B., Allers, T., Soppa, J., and Marchfelder, A. (2011), 'The archaeal Lsm protein binds to small RNAs', *J Biol Chem,* 285 (45), 34429-38.

Franze de Fernandez, M. T., Eoyang, L., and August, J. T. (1968), 'Factor fraction required for the synthesis of bacteriophage Qbeta-RNA', *Nature,* 219 (5154), 588-90.

Fraser, M. M., Watson, P. M., Fraig, M. M., Kelley, J. R., Nelson, P. S., Boylan, A. M., Cole, D. J., and Watson, D. K. (2005), 'CaSm-mediated cellular transformation is associated with altered gene expression and messenger RNA stability', *Cancer Res,* 65 (14), 6228-36.

Fromont-Racine, M., Rain, JC., and Legrain, P. (1997), 'Toward a functional analysis of the yeast genome through exhaustive two-hybrid screens.', *Nat Genetics,* 16.

Fromont-Racine, M., Mayes, A. E., Brunet-Simon, A., Rain, J. C., Colley, A., Dix, I., Decourty, L., Joly, N., Ricard, F., Beggs, J. D., and Legrain, P. (2000), 'Genome-wide protein interaction screens reveal functional networks involving Sm-like proteins', *Yeast,* 17 (2), 95-110.

Galao, R. P., Chari, A., Alves-Rodrigues, I., Lobao, D., Mas, A., Kambach, C., Fischer, U., and Diez, J. (2010), 'LSm1-7 complexes bind to specific sites in viral RNA genomes and regulate their translation and replication', *RNA,* 16 (4), 817-27.

Garneau, Nicole L., Wilusz, Jeffrey, and Wilusz, Carol J (2007), 'The highways and byways of mRNA decay', *Nat Rev Mol Cell Biol,* 8, 113-26.

Gottesman, S. and Storz, G. (2010), 'Bacterial Small RNA Regulators: Versatile Roles and Rapidly Evolving Variations', *Cold Spring Harb Perspect Biol.*

He, W. and Parker, R. (2001), 'The yeast cytoplasmic LsmI/Pat1p complex protects mRNA 3' termini from partial degradation', *Genetics,* 158 (4), 1445-55.

Kambach, Christian, Walke, Stefan, Young, Robert, Avis, Johanna M, de la Fortelle, Eric , Raker, Veronica A, Luerhmann, Reinhard, Li, Jade, and Nagai, Kiyoshi (1999), 'Crystal Structures of Two Sm Protein Complexes and Their Implications for the Assembly of the Spliceosomal snRNPs', *Cell,* 96, 375-87.

Karaduman, R., Fabrizio, P., Hartmuth, K., Urlaub, H., and Luerhmann, R. (2006), 'RNA structure and RNA-Protein interactions in Purified Yeast U6 snRNPs', *J Mol Biol,* 356, 1248-62.

Karaduman, R., Dube, P., Stark, H., Fabrizio, P., Kastner, B., and Luhrmann, R. (2008), 'Structure of yeast U6 snRNPs: arrangement of Prp24p and the LSm complex as revealed by electron microscopy', *RNA,* 14 (12), 2528-37.

Kelley, J. R., Fraser, M. M., Schweinfest, C. W., Vournakis, J. N., Watson, D. K., and Cole, D. J. (2001), 'CaSm/gemcitabine chemo-gene therapy leads to prolonged survival in a murine model of pancreatic cancer', *Surgery,* 130 (2), 280-8.

Kelley, J. R., Brown, J. M., Frasier, M. M., Baron, P. L., Schweinfest, C. W., Vournakis, J. N., Watson, D. K., and Cole, D. J. (2000), 'The cancer-associated Sm-like oncogene: a novel target for the gene therapy of pancreatic cancer', *Surgery,* 128 (2), 353-60.

Khusial, P., Plaag, R., and Zieve, GW. (2005), 'LSm proteins form heptameric rings that bind to RNA via repeating motifs', *Trends Biochem Sci* 30 (9).

Kufel, J., Bousquet-Antonelli, C., Beggs, J. D., and Tollervey, D. (2004), 'Nuclear pre-mRNA decapping and 5' degradation in yeast require the Lsm2-8p complex', *Mol Cell Biol,* 24 (21), 9646-57.

Kufel, J., Allmang, C., Verdone, L., Beggs, J. D., and Tollervey, D. (2002), 'Lsm proteins are required for normal processing of pre-tRNAs and their efficient association with La-homologous protein Lhp1p', *Mol Cell Biol,* 22 (14), 5248-56.

Kufel, J., Allmang, C., Verdone, L., Beggs, J., and Tollervey, D. (2003a), 'A complex pathway for 3' processing of the yeast U3 snoRNA', *Nucleic Acids Res,* 31 (23), 6788-97.

Kufel, J., Allmang, C., Petfalski, E., Beggs, J., and Tollervey, D. (2003b), 'Lsm Proteins are required for normal processing and stability of ribosomal RNAs', *J Biol Chem,* 278 (4), 2147-56.

Lease, R. A. and Woodson, S. A. (2004), 'Cycling of the Sm-like protein Hfq on the DsrA small regulatory RNA', *J Mol Biol,* 344 (5), 1211-23.

Lefebvre, S., Burglen, L., Reboullet, S., Clermont, O., Burlet, P., Viollet, L., Benichou, B., Cruaud, C., Millasseau, P., Zeviani, M., and et al. (1995), 'Identification and characterization of a spinal muscular atrophy-determining gene', *Cell,* 80 (1), 155-65.

Lerner, M. R. and Steitz, J. A. (1979), 'Antibodies to small nuclear RNAs complexed with proteins are produced by patients with systemic lupus erythematosus', *Proc Natl Acad Sci U S A,* 76 (11), 5495-9.

Li, Z., Lee, I., Moradi, E., Hung, N. J., Johnson, A. W., and Marcotte, E. M. (2009), 'Rational extension of the ribosome biogenesis pathway using network-guided genetics', *PLoS Biol,* 7 (10), e1000213.

Licht, K., Medenbach, J., Luerhmann, R., Kambach, C., and Bindereif, A. (2008), '3'-cyclic phosphorylation of U6 snRNA leads to recruitment of recycling factor p110 through LSm proteins', *RNA,* 14 (8), 1-7.

Lilley, D. M. (2005), 'Structure, folding and mechanisms of ribozymes', *Curr Opin Struct Biol,* 15 (3), 313-23.

Ling, S. H., Decker, C. J., Walsh, M. A., She, M., Parker, R., and Song, H. (2008), 'Crystal structure of human Edc3 and its functional implications', *Mol Cell Biol,* 28 (19), 5965-76.

Link, T. M., Valentin-Hansen, P., and Brennan, R. G. (2009), 'Structure of Escherichia coli Hfq bound to polyriboadenylate RNA', *Proc Natl Acad Sci U S A,* 106 (46), 19292-7.

Liu, Y., Wu, N., Dong, J., Gao, Y., Zhang, X., Mu, C., Shao, N., and Yang, G. (2010), 'Hfq is a global regulator that controls the pathogenicity of Staphylococcus aureus', *PLoS One,* 5 (9):e13069.

Livny, J. and Waldor, M. K. (2007), 'Identification of small RNAs in diverse bacterial species', *Curr Opin Microbiol,* 10 (2), 96-101.

Luhrmann, R., Kastner, B., and Bach, M. (1990), 'Structure of spliceosomal snRNPs and their role in pre-mRNA splicing', *Biochim Biophys Acta,* 1087 (3), 265-92.

Lyng, H., Brovig, R. S., Svendsrud, D. H., Holm, R., Kaalhus, O., Knutstad, K., Oksefjell, H., Sundfor, K., Kristensen, G. B., and Stokke, T. (2006), 'Gene expressions and copy numbers associated with metastatic phenotypes of uterine cervical cancer', *BMC Genomics,* 7, 268.

Ma, Y., Dostie, J., Dreyfuss, G., and Van Duyne, G. D. (2005), 'The Gemin6-Gemin7 heterodimer from the survival of motor neurons complex has an Sm protein-like structure', *Structure,* 13 (6), 883-92.

Majdalani, N., Vanderpool, C. K., and Gottesman, S. (2005), 'Bacterial small RNA regulators', *Crit Rev Biochem Mol Biol,* 40 (2), 93-113.

Mas, A., Alves-Rodrigues, I., Noueiry, A., Ahlquist, P., and Diez, J. (2006), 'Host deadenylation-dependent mRNA decapping factors are required for a key step in brome mosaic virus RNA replication', *J Virol,* 80 (1), 246-51.

Mattick, J. S. (2001), 'Non-coding RNAs: the architects of eukaryotic complexity', *EMBO Rep,* 2 (11), 986-91.

Mattick, J. S. and Makunin, I. V. (2006), 'Non-coding RNA', *Hum Mol Genet,* 15 Spec No 1, R17-29.

Mayes, AE., Verdone, L., Legraine, P., and Beggs, JD. (1999), 'Characerization of Sm-like proteins in yeast and their association with U6 snRNA ', *EMBO J,* 18 (15), 4321-31.

Moll, I., Leitsch, D., Steinhauser, T., and Blasi, U. (2003), 'RNA chaperone activity of the Sm-like Hfq protein', *EMBO Rep,* 4 (3), 284-9.

Morita, T., Maki, K., and Aiba, H. (2005), 'RNase E-based ribonucleoprotein complexes: mechanical basis of mRNA destabilization mediated by bacterial noncoding RNAs', *Genes Dev,* 19 (18), 2176-86.

Morita, T., Mochizuki, Y., and Aiba, H. (2006), 'Translational repression is sufficient for gene silencing by bacterial small noncoding RNAs in the absence of mRNA destruction', *Proc Natl Acad Sci U S A,* 103 (13), 4858-63.

Mura, C., Phillips, M., Kozhukhovsky, A., and Eisenberg, D. (2003), 'Structure and assembly of an augmented Sm-like archaeal protein 14-mer', *Proc Natl Acad Sci U S A,* 100 (8), 4539-44.

Naidoo, N., Harrop, SJ., Sobti, M., Haynes, PA., Szymczyna, BR., Williamson, JR., Curmi, PMG., and Mabbutt, BC. (2008), 'Crystal Structure of Lsm3 Octamer from Saccharomyces cerevisiae: Implications for Lsm Ring Organisation and Recruitment', *J Mol Biol,* 377, 1357-71.

Nissan, T., Rajyaguru, P., She, M., Song, H., and Parker, R. (2010), 'Decapping activators in Saccharomyces cerevisiae act by multiple mechanisms', *Mol Cell,* 39 (5), 773-83.

Noueiry, A. O., Diez, J., Falk, S. P., Chen, J., and Ahlquist, P. (2003), 'Yeast Lsm1p-7p/Pat1p deadenylation-dependent mRNA-decapping factors are required for brome mosaic virus genomic RNA translation', *Mol Cell Biol,* 23 (12), 4094-106.

Parker, R. and Sheth, U. (2007), 'P Bodies and the control of mRNA Translation and Degradation', *Mol Cell,* 25 (5), 635-46.

Patel, S. B. and Bellini, M. (2008), 'The assembly of a spliceosomal small nuclear ribonucleoprotein particle', *Nucleic Acids Res,* 36 (20), 6482-93.

Peng, R. and Gallwitz, D. (2004), 'Multiple SNARE interactions of an SM protein: Sed5p/Sly1p binding is dispensable for transport', *EMBO J,* 23 (20), 3939-49.

Pomeranz Krummel, D. A., Oubridge, C., Leung, A. K., Li, J., and Nagai, K. (2009), 'Crystal structure of human spliceosomal U1 snRNP at 5.5 A resolution', *Nature,* 458 (7237), 475-80.

Pozzoli, U., Sironi, M., Cagliani, R., Comi, G. P., Bardoni, A., and Bresolin, N. (2002), 'Comparative analysis of the human dystrophin and utrophin gene structures', *Genetics,* 160 (2), 793-8.

Proudfoot, N. J., Furger, A., and Dye, M. J. (2002), 'Integrating mRNA processing with transcription', *Cell,* 108 (4), 501-12.

Rader, S. D. and Guthrie, C. (2002), 'A conserved Lsm-interaction motif in Prp24 required for efficient U4/U6 di-snRNP formation', *RNA,* 8 (11), 1378-92.

Raker, VA., Hartmuth, K., Kastner, B., and Luhrmann, R. (1999), 'Spliceosomal U snRNP core assembly: Sm proteins assemble onto an Sm site RNA nonanucleotide in a specific and thermodynamically stable manner', *Mol Cell Biol,* 19 (10), 6554-65.

Reijns, M. A., Auchynnikava, T., and Beggs, J. D. (2009), 'Analysis of Lsm1p and Lsm8p domains in the cellular localization of Lsm complexes in budding yeast', *FEBS J,* 276 (13), 3602-17.

Reijns, M. A., Alexander, R. D., Spiller, M. P., and Beggs, J. D. (2008), 'A role for Q/N-rich aggregation-prone regions in P-body localization', *J Cell Sci,* 121 (Pt 15), 2463-72.

Rosen, J., He, M., Umbricht, C., Alexander, H. R., Dackiw, A. P., Zeiger, M. A., and Libutti, S. K. (2005), 'A six-gene model for differentiating benign from malignant thyroid tumors on the basis of gene expression', *Surgery,* 138 (6), 1050-6; discussion 56-7.

Ryan, D. E., Stevens, S. W., and Abelson, J. (2002), 'The 5' and 3' domains of yeast U6 snRNA: Lsm proteins facilitate binding of Prp24 protein to the U6 telestem region', *RNA,* 8 (8), 1011-33.

Salgado-Garrido, J., Bragado-Nielsson, E., Kandels-Lewis, S., and Seraphin, B. (1999), 'Sm and Sm-like proteins assemble in two related complexes of deep evolutionary origin', *EMBO J,* 18 (12), 3451-62.

Scheller, N., Mina, L. B., Galao, R. P., Chari, A., Gimenez-Barcons, M., Noueiry, A., Fischer, U., Meyerhans, A., and Diez, J. (2009), 'Translation and replication of hepatitis C virus genomic RNA depends on ancient cellular proteins that control mRNA fates', *Proc Natl Acad Sci U S A,* 106 (32), 13517-22.

Schumacher, MA., Pearson, RF., Moller, T., Valentin-Hansen, P., and Brennan, RG. (2002), 'Structures of the pleiotropic translational regulator Hfq and an Hfq-RNA complex: a bacterial Sm-like protein', *EMBO J,* 21 (13), 3546-56.

Schweinfest, C. W., Graber, M. W., Chapman, J. M., Papas, T. S., Baron, P. L., and Watson, D. K. (1997), 'CaSm: an Sm-like protein that contributes to the transformed state in cancer cells', *Cancer Res,* 57 (14), 2961-5.

Selenko, P., Sprangers, R., Stier, G., Buhler, D., Fischer, U., and Sattler, M. (2001), 'SMN tudor domain structure and its interaction with the Sm proteins', *Nat Struct Biol,* 8 (1), 27-31.

Sheth, U. and Parker, R. (2003), 'Decapping and decay of messenger RNA occur in cytoplasmic processing bodies', *Science,* 300 (5620), 805-8.

Sobti, M., Cubeddu, L., Haynes, P. A., and Mabbutt, B. C. (2010), 'Engineered rings of mixed yeast Lsm proteins show differential interactions with translation factors and U-rich RNA', *Biochemistry,* 49 (11), 2335-45.

Song, M. G. and Kiledjian, M. (2007), '3' Terminal oligo U-tract-mediated stimulation of decapping', *RNA,* 13 (12), 2356-65.

Spiller, M. P., Boon, K. L., Reijns, M. A., and Beggs, J. D. (2007), 'The Lsm2-8 complex determines nuclear localization of the spliceosomal U6 snRNA', *Nucleic Acids Res,* 35 (3), 923-9.

Storz, G., Opdyke, J. A., and Zhang, A. (2004), 'Controlling mRNA stability and translation with small, noncoding RNAs', *Curr Opin Microbiol,* 7 (2), 140-4.

Streicher, K. L., Yang, Z. Q., Draghici, S., and Ethier, S. P. (2007), 'Transforming function of the LSM1 oncogene in human breast cancers with the 8p11-12 amplicon', *Oncogene,* 26 (14), 2104-14.

Sukhodolets, M. V. and Garges, S. (2003), 'Interaction of Escherichia coli RNA polymerase with the ribosomal protein S1 and the Sm-like ATPase Hfq', *Biochemistry,* 42 (26), 8022-34.

Tharun, S., He, W., Mayes, A. E., Lennertz, P., Beggs, J. D., and Parker, R. (2000), 'Yeast Sm-like proteins function in mRNA decapping and decay', *Nature,* 404 (6777), 515-8.

Thore, S., Mayer, C., Sauter, C., Weeks, S., and Suck, D. (2003), 'Crystal structures of the Pyrococcus abyssi Sm core and its complex with RNA. Common features of RNA binding in archaea and eukarya', *J Biol Chem,* 278 (2), 1239-47.

Tomasevic, N. and Peculis, B. A. (2002), 'Xenopus LSm proteins bind U8 snoRNA via an internal evolutionarily conserved octamer sequence', *Mol Cell Biol,* 22 (12), 4101-12.

Toro, I., Basquin, J., Teo-Dreher, H., and Suck, D. (2002), 'Archaeal Sm proteins form heptameric and hexameric complexes: crystal structures of the Sm1 and Sm2 proteins from the hyperthermophile Archaeoglobus fulgidus', *J Mol Biol,* 320 (1), 129-42.

Toro, I., Thore, Stephane , Mayer, Claudine, Basquin, Jerome, Seraphin, Bertrand, and Suck, Dietrich (2001), 'RNA binding in an Sm core domain: X-ray structure and functional analysis of an archeal Sm protein complex', *EMBO J,* 20 (9), 2293-303.

Tritschler, F., Eulalio, A., Truffault, V., Hartmann, M. D., Helms, S., Schmidt, S., Coles, M., Izaurralde, E., and Weichenrieder, O. (2007), 'A divergent Sm fold in EDC3 proteins mediates DCP1 binding and P-body targeting', *Mol Cell Biol,* 27 (24), 8600-11.

Tsui, H. C., Leung, H. C., and Winkler, M. E. (1994), 'Characterization of broadly pleiotropic phenotypes caused by an hfq insertion mutation in Escherichia coli K-12', *Mol Microbiol,* 13 (1), 35-49.

Tucker, M., Valencia-Sanchez, M. A., Staples, R. R., Chen, J., Denis, C. L., and Parker, R. (2001), 'The transcription factor associated Ccr4 and Caf1 proteins are components of the major cytoplasmic mRNA deadenylase in Saccharomyces cerevisiae', *Cell,* 104 (3), 377-86.

Urlaub, H., Raker, V. A., Kostka, S., and Luhrmann, R. (2001), 'Sm protein-Sm site RNA interactions within the inner ring of the spliceosomal snRNP core structure', *EMBO J,* 20 (1-2), 187-96.

Verdone, L., Galardi, S., Page, D., and Beggs, J. D. (2004), 'Lsm proteins promote regeneration of pre-mRNA splicing activity', *Curr Biol,* 14 (16), 1487-91.

Veretnik, S., Wills, C., Youkharibache, P., Valas, R. E., and Bourne, P. E. (2009), 'Sm/Lsm genes provide a glimpse into the early evolution of the spliceosome', *PLoS Comput Biol,* 5 (3), e1000315.

Wahl, M. C., Will, C. L., and Luhrmann, R. (2009), 'The spliceosome: design principles of a dynamic RNP machine', *Cell,* 136 (4), 701-18.

Wan, L., Battle, D. J., Yong, J., Gubitz, A. K., Kolb, S. J., Wang, J., and Dreyfuss, G. (2005), 'The survival of motor neurons protein determines the capacity for snRNP assembly: biochemical deficiency in spinal muscular atrophy', *Mol Cell Biol,* 25 (13), 5543-51.

Wassarman, K. M., Repoila, F., Rosenow, C., Storz, G., and Gottesman, S. (2001), 'Identification of novel small RNAs using comparative genomics and microarrays', *Genes Dev,* 15 (13), 1637-51.

Weber, G., Trowitzsch, S., Kastner, B., Luhrmann, R., and Wahl, M. C. (2010), 'Functional organization of the Sm core in the crystal structure of human U1 snRNP', *EMBO J,* 29 (24), 4172-84.

Wen, Y. and Shatkin, A. J. (1999), 'Transcription elongation factor hSPT5 stimulates mRNA capping', *Genes Dev,* 13 (14), 1774-9.

Will, C. L. and Luhrmann, R. (2001), 'Spliceosomal UsnRNP biogenesis, structure and function', *Curr Opin Cell Biol,* 13 (3), 290-301.

Wolin, S. L. and Cedervall, T. (2002), 'The La protein', *Annu Rev Biochem,* 71, 375-403.

Yan, Y., Rubinchik, S., Wood, A. L., Gillanders, W. E., Dong, J. Y., Watson, D. K., and Cole, D. J. (2006), 'Bystander effect contributes to the antitumor efficacy of CaSm antisense gene therapy in a preclinical model of advanced pancreatic cancer', *Mol Ther,* 13 (2), 357-65.